Personalized Nutrition
Translating Nutrigenetic/Nutrigenomic Research into Dietary Guidelines

World Review of Nutrition and Dietetics

Vol. 101

Series Editor

Artemis P. Simopoulos

The Center for Genetics, Nutrition and Health, Washington, D.C., USA

Advisory Board

Regina C. Casper USA
Uri Goldbourt Israel
C. Gopalan India
Tomohito Hamazaki Japan
Federico Leighton Chile
Michel de Lorgeril France
Edwin C.M. Mariman The Netherlands
Victor A. Rogozkin Russia

Marjanne Senekal South Africa
Leonard Storlien Australia
Changhao Sun China
Antonio Velazquez Mexico
Mark L. Wahlqvist Australia
Paul Walter Switzerland
Bruce A. Watkins USA

Personalized Nutrition

Translating Nutrigenetic/Nutrigenomic Research into Dietary Guidelines

Volume Editors

Artemis P. Simopoulos
The Center for Genetics, Nutrition and Health, Washington, D.C., USA

John A. Milner
National Institutes of Health, Health and Human Services, Rockville, MD

19 figures and 15 tables, 2010

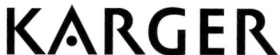

Basel · Freiburg · Paris · London · New York · Bangalore ·
Bangkok · Shanghai · Singapore · Tokyo · Sydney

Artemis P. Simopoulos
The Center for Genetics
Nutrition and Health
Washington, D.C., USA

John A. Milner
Nutritional Science Research Group
Division of Cancer Prevention
National Cancer Institute
National Institutes of Health
Health and Human Services
Rockville, MD

Library of Congress Cataloging-in-Publication Data

International Society of Nutrigenetics/Nutrigenomics. Congress (3rd : 2009 : National Institutes of Health)
 Personalized nutrition : translating nutrigenetic/nutrigenomic research into dietary guidelines / volume editors, Artemis P. Simopoulos, John A. Milner.
       p. ; cm. -- (World review of nutrition and dietetics, ISSN 0084-2230 ; v. 101)
 Includes bibliographical references and indexes.
 ISBN 978-3-8055-9427-1 (hard cover : alk. paper)
 1. Nutrition--Genetic aspects--Congresses. I. Simopoulos, Artemis P., 1933- II. Milner, J. A. (John A.) III. Title. IV. Series: World review of nutrition and dietetics, v. 101. 0084-2230 ;
 [DNLM: 1. Diet Therapy--methods--Congresses. 2. Nutrigenomics--Congresses. 3. Nutritional Physiological Phenomena--genetics--Congresses. WB 400 I6145p 2010]
 QP144.G45I58 2009
 612.3--dc22
                                                    2010009355

Bibliographic Indices. This publication is listed in bibliographic services, including Current Contents® and PubMed/MEDLINE.

Disclaimer. The statements, opinions and data contained in this publication are solely those of the individual authors and contributors and not of the publisher and the editor(s). The appearance of advertisements in the book is not a warranty, endorsement, or approval of the products or services advertised or of their effectiveness, quality or safety. The publisher and the editor(s) disclaim responsibility for any injury to persons or property resulting from any ideas, methods, instructions or products referred to in the content or advertisements.

Drug Dosage. The authors and the publisher have exerted every effort to ensure that drug selection and dosage set forth in this text are in accord with current recommendations and practice at the time of publication. However, in view of ongoing research, changes in government regulations, and the constant flow of information relating to drug therapy and drug reactions, the reader is urged to check the package insert for each drug for any change in indications and dosage and for added warnings and precautions. This is particularly important when the recommended agent is a new and/or infrequently employed drug.

All rights reserved. No part of this publication may be translated into other languages, reproduced or utilized in any form or by any means electronic or mechanical, including photocopying, recording, microcopying, or by any information storage and retrieval system, without permission in writing from the publisher.

© Copyright 2010 by S. Karger AG, P.O. Box, CH–4009 Basel (Switzerland)
www.karger.com
Printed in Switzerland on acid-free and non-aging paper (ISO 9706) by Reinhardt Druck, Basel
ISSN 0084–2230
ISBN 978–3–8055–9427–1
e-ISBN 978–3–8055–9428–8

Contents

VII List of Contributors

XI Preface
Simopoulos, A.P. (Washington, D.C.); Milner, J.A. (Bethesda, Md.)

1 **Opportunities and Challenges in Nutrigenetics/Nutrigenomics and Health**
De Caterina, R. (Pisa)

8 **Genome-Wide Association Studies and Diet**
Ferguson, L.R. (Auckland)

15 **Copy Number Variation, Eicosapentaenoic Acid and Neurological Disorders. With Particular Reference to Huntington's Disease and Associated CAG Repeats, and to Myalgic Encephalomyelitis and Viral Infection**
Puri, B.K. (London); Manku, M.S. (Oxford)

21 **Nutrigenetics: A Tool to Provide Personalized Nutritional Therapy to the Obese**
Marti, A.; Goyenechea, E.; Martínez, J.A. (Pamplona)

34 **Xenobiotic Metabolizing Genes, Meat-Related Exposures, and Risk of Advanced Colorectal Adenoma**
Ferrucci, L.M. (Bethesda, Md./New Haven, Conn.); Cross, A.J. (Bethesda, Md.); Gunter, M.J.; Ahn, J. (New York, N.Y.); Mayne, S.T.; Ma, X. (New Haven, Conn.); Chanock, S.J.; Yeager, M.; Graubard, B.I.; Berndt, S.I.; Huang, W.-Y. (Bethesda, Md.); Hayes, R.B. (New York, N.Y.); Sinha, R. (Bethesda, Md.)

46 **Strategies to Improve Detection of Hypertension Genes**
Hunt, S.C. (Salt Lake City, Utah)

56 **Diet, Nutrition and Modulation of Genomic Expression in Fetal Origins of Adult Disease**
Jackson, A.A.; Burdge, G.C.; Lillycrop, K.A. (Southampton)

73 **Choline: Clinical Nutrigenetic/Nutrigenomic Approaches for Identification of Functions and Dietary Requirements**
Zeisel, S.H. (Chapel Hill, N.C.)

84 **Dietary Polyphenols, Deacetylases and Chromatin Remodeling in Inflammation**
Rahman, I.; Chung, S. (Rochester, N.Y.)

95 **Dietary Manipulation of Histone Structure and Function**
Ho, E.; Dashwood, R.H. (Corvallis, Oreg.)

103 Changes in Human Adipose Tissue Gene Expression during Diet-Induced Weight Loss
Svensson, P.-A.; Gummesson, A.; Carlsson, L.M.S.; Sjöholm, K. (Gothenburg)

115 Toxicogenomics and Studies of Genomic Effects of Dietary Components
Thompson, K. (Silver Spring, Md.)

123 Dietary Methyl Deficiency, microRNA Expression and Susceptibility to Liver Carcinogenesis
Starlard-Davenport, A.; Tryndyak, V. (Jefferson, Ariz.); Kosyk, O. (Chapel Hill, N.C.); Ross, S.R. (Bethesda, Md.); Rusyn, I. (Chapel Hill, N.C.); Beland, F.A.; Pogribny, I.P. (Jefferson, Ariz.)

131 Redox Dysregulation and Oxidative Stress in Schizophrenia: Nutrigenetics as a Challenge in Psychiatric Disease Prevention
Do, K.Q.; Conus, P.; Cuenod, M. (Lausanne)

154 Nutrigenomics and Agriculture: A Perspective
Spence, J.T. (Beltsville, Md.)

160 Opportunities and Challenges in Nutrigenetics/Nutrigenomics: Building Industry-Academia Partnerships
Gillies, P.J. (Wilmington, De.); Kris-Etherton, P.M. (University Park, Pa.)

169 Tailoring Foods to Match People's Genes in New Zealand: Opportunities for Collaboration
Ferguson, L.R.; Hu, R.; Lam, W.J.; Munday, K.;Triggs, C.M. (Auckland)

176 Author Index
177 Subject Index

List of Contributors

Jiyoung Ahn
Division of Epidemiology
Department of Environmental Medicine
New York University School of Medicine
New York, NY 10016 (USA)

Frederick A. Beland
Division of Biochemical Toxicology
National Center for Toxicological Research
3900 NCTR Rd.
Jefferson, AR 72079 (USA)

Sonja I. Berndt
Division of Cancer Epidemiology and
Genetics
National Cancer Institute
National Institutes of Health
Department of Health and Human
Services
Bethesda, MD 20892 (USA)

Graham C. Burdge
Institute of Human Nutrition
University of Southampton School of Medicine
IDS Building, MP88
Southampton General Hospital
Tremona Road
Southampton SO16 6YD (UK)

Lena MS Carlsson
Sahlgrenska Center for Cardiovascular and
Metabolic Research
Department of Molecular and Clinical
Medicine
The Sahlgrenska Academy at University of
Gothenburg
SOS-sekr, Vita Stråket 15
SE-413 45 Gothenburg (Sweden)

Stephen J. Chanock
Division of Cancer Epidemiology and
Genetics
National Cancer Institute
National Institutes of Health
Department of Health and Human
Services
Bethesda, MD 20892 (USA)

Sangwoon Chung
Department of Environmental Medicine
Lung Biology and Disease Program
University of Rochester Medical Center
MRBX 3.11106, Box 850
601 Elmwood Ave.
Rochester, NY 14642 (USA)

Philippe Conus
Department of Psychiatry
Lausanne University Hospital
Site de Cery
CH-1008 Prilly-Lausanne (Switzerland)

Amanda J. Cross
Division of Cancer Epidemiology and
Genetics
National Cancer Institute
National Institutes of Health
Department of Health and Human
Services
Bethesda, MD 20892 (USA)

Michel Cuenod
Center for Psychiatric Neuroscience
Department of Psychiatry
Lausanne University Hospital
Site de Cery
CH-1008 Prilly-Lausanne (Switzerland)

Roderick H. Dashwood
Linus Pauling Institute
Oregon State University
571 Weniger Hall
Corvallis, OR 97331 (USA)

Raffaele De Caterina
Chair and Postgraduate School of Cardiology
"G. d'Annunzio" University – Chieti
C/o Ospedale SS. Annunziata
Via dei Vestini
I-66013 Chieti (Italy)

Kim Q. Do
Center for Psychiatric Neuroscience
Department of Psychiatry
Lausanne University Hospital
Site de Cery
CH-1008 Prilly-Lausanne (Switzerland)

Leah M. Ferrucci
Division of Cancer Epidemiology and Genetics
National Cancer Institute
National Institutes of Health
Department of Health and Human Services,
Bethesda, MD 20892 (USA)

Lynnette R. Ferguson
Discipline of Nutrition
Faculty of Medical and Health Sciences
The University of Auckland
Private Bag 92019
1142 Auckland (New Zealand)

Estibaliz Goyenechea
Institute of Nutrition and Food Sciences
University of Navarra
E-31080 Pamplona (Spain)

Marc J. Gunter
Department of Epidemiology and Population Health
Albert Einstein College of Medicine
Bronx
New York, NY 10461 (USA)

Barry I. Graubard
Division of Cancer Epidemiology and Genetics
National Cancer Institute
National Institutes of Health
Department of Health and Human Services
Bethesda, MD 20892 (USA)

Anders Gummesson
Sahlgrenska Center for Cardiovascular and
Metabolic Research
Department of Molecular and Clinical Medicine
The Sahlgrenska Academy at University of
Gothenburg
SOS-sekr, Vita Stråket 15
SE-413 45 Gothenburg (Sweden)

Peter J. Gillies
DuPont Applied BioSciences
DuPont Experimental Station, E328/267
Wilmington, DE 19880-0328 (USA)

Richard B. Hayes
Division of Epidemiology
Department of Environmental Medicine
New York University School of Medicine
New York, NY 10016 (USA)

Emily Ho
Department of Nutrition & Exercise Sciences
Oregon State University
117 Milam Hall
Corvallis, OR 97331 (USA)

Rong Hu
Discipline of Nutrition,
Faculty of Medical and Health Sciences,
The University of Auckland
NZ-1142 Auckland (New Zealand)

Wen-Yi Huang
Division of Cancer Epidemiology and Genetics
National Cancer Institute
National Institutes of Health
Department of Health and Human Services
Bethesda, MD 20892 (USA)

Steven C. Hunt
Cardiovascular Genetics Division
Department of Internal Medicine
University of Utah
420 Chipeta Way, Room 1160
Salt Lake City, Utah 84108 (USA)

Alan A. Jackson
Institute of Human Nutrition,
Southampton General Hospital (MP 113)
Tremona Road
Southampton SO16 6YD (UK)

Penny M. Kris-Etherton
The Pennsylvania State University
University Park, PA 16802-1294 (USA)

Oksana Kosyk
Department of Environmental Sciences and Engineering
University of North Carolina
135 Dauer Dr.
Chapel Hill, NC 27599 (USA)

Wen Jiun Lam
Discipline of Nutrition,
Faculty of Medical and Health Sciences
The University of Auckland
NZ-1142 Auckland (New Zealand)

Karen A. Lillycrop
Developmental and Cell Biology
University of Southampton
Southampton SO16 7PX (UK)

John A. Milner
Nutritional Science Research Group
Division of Cancer Prevention
National Cancer Institute
National Institutes of Health
Health and Human Services
6130 Executive Boulevard
Executive Plaza North Suite 3164
Rockville, MD 20892 (USA)

Karen Munday
Institute of Food, Nutrition and Health
Massey University,
NZ- 4474 Palmerston North (New Zealand)

Xiaomei Ma
Yale School of Public Health
New Haven, CT 06520-8034 (USA)

Mehar S. Manku
Amarin Neuroscience
Oxford OX4 4GA (UK)

Amelia Marti
Institute of Nutrition and Food Sciences
University of Navarra
E-31080 Pamplona (Spain)

J. Alfredo Martínez
Institute of Nutrition and Food Sciences
University of Navarra
E-31080 Pamplona (Spain)

Susan T. Mayne
Yale School of Public Health,
New Haven, CT 06520-8034 (USA)

Igor P. Pogribny
Division of Biochemical Toxicology,
National Center for Toxicological Research
3900 NCTR Rd.
Jefferson, AR 72079 (USA)

Irfan Rahman
Department of Environmental Medicine
Lung Biology and Disease Program
University of Rochester Medical Center
MRBX 3.11106, Box 850
601 Elmwood Ave.
Rochester, NY 14642 (USA)

Basant K. Puri
MRI Unit
Imaging Sciences Department
MRC Clinical Sciences Centre
Imperial College London
Hammersmith Hospital
London W12 0HS (UK)

Sharon R. Ross
Nutritional Science Research Group
Division of Cancer Prevention
National Cancer Institute
National Institutes of Health
Department of Health and Human Services
6130 Executive Blvd.
Bethesda, MD 20892-7328 (USA)

Ivan Rusyn
Department of Environmental Sciences and Engineering
University of North Carolina
135 Dauer Dr.
Chapel Hill, NC 27599 (USA)

Artemis P. Simopoulos
The Center for Genetics, Nutrition and Health
2001 S Street, N.W.
Suite 530
Washington, DC 20009 (USA)

Rashmi Sinha
Division of Cancer Epidemiology and Genetics
National Cancer Institute
National Institutes of Health
Department of Health and Human Services
Bethesda, MD 20892 (USA)

Kajsa Sjöholm
Sahlgrenska Center for Cardiovascular and Metabolic Research
Department of Molecular and Clinical Medicine
The Sahlgrenska Academy at University of Gothenburg
SOS-sekr, Vita Stråket 15
SE-413 45 Gothenburg (Sweden)

Joseph T. Spence, Ph.D.
Beltsville Agricultural Research Center
Building 003, Room 238
10300 Baltimore Avenue
Beltsville, MD 20705 (USA)

Athena Starlard-Davenport
Division of Biochemical Toxicology,
National Center for Toxicological Research
3900 NCTR Rd.
Jefferson, AR 72079 (USA)

Per-Arne Svensson
Sahlgrenska Center for Cardiovascular and Metabolic Research
Department of Molecular and Clinical Medicine
The Sahlgrenska Academy at University of Gothenburg
SOS-sekr, Vita Stråket 15
SE-413 45 Gothenburg (Sweden)

Karol Thompson
US Food and Drug Administration
Life Science Building 64, Rm 2036
10903 New Hampshire Ave
Silver Spring, MD 20993-0002 (USA)

Christopher M. Triggs
Department of Biostatistics, Nutrigenomics
The University of Auckland
NZ-1142 Auckland (New Zealand)

Volodymyr Tryndyak
Division of Biochemical Toxicology,
National Center for Toxicological Research
3900 NCTR Rd.
Jefferson, AR 72079 (USA)

Meredith Yeager
Division of Cancer Epidemiology and Genetics
National Cancer Institute
National Institutes of Health
Department of Health and Human Services
Bethesda, MD 20892 (USA)

Steven Zeisel
Gillings School of Global Public Health
and School of Medicine
University of North Carolina at Chapel Hill
Nutrition Research Institute at Kannapolis
500 Laureate Way
Kannapolis, NC 28081-4332 (USA)

Preface

Volume 101 in the series *World Reviews of Nutrition and Dietetics* consists of selected papers presented at the Third Congress of the International Society of Nutrigenetics/Nutrigenomics (ISNN). The congress was held at the National Institutes of Health (NIH) campus in Bethesda (Md., USA) on October 21–23, 2009. The congress was truly international, with speakers and participants from 14 countries of North and South America, Europe, Asia and Africa. The congress was co-chaired by Dr. John Milner of the National Cancer Institute, NIH, and Dr. Artemis P. Simopoulos, President of the ISNN. The congress's focus was that 'research and its translation into medical practice and dietary recommendations must be based on a solid foundation of knowledge derived from studies on nutrigenetics and nutrigenomics'. The congress consisted of 7 sessions. In keeping with the theme of the congress, sessions I and II addressed 'Frontiers in Nutrigenetics', session III focused on 'Frontiers in Epigenetics', session IV addressed the 'Impact of Transcriptomics on Nutrigenomics', session V centered on 'Non-coding RNAs and Post-translational Gene Regulation', session VI was called 'Moving Beyond Genomics', and session VII was titled on 'Frontiers in Nutrigenetics/Nutrigenomics. Building Partnerships: the Challenges and Opportunities Facing Governments, International Organizations, Academia and Industry'.

Dr. Simopoulos and Dr. Milner opened the congress and welcomed everyone. The keynote address was given by Dr. Raffaele De Caterina, Vice-President of the ISNN who spoke on 'Opportunities and Challenges in Nutrigenetics/Nutrigenomics and Health.' Dr. De Caterina emphasized that, like drugs, nutrients have the ability to interact and modulate molecular mechanisms underlying an organism's physiological functions. Awareness of the different effects of nutrients according to our genetic constitution (nutrigenetics) and how nutrients may affect gene expression (nutrigenomics) is prompting a revolution in the field of nutrition. Nutritional sciences have always studied the effects of nutrients in terms of 'average' responses, without bothering much about inter-individual variability and the underlying causes. The creation of nutrigenetics and nutrigenomics, with distinct approaches to elucidate the interaction between diet and genes, but with the common ultimate goal of optimizing health through personalized diet, provides powerful approaches to unravel the complex relationships among nutritional molecules, genetic variants and the biological system. Translated as the simple concept of 'personalized nutrition' the promise of nutrigenetics/nutrigenomics is a major step forward in the understanding of individual responses to a component nutrient or to our changing environment. Referring to the future, Dr. De Caterina stated two major challenges. One is the reluctance to embrace this concept, primarily due to the fear of being unable to manage the overwhelming quantity and complexity of biological data that will require interpretation and – to a large extent – simplification to be translated into practical messages. The danger of the consequent simplification would be to take the results of a single study on a very specific outcome, very often on intermediate (surrogate) endpoints, and to infer that such results are applicable to the complexity of a living organism, where no single organ or tissue is independent of the others. The second challenge is the need to be aware that the area of 'personalized nutrition' is seen by disguised amateurs as a golden opportunity for marketing enterprises before solid knowledge in any specific area is acquired. Although the first challenge is manageable by the ever-increasing availability of biomedical and statistical tools and the wisdom necessary in health inference – a general problem in medical science – the second challenge requires great attention and wisdom and poses important ethical and scientific issues. A scientific society, such as the ISNN, devoted to the study of nutrigenetics/nutrigenomics can indeed serve the commendable roles of (1) promoting science and favoring scientific communication and (2) permanently working as a 'clearing house' to prevent disqualifying logical jumps, correct or stop unwarranted claims, and prevent the creation of unwarranted expectations in patients and in the general public.

In the next paper Dr. Lynnette Ferguson focuses on 'Genome-Wide Association Studies and Diet'. Dr. Ferguson points out that genome-wide association studies (GWAS) are not only validating genes and single-nucleotide polymorphisms (SNPs) that have been anticipated by knowledge of biochemical pathways, but are also revealing new gene-disease associations not anticipated from prior knowledge (e.g. Crohn's disease). Dr. Ferguson emphasizes that current GWAS methods need to be complemented with innovative methodologies in order to characterize the impact of food and to take the field to another level of value for human diet, development and optimized health through personalized nutrition.

Genetic variants are caused by SNPs through substitutions, additions or deletions. Copy number variants are the most recent discovery that accounts for genetic variation in humans and may be responsible for much more individuality than previously considered. In their paper, 'Copy Number Variation, Eicosapentaenoic Acid and Neurological Disorders' Dr. Basant Puri and Dr. Mehar Manku discuss the way in which the clinical response of neurological disorders to treatment with the semi-synthetic omega-3 long-chain polyunsaturated fatty acid derivative ethyl-eicosapentaenoic acid (ethyl-EPA) varies according to copy number variation. Two examples of neurological disorders are given, namely Huntington's disease, which is caused by increased CAG repeats at 4p16.3, and myalgic encephalomyelitis, which has recently been associated with evidence of retroviral infection with XMRV. These findings are likely to apply to other neurological disorders and indeed also to the differential response to ethyl-EPA of psychiatric disorders, such as depression and schizophrenia.

Obesity is a multigenetic and multifactorial condition in which SNPs involved in the regulation of food intake (e.g. MC4R, LEP, LEPLR, POMC, FTO) fat metabolism and thermogenesis (e.g. PPARG, ADBRs, UCPs) inflammation, and signaling (e.g. IL-6, ADIPOQ, CD36) induce different responses to energy-restricted diets, or macronutrient content (fat or fiber) during weight loss, along with beneficial effects on elements such as insulin sensitivity, lipid biomarkers and satiety. Dr. Amelia Marti and colleagues in their paper 'Nutrigenetics: A Tool to Provide Personalized Nutritional Therapy for the Obese' present an extensive review of the field. Their review includes observational studies that showcase gene-nutrient interactions on weight gain and international studies on genetic modification effects following weight loss and maintenance.

There have been many studies on the relationship between diet and various forms of cancer. Among those that have been studied extensively are the carcinogenic actions of compounds during cooking of meat, such as heterocyclic amines (HCAs), polycyclic aromatic hydrocarbons (PAHs) and N-nitroso compounds (NOCs). In their paper 'Xenobiotic Metabolizing Genes, Meat-Related Exposures, and Risk of Advanced Colorectal Adenoma,' Dr. Leah Ferrucci and colleagues evaluate SNPs in xenobiotic metabolizing enzyme genes and possible alteration in the activation/detoxification of HCAs, PAHs and NOCs. A number of possible interactions are noted between certain SNPs in relation to colorectal adenoma. The authors conclude that common variants in xenobiotic metabolizing enzyme genes may modify the association of HCAs, PAHs and NOCs and advanced colorectal adenoma, but further investigations in other populations are needed.

Animal models with kidney transplants have unequivocally shown that hypertension follows the kidney. There is also evidence for differential, possibly additive, influences of central versus kidney-specific hormonal blood pressure control of salt balance. In any homeostatic system, such as salt balance, multiple factors are involved in counteracting any factor that perturbs the system. These compensating factors, if working efficiently, should return the system back to balance. Should environmental or genetic effects prevent appropriate compensation over the long term, hypertension will likely develop. However, there are also likely to be genetic initiating factors that would lead to hypertension if not adequately compensated and that may be strong enough so that complete compensation is not attained. Dr. Steven Hunt in his paper 'Strategies to Improve Detection of Hypertension Genes' points out that when studying the genetics of the initiating factors, associations will be masked by the degree of compensation and perhaps not even found if compensation is nearly complete. Detecting the genetic initiators may require studying associations after acute interventions and prior to long-term compensation. Detection also may depend on the genetic backgrounds of the subjects being studied: subjects with few hypertension genes may show little association with any particular gene, whereas subjects with many hypertension-susceptibility genes may show strong associations. Although some genes have been consistently related to elevated blood pressure and hypertension, the observed effects of these genes are small and difficult to replicate. These common genes have almost always been related to renal electrolyte handling, similar to mechanisms of the rarer monogenic hypertension disorders. Several large studies now have the power to detect hypertension genes with smaller effect sizes and to assess interactions with diet and other environmental risk factors for hypertension. Intervention studies appear to magnify the baseline effects of genes so that they are more easily detected. In addition to genetic interactions with dietary salt on blood pressure, there appear to be important but less understood genetic interactions with dietary fat and cholesterol on blood pressure pathways. Multiple interventions – including less dietary salt, increased dietary potassium, increased intake of fruits and vegetables, lower fat intake, weight loss and drug treatment – appear to help reduce blood pressure to a greater extent in subjects genetically susceptible to hypertension than those not as susceptible. It appears that those at highest genetic risk of hypertension show a greater improvement in blood pressure for interventions that target the defective genetic pathways than do those at low risk. There remains an urgent need for the addition of dietary and pharmacologic interventions to genetic studies and vice versa, so that biological mechanisms may be uncovered, represented by these statistical interactions, and additional interactions discovered. Knowledge arising from such studies may be used to design specific dietary, exercise, weight loss and drug interventions for the subset of patients that will benefit the most from that intervention.

For the past century, broad social development has been reflected in changes in height. There is convincing evidence from population studies that achieved height marks a significantly increased risk for some cancers. Major cancers are associated with increased adiposity, especially with centrally deposited fat for some. Thus, findings of epidemiological studies of the relationship between prenatal growth and risk for specific cancers, metabolic disease and cardiovascular disease suggest that early life environment is a causal component in the etiology of these conditions. Mechanistic studies provide some evidence that explains how variations of diet within the normal range of consumption in early life can set later susceptibility through processes such as DNA methylation and covalent modifications to histones. Dr. Alan Jackson and colleagues in their paper 'Diet, Nutrition and Modulation of Genomic Expression in Fetal Origins of Adult Disease' state that nutrient interventions in laboratory animals during pregnancy and/or lactation show that there is developmental plasticity to environmental stimuli that induces a phenotype that confers survival advantage in the short term but increases susceptibility to pathology in the longer term. These influences can be modified by the dietary pattern during the weaning period, demonstrating an important interaction between prenatal nutrition and food consumption during later life. This is further implied by the common role for altered epigenetic regulation of specific genes and of altered Dnmt activity. Thus, risk of these seemingly heterogeneous patterns of ill health may reflect a continuum of developmental changes that operate through the same enzymes and pathways that induce epigenetic regulation of specific genes. Risk of specific diseases may reflect the nature and/or magnitude of the environmental exposure during early life. It is not known how these environmental cues may be targeted in a manner that induces altered epigenetic regulation of specific genes or of individual CpG dinucleotides and so lead to increased risk of different disease processes. However, such specificity is implied by emerging evidence that the magnitude of the maternal nutritional challenge and the relative amount of specific nutrients in the maternal diet induce directionally opposite changes in the physiology and epigenotype of the offspring. Overall, these findings support the concept that a range of prenatal nutritional environments, from constraint to abundance, may induce risk of ultimate different pathological processes. The induced epigenetic changes are likely to be permissive for altered gene expression and hence determine the interaction between an organism and its environment over the life course and, in turn, determine whether increased risk due to the early-life environment becomes disease in later life.

Dr. Steven H. Ziesel in his manuscript 'Choline: Clinical Nutrigenetic/Nutrigenomic Approaches for Identification of Functions and Dietary Requirements' points out that whereas GWAS examine correlations between variants and diseases in terms of thousands of subjects are a mainstay of nutrigenetics/nutrigenomics, less common are the studies that examine the effects of genetic variants on nutritional phenotypes using clinical studies involving smaller numbers of studies – clinical nutrigenetics/nutrigenomics. Dr. Ziesel noted in his and other studies with choline as an example of clinical nutrigenetics. In animal models, there is a critical period during pregnancy when dietary choline intake modulates fetal brain development with structural and functional consequences that last throughout the entire life of the offspring. Maternal intake of diets low in choline negatively impacts the proliferation and survival of neuronal and glial progenitor cells in the fetal hippocampus, septum and cortex, whereas maternal diets high in choline exert the opposite effects on brain development, increasing progenitor cell proliferation and survival and enhancing memory function. One mechanism mediating these changes involves the epigenetic modification of genes in fetal brain that are important regulators of cell division, apoptosis and neural differentiation.

The following paper, by Dr. Irfan Rahman and Dr. Sangwoon Chung, is entitled 'Dietary Polyphenols, Deacetylases and Chromatin Remodeling in Inflammation'. The therapeutic benefits of fruits and vegetables, tea and wine are mostly attributed to the presence of phenolic compounds. Naturally occurring dietary polyphenols such as curcumin (diferuloylmethane) an active component of the spice turmeric and resveratrol (phytoalexin), a flavanoid found in red wine, can directly scavenge reactive oxygen species and modulate signaling pathways mediated by NF-κB and MAP kinase pathways and up-regulate glutathione/phase II enzyme biosynthesis via activation of Nrf2. They also down-regulate the expression of pro-inflammatory mediators, matrix metalloproteinases, adhesion molecules, and growth-factor receptor genes by inhibiting histone acetyltransferase activity and activating histone deacetylase (HDAC)/sirtuins(SIRTs). The expression of NF-κB-dependent pro-inflammatory genes in response to oxidative stress is regulated by the acetylation-deacetylation status of histones bound to the DNA. It has been reported in severe asthma and in chronic obstructive pulmonary disease (COPD) patients, that oxidative stress not only activates the NF-κB pathway but also alters the histone acetylation and deacetylation balance via post-translational modification of HDACs. Corticosteroids have been one of the major modes of therapy against respiratory diseases such as asthma and COPD. Failure of corticosteroids to ameliorate such disease conditions has been attributed to their failure to recruit either HDAC2 or SIRT1 or to the presence of an oxidatively/post-translationally modified HDAC2/SIRT1 in asthmatics and COPD patients. Dietary polyphenols such as curcumin, resveratrol and catechins have been reported to modulate epigenetic alterations in various experimental models. The anti-inflammatory properties of curcumin, resveratrol and catechins may be due to their ability to induce HDACs/SIRT1 activity, and thereby restore the efficacy of glucocorticoids or overcome its resistance. Thus, these polyphenolic compounds have value as antioxidant, anti-inflammatory and adjuvant therapies with steroids against chronic inflammatory epigenetically regulated diseases. The current knowledge on the mechanism of action of these polyphenols in the light of deacetylases in regulation of chromatin remodeling in inflammation is extensively presented.

Dr. Emily Ho and Dr. Roderick Dashwood in their manuscript 'Dietary Manipulation of Histone Structure and Function' point out that the influence of epigenetic alterations during cancer has gained increasing attention and has resulted in a paradigm shift in our understanding of mechanisms leading to cancer susceptibility. The reversible acetylation of histones is an important mechanism of gene regulation. Targeting the epigenome, including the use of HDAC inhibitors, is a novel strategy for cancer chemoprevention. The authors have found that sulforaphane, a compound found in cruciferous vegetables, inhibits HDAC activity in human colorectal and prostate cancer cells. The ability of sulforaphane to target aberrant acetylation patterns, in addition to effects on phase 2 enzymes, may make it an effective chemoprevention agent. Other dietary agents such as butyrate, allyl sulfides and organoselenium compounds have also shown promise as HDAC inhibitors. These studies are significant because of the potential to qualify or change recommendations for high-risk cancer patients, thereby increasing their survival through simple dietary choices, such as incorporating easily accessible foods into a patient's diet. The findings provide a scientific foundation for future large-scale human clinical intervention studies with dietary agents that affect the epigenome.

The adipose tissue plays a key role in energy storage but is also a major endocrine organ, communicating with the brain and peripheral tissues through mediators known as adipokines. Adipose tissue function has been implicated in the development of obesity-related diseases such as diabetes, cardiovascular disease and cancer.

Thus, regulation of genes in adipose tissue may be important in the pathogenesis of obesity and obesity-related diseases. In their paper 'Changes in Human Adipose Tissue Gene Expression during Diet-Induced Weight Loss,' Dr. Per-Arne Svensson and colleagues state that changes in energy availability have profound effects on adipose tissue metabolism. Expression profiling of human adipose tissue has been used extensively to gain insights into genes and mechanisms implicated in the development of obesity and related metabolic disease. The study of expression profiles from adipose tissue during caloric restriction is a valuable tool to gain such insights. In their review, the authors summarize the major findings from human adipose tissue expression profiling studies performed on subjects undergoing diet-induced weight loss treatment, and the current knowledge on 3 different genes/groups of genes that are regulated in human adipose tissue by diet-induced weight loss.

Dr. Karol Thompson in her manuscript 'Toxicogenomics and Studies of Genomic Effects of Dietary Components' points out that toxicogenomics analyses are recognized to be of value in assessments of the clinical relevance of adverse events that are observed in animal models. Resources have been developed to help interpret gene expression profiles within the context of a study. Reference compound datasets and pathway mapping tools provide a basis for differentiating pharmacologic from toxicologic effects. From large sets of gene expression data from control groups in toxicogenomics studies, the normal range of variability of individual genes and the contribution of study factors to baseline variability can be assessed. Sources of biological and technical noise can be controlled using performance standards and metrics that have been developed for rat and human samples. These resources, in content or design, have crossover applications of interest and utility to nutrigenomics research.

Altered expression of microRNAs is frequently detected during tumor development; however, it has not been established if variations in the expression of specific microRNAs are associated with differences in the susceptibility to tumorigenesis. Dr. Athena Starlard-Davenport and colleagues in their manuscript 'Dietary Methyl Deficiency, microRNA Expression and Susceptibility to Liver Carcinogenesis' report that inbred male mice (C57BL/6J and DBA/2J) were fed a lipogenic methyl-deficient diet, which causes liver injury that progresses to liver tumors. Differentially expressed microRNAs were identified by µParaflo microRNA microarray analysis and validated by quantitative reverse transcription PCR. They identified 74 significantly up- or down-regulated microRNAs, including miR-29c, miR-34a, miR-122, miR-155, miR-200b, miR-200c and miR-221, in the livers of mice fed a methyl-deficient diet for 12 weeks as compared to their age-matched control mice. The targets for these microRNAs are known to affect cell proliferation, apoptosis, lipid metabolism, oxidative stress, DNA methylation and inflammation. Interestingly, DBA/2J mice, which develop more extensive hepatic steatosis-specific pathomorphological changes, had a greater extent of miR-29c, miR-34a, miR-155 and miR-200b expression. These results demonstrate that alterations in expression of microRNAs are a prominent event during early stages of liver carcinogenesis induced by methyl deficiency. More importantly, the data link alterations in microRNA expression to the pathogenesis of liver cancer and strongly suggest that differences in the susceptibility to liver carcinogenesis may be determined by the differences in the microRNA expression response.

A developmental dysregulation of glutathione (GSH) synthesis of genetic origin leading to oxidative stress, when combined with environmental risk factors generating reactive oxygen species, can play a critical role in inducing schizophrenia phenotypes. GSH, a major redox regulator and antioxidant, is essential for protection against cellular oxidative damage. Dr. Kim Do and colleagues in their paper 'Redox Dysregulation and Oxidative Stress in Schizophrenia: Nutrigenetics as a Challenge in Psychiatric Diseases Prevention' review the results obtained through a reverse translational approach showing redox dysregulation of genetic origin in schizophrenia patients. Patients have decreased GSH levels in cerebrospinal fluid and prefrontal cortex and abnormal GSH synthesis: a GAG trinucleotide repeat polymorphism in the rate-limiting GSH synthesizing glutamate-cysteine ligase (GCL) catalytic subunit (GCLC) gene is associated with the disease. The associated genotypes correlate with decreased GCLC mRNA, protein expressions, GCL activity and GSH content. As demonstrated in various models, such redox dysregulation underlies structural and functional connectivity anomalies and behavioral deficits. In a clinical trial, the GSH precursor N-acetyl cysteine improved both negative symptoms and auditory evoked potentials. Thus, a genetic GSH synthesis impairment represents one major risk factor in schizophrenia. Redox dysregulation may constitute a 'hub' where genetic and environmental vulnerability factors converge and their timing during neurodevelopment might influence disease phenotypes.

The relationship between nutrition and food production is one that must be considered in any discussion of the value of nutrigenomics. The goal of the development of individualized dietary guidance is dependent on the availability and composition of the agricultural commodities that make up the food supply. Dr. Joseph Spence in the chapter 'Nutrigenomics and Agriculture: A Perspective' explores the recent example of genomic prediction in dairy cattle. The lessons learned in application of the genome-based technologies are related to the development of dietary guidance for humans. An examination of the success of genetic prediction suggests that the identification of individuals at risk for nutritionally related diseases is possible and could form the basis for individualized nutritional advice and guidance. Potential problems in the development of such advice and how an individual might use that information to change their diet are of concern. The use of genomic tools to identify individuals at risk of nutritionally related diseases and to develop individualized dietary advice are possible but is not without pitfalls and problems that will need to be addressed.

Dr. Peter Gillies and Dr. Penny M. Kris-Etherton in their paper 'Opportunities and Challenges in Nutrigenetics/Nutrigenomics: Building Industry-Academia Partnerships' state that the intersection of industry and academia creates a Venn space wherein knowledge, experience and nutrigenomic technology can be leveraged to produce healthier foods and dietary supplements. Notably, such products are expected to have unprecedented nutritional pharmacology based on emerging principles of molecular nutrition. As the health-promoting properties of functional foods and dietary supplements increase, so does the need to resolve the 'nutrient-drug' debate. In this regard, the translational science of nutrigenomics involves everything from DNA to the FDA, and everybody from the private to the public sectors. The complexity and expense of this science, coupled with its potential for commercial application, inevitably draws industry and academia closer together as collaborators and partners. Although such ties are viewed by some as suspicious, fraught with bias and rife with conflict of interest, relationships based on shared ethical values, rigorous science and carefully selected projects, can be transparent and mutually beneficial. The experience of DuPont and the Pennsylvania State University is offered as a heuristic example of a successful industry-academic partnership and is presented herein in the context of omega-3 fatty acid research and molecular nutrition.

Another collaborative approach is presented by Dr. Lynnette Ferguson and colleagues in their manuscript 'Tailoring Foods to Match People's Genes in New Zealand: Opportunities for Collaboration'. They point out that Nutrigenomics New Zealand is tasked with developing the necessary competence for the development of gene-specific personalized foods (i.e. nutrigenetics). Initial work considers the response of 1 gene or gene variant, usually in the form of a SNP, to individual nutrients. The authors use Crohn's disease as proof of principle. Knowledge of key human Crohn's disease SNPs is incorporated into the design of isogenic cell lines, with and without the variant SNP of interest. Food extracts and components are tested for their ability to restore the normal phenotype in cellular models, before more selective testing in relevant animal models. In parallel, New Zealand Crohn's disease and control populations are tested for key genetic variants, and this information is compared with detailed dietary analysis. For example, a range of different foods show different tolerances in individuals carrying variants in an important Crohn's disease gene, NOD2. A substantial component of the program relies on high-quality data management, bioinformatics and biostatistics. International linkages will be essential for enhanced success of this program. In particular, testing hypotheses on gene-diet interactions will require large numbers of individuals in collaborative studies, with coordinated dietary and genotyping methods, to ensure that conclusions are adequately powered.

These proceedings should be of interest not only to scientists carrying out nutrigenetics/nutrigenomics research in academia, government and industry, but also to anyone interested in the future of personalized medicine, personalized nutrition and the future of agriculture. Such people would include physicians, geneticists, nutritionists, dieticians, food scientists, agriculturists in animal husbandry and horticulture, plant pathologists and persons interested in policy development in academia, industry and government.

Artemis P. Simopoulos, Washington, D.C.
John A. Milner, Bethesda, Md.

Conference Organization

Conference Co-Chairs

Artemis P. Simopoulos, MD (USA)
John A. Milner, MD (USA)

Planning Committee

Cindy D. Davis, NCI, NIH
Joseph Hibbelin, NIAAA, NIH
David Klurfeld, ARS, USDA
John Paul SanGiovanni, NEI, NIH
Pamela Starke-Reed, NIDDK, NIH

Conference Sponsors

National Cancer Institute
National Eye Institute
National Institute on Alcohol Abuse and Alcoholism
Eunice Kennedy Shriver National Institute of Child Health and Human Development
Division of Nutrition Research Coordination
Office of Dietary Supplements
U.S. Department of Agriculture
U.S. Food and Drug Administration
The Center for Genetics Nutrition and Health
Nutrilite Health Institute
National Dairy Council

Opportunities and Challenges in Nutrigenetics/Nutrigenomics and Health

Raffaele De Caterina

G. d'Annunzio University, Chieti and CNR Institute of Clinical Physiology, Pisa, Italy

Looking into the crystal ball to predict the future is always a risky operation. We are, however, confronted by this challenge when asked to provide, for others and ourselves, a vision of the evolution of a scientific area. As the essayist Jonathan Swift wrote: 'Vision is the art of seeing things invisible.' It is the attempt to imagine what is behind the curtain of current knowledge and wisdom. Nutrigenetics/nutrigenomics is a novel area of scientific research, its roots do not run deep in a glorious past but instead it looks towards the future. The symbol of the recently founded International Society of Nutrigenetics/Nutrigenomics (ISNN) is a tree bearing fruit, reflecting this sense of optimism. But it is a tree in springtime, when the fruits are foreseeable, but not yet within reach.

In this brief introductory chapter I will analyze some of the current needs of this new discipline. I will try to delineate the unique opportunities, and anticipate at least some of the challenges ahead.

Why Nutrigenetics/Nutrigenomics?

As living organisms, we are all the product of the interaction of our genes with our environment. Both genes and environment are essential components of life. Contrary to monogenic diseases, where a mutation in one single gene can be the sole cause and the 'essence' of a disease (e.g. sickle cell anemia), most global acquired diseases, such as coronary heart disease and cancer, are under the influence of a very large number of genes, and are always profoundly influenced by the environment. Therefore, acquired chronic diseases are paradigmatic examples of gene-environment interactions, where it is difficult to say which is predominant. Although family history can often be found in patients suffering an acute myocardial infarction, siblings in the same family are often unaffected, illustrating the principle that in such cases we inherit propensities, not inevitabilities.

Whatever the relative proportions of genetic and environmental factors that we may try to evaluate in such cases, the fact is that genes and environment are not entities in isolation, but they deeply interact with each other. The influence is bidirectional, in the sense that genes can affect factors that we recognize as environmentally modifiable (e.g. serum cholesterol), and environmental factors can affect gene expression. Nutrients are most likely the main environmental factors which we are exposed to, and they also interact with our genes bidirectionally. Coronary heart disease, which is now the leading cause of death and disability worldwide [1], is a case in point. In 52 countries spread across every inhabited continent, a study of the occurrence of a first myocardial infarction estimated that 9 known risk factors (smoking, history of hypertension or diabetes, waist/hip ratio, dietary patterns, physical activity, consumption of alcohol, blood apolipoproteins, and psychosocial factors) account for 90% of the population-attributable risk in men and 94% in women [2].

Three considerations appear to me extremely relevant here: (1) the above risk factors, including dietary pattern and the propensity for alcohol consumption, are all under genetic influence; (2) all these factors are modifiable, they are not at all inevitable; (3) six of these nine risk factors are influenced by the diet (or are themselves dietary patterns) and they interact with physical activity, which in the above analysis was also accounted for as an independent factor. Thus, nutritional factors, which were the first example given in molecular biology for ways to control gene expression (see the operon theory by Jacob and Monod [3]) are the best example I can give of how the environment influences our genes, and are themselves influenced by our genes. Indeed the terms 'nutrigenetics' (how the genetic constitution modulates the response to nutrients) and 'nutrigenomics' (how nutrients affect gene expression) are themselves intertwined, and are largely understandable as two faces of the same coin [4].

Opportunities

Nutrigenetics/nutrigenomics has an increasing public profile and is attracting the attention of the media. In its 2007 special report into nutrition, *The Economist*, a current affairs magazine, carried the following text:

Some people eat three-egg omelettes topped with slivers of bacon and show no sign of a spike in cholesterol. Some people indulge in one chocolate bar after another and stay as thin as a rake. Many, however, are less fortunate. Current research suggests that the culprit may be found in one's genes. Differences in genetic make-up may not only determine the ability to metabolize certain nutrients, such as fats and lactose, but also susceptibility to disease.

The good news is that, within five years or so, researchers should learn how to modify people's diets to thereby prevent or delay the onset of a possible illness. At least, that is the goal of nutritional genomics, a new field that studies how genes and diet interact [5].

In this way, the media reflects and drives public interest in nutrigenetics/nutrigenomics, seeing it as holding the promise of personalized nutrition where each individual's diet is devised to best interact with his or her genetic make-up. This is the unique opportunity of this new discipline as it deepens its roots in nutrition, preventive medicine, clinical disciplines, genetics and molecular biology and systems biology. It gives rise to the possibility of exploiting subcellular, cellular and preclinical animal models and also to provide a unique way of synthesis, a unique new idea.

Thomas Aquinas, the 13th century theologian and philosopher, stated: 'The essence of the human being is to take two concepts which are themselves abstract, then to put them together to form a new abstract concept which is unlike the two original ones.' This applies to the combination of the concepts that give rise to an entirely new individual entity. Nutrigenetics/nutrigenomics is indeed a single leap forward of the imagination, opening a new area of investigation with enormous potential consequences.

Although nutrition obviously predates pharmaceutics in human history, interestingly nutrigenetics is an expansion of concepts seen in pharmacogenetics: an attempt to better understand the reasons underlying variability of individual responses to the environment. Thus, nutrigenetics is an attempt to make sense of the inter-individual variation in our responses to diet – the main environmental factor – in the way that we are now approaching an understanding of why people react differently to the same antiplatelet drug [6] in terms of inhibition of platelet function and how this translates into a greater or lesser protective effect against myocardial infarction. Indeed, we now have excellent examples of genetic variants affecting the *probability* of a disease, and of nutrients able to modify such probability. For example, insertion/deletion gene variants in the promoter region of 5-lipoxygenase, affecting the production of leukotrienes, are related to the risk of increased intima-media thickness in the carotid arteries (a proxy for the burden of atherosclerosis), but such genetic influence can be totally abrogated by increased intake of omega-3 fatty acids, known sources of weaker leukotrienes and alternatives to the main eicosanoids derived from omega-6 fatty acids [7, 8]. And we have, likewise, examples of direct control by nutrients of gene expression, examples being – from my own personal interest – the modulation of expression of adhesion molecules and of the inflammatory enzyme cyclooxygenase-2 by omega-3 fatty acids [9, 10].

The background science is there, but how close are we to the goal of implementing personalized nutrition based on genetic knowledge? We are not there yet. I will briefly explain why.

We already now know, by-and-large, how to modify people's diets to prevent or delay the onset of a possible illness, but we know this in terms of 'average' responses of groups of subjects to a given change in the diet. We also have excellent cases where dietary habits that can be good for some can be bad for others, for example, in attempts at understanding the responses of lipid metabolism to the intake of polyunsaturated fatty acids [11].

However, most such studies have not yet come full circle to establish a solid ground for health claims. The reasons are:
– Most studies performed have been either complex nutritional interventions or they isolated the effect of a single nutritional component. So far there has never been a combination of the 2 approaches with the same aim. The result is that,

with the first approach, we cannot ascribe the effect observed to one single dietary factor, and with the second, we cannot exclude the abrogation or the reversal of the effect by contrasting effects from other nutrients, due to scarce or actually absent knowledge on the effects of interactions with other dietary components.
- There is usually in such studies little or no knowledge of the overall effect on the organism. We study single outcomes, thought to be related to a more general endpoint (I use the terms 'outcomes' and 'endpoint' deliberately), but we have not proved so far the effect on the general endpoint itself.

Challenges

As researchers in a new discipline, those working in nutrigenetics/nutrigenomics are energized by the excitement of navigating uncharted waters, but we must not allow our enthusiasm to blind us to the problems. Sailors venturing into the Arctic sea know that most of the dangers lie below the surface, and because these dangers are not readily visible there is a risk of trivializing them, rendering them more insidious. It is important at the very beginning of the life of a new discipline to recognize and manage upfront these difficulties, as if they are left unchecked they may undermine the credibility of the entire field.

I see major challenges in the following areas:
- relying on surrogate/intermediate endpoints;
- issuing premature health claims;
- underestimating the financial interests involved;
- misjudging ethical and legal implications.

Surrogate Endpoints
We need surrogate endpoints. At the beginning of a clinical investigation we need readily measurable and obtainable parameters that give us a sense of where that research topic is going. In the two examples given before [7, 8], the measurement of the intima-media thickness as a proxy for atherosclerosis is logical, understandable, and supported by good evidence of its relationship to more concrete endpoints. For the relationship of polyunsaturated fatty acid intake to the blood levels of HDL cholesterol, in the other example given above [11], HDL cholesterol is a lipid parameter related to the firmer endpoint of coronary heart disease morbidity and mortality.

However, in addition to often being of little importance to patients, surrogates may lead to misleading and erroneous conclusions [12]. Endpoints are indeed a first approximation to the disease we are trying to prevent, but they must be substantiated at some point with firmer evaluations. The history of clinical pharmacology is replete with examples of drugs found to be effective in large-scale trials on some intermediate outcome and then proven in the end to cause harm rather than benefit on the same disease process that is known to be related to the intermediate outcome investigated.

An example is hormone replacement therapy, which was found to favorably affect atherosclerosis progression and yet caused increased – rather than decreased – cardiovascular deaths because of an unexpectedly high excess risk of thrombosis [13]. There is also the more recent unfortunate story of the cholesterol ester transfer protein inhibitor torcetrapib, found to be very effective in raising HDL-cholesterol, and yet causing more harm than benefit in treated patients, likely due to some unanticipated off-target detrimental effect of the specific drug used [14]. How much of the currently performed nutrigenetic/nutrigenomic research goes down the road to the point of showing the ultimate health consequences of personalized nutrition? I would assert that no such examples yet exist. There must be a way to come to full circle to demonstrate the clinical relevance of operating differentially in different patient categories. Until this process is completed, it is premature to make health claims.

Premature Health Claims
As a consequence of the current weaknesses in evidence, most of the other challenges come from the temptation to rapidly exploit the burgeoning amount of knowledge being acquired for rushed, unwarranted health claims, linked immediately to financial interests. While industrial interests can help the development of sound scientific research, they can also thwart it, ultimately discrediting it. It is easy to understand the willingness of manufacturers to sell their genetic tests even if doctors do not know what to do with them [15]. Similarly, it is easy to anticipate (actually, to witness) the creation of companies wishing to ride the horse of the trendy business of personalized nutrition, selling recipes claiming to be 'good for you' and 'based on the latest scientific developments'. This is a huge problem that has to be faced properly.

Ethical and Legal Implications
Last, but not least, there are ethical and legal implications in the area of genetic testing [16] and of nutrigenetics [17] that need to be known and carefully approached. These involve:
– the management of genetic information;
– consent, confidentiality, familial consequences, testing children;
– non-medical uses of information by employers and insurers.

The handling of genetic information is an area fraught with difficulty. For example, we know that a mutation in apolipoprotein E (e4/e4) that is found in 14% of the UK and US populations is linked to an increased risk of early cardiovascular disease, and such risk can be modified with diet. This genotype is, however, also linked with a 60% increased risk of developing Alzheimer's disease, where it is not clear whether changing dietary fat intake favorably or unfavorably affects the risk of Alzheimer's disease.

We must also consider the fact that, in general, it is well established that having a healthy diet and lifestyle are of paramount importance. We should therefore not risk diluting these messages with premature speculation and resist the temptation to raise expectations that may later prove unrealistic. It is also important not to frighten people with results of genetic tests showing they have increased risk for a condition that could be modifiable with an expensive and at this time still unproven 'personalized' diet. In other words, we should continue looking at what we have already on our shelves, where there are already dietary choices known to be healthier than others, independent of any knowledge of individuals' genetic constitution. These include foods derived from organic and free-range animal farming (which not just affect our genes, but also involve ethical choices), low-fat products, products with a low glycemic index, increased intake of fish, fruits and vegetables, friendly bacteria products, folic acid to prevent neural tube defects and severe cases of hyperhomocysteinemia, vitamins for children and older age groups to combat absolute or relative deficiencies.

How to Deal with the Challenges

Meeting these challenges is a daunting prospect and fighting this battle will be difficult, more so if those in the field act only individually. It is for this reason that there is a great need for a scientific society with the mission to select and give voice to sound scientific information in an extremely complex, crowded and 'polluted' arena. The ISNN aims to act as a clearing house for media and scientific information, and place itself in an intermediate position between investigators and industry. In his welcome note on the organization's website, society president Dr. Artemis P. Simopoulos wrote that the purpose of the ISNN is to 'increase understanding through research and education of professionals and the general public of the role of genetic variation and dietary response and the role of nutrients in gene expression' [18]. Dr. Simopoulos continued that important aims of the ISNN include serving as a clearing-house for the media in disseminating facts regarding the role of genetic variation and dietary response and the role of nutrients in gene expression, assisting in interpreting the new facts into sound nutritional advice for the public, and establishing science and education committees. The ISNN provides an opportunity for an ethical alliance of scientists motivated by genuine science to advance knowledge, but also to act as a transmission chain to the public.

We are humbled by the magnitude of the task, but also proud and thrilled by the opportunities and the challenges ahead.

References

1 World Health Organization. World Health Statistics 2009. www.who.int/whosis/whostat/2009/en/print.html (accessed January 13, 2010).
2 Yusuf S, Hawken S, Ounpuu S, Dans T, Avezum A, Lanas F, McQueen M, Budaj A, Pais P, Varigos J, Lisheng L: Effect of potentially modifiable risk factors associated with myocardial infarction in 52 countries (the INTERHEART study): case-control study. Lancet 2004;364:937–952.
3 Jacob F, Perrin D, Sanchez C, Monod J: Operon: a group of genes with the expression coordinated by an operator. C R Hebd Seances Acad Sci 1960; 250: 1727–1729.
4 Mutch DM, Wahli W, Williamson G: Nutrigenomics and nutrigenetics: the emerging faces of nutrition. FASEB J 2005;19:1602–1616.
5 Nutrition: Special Report. The Economist, July 22, 2007.

6 Collet JP, Hulot JS, Pena A, Villard E, Esteve JB, Silvain J, Payot L, Brugier D, Cayla G, Beygui F, Bensimon G, Funck-Brentano C, Montalescot G: Cytochrome P450 2C19 polymorphism in young patients treated with clopidogrel after myocardial infarction: a cohort study. Lancet 2009;373:309–317.

7 Dwyer JH, Allayee H, Dwyer KM, Fan J, Wu H, Mar R, Lusis AJ, Mehrabian M: Arachidonate 5-lipoxygenase promoter genotype, dietary arachidonic acid, and atherosclerosis. N Engl J Med 2004;350:29–37.

8 De Caterina R, Zampolli A: From asthma to atherosclerosis; 5-lipoxygenase, leukotrienes, and inflammation. N Engl J Med 2004;350:4–7.

9 De Caterina R, Cybulsky MI, Clinton SK, Gimbrone MA Jr, Libby P: The omega-3 fatty acid docosahexaenoate reduces cytokine-induced expression of proatherogenic and proinflammatory proteins in human endothelial cells. Arterioscler Thromb 1994;14:1829–1836.

10 Massaro M, Habib A, Lubrano L, Del Turco S, Lazzerini G, Bourcier T, Weksler BB, De Caterina R: The omega-3 fatty acid docosahexaenoate attenuates endothelial cyclooxygenase-2 induction through both NADP(H) oxidase and PKC epsilon inhibition. Proc Natl Acad Sci USA 2006;103:15184–15189.

11 Ordovas JM, Corella D, Cupples LA, Demissie S, Kelleher A, Coltell O, Wilson PW, Schaefer EJ, Tucker K: Polyunsaturated fatty acids modulate the effects of the APOA1 G-A polymorphism on HDL-cholesterol concentrations in a sex-specific manner: the Framingham Study. Am J Clin Nutr 2002;75:38–46.

12 DeMaria AN: Clinical trials and clinical judgment. J Am Coll Cardiol 2008;51:1120–1122.

13 Manson JE, Martin KA: Clinical practice: postmenopausal hormone-replacement therapy. N Engl J Med 2001;345:34–40.

14 Barter PJ, Caulfield M, Eriksson M, Grundy SM, Kastelein JJ, Komajda M, Lopez-Sendon J, Mosca L, Tardif JC, Waters DD, Shear CL, Revkin JH, Buhr KA, Fisher MR, Tall AR, Brewer B: Effects of torcetrapib in patients at high risk for coronary events. N Engl J Med 2007;357:2109–2122.

15 Hunter DJ, Khoury MJ, Drazen JM: Letting the genome out of the bottle: will we get our wish? N Engl J Med 2008;358:105–107.

16 Simopoulos AP: Genetic screening: programs, principles, and research – thirty years later. Reviewing the recommendations of the Committee for the Study of Inborn Errors of Metabolism (SIEM). Public Health Genomics 2009;12:105–111.

17 Capron A, Bice S: Learning from the past and looking to the future. J Nutrigenet Nutrigenomics 2009;2:85–90.

18 Simopoulos AP: ISNN Home. http://www.isnn.info (accessed January 13, 2010).

Raffaele De Caterina, MD, PhD
Chair and Postgraduate School of Cardiology, G. d'Annunzio University, Chieti, c/o Ospedale SS. Annunziata
Via dei Vestini
IT–66013 Chieti (Italy)
Tel. +39 0871 41512, Fax +39 0871 402817, E-Mail rdecater@unich.it

Genome-Wide Association Studies and Diet

Lynnette R. Ferguson

Discipline of Nutrition, FM & HS, University of Auckland, and Nutrigenomics New Zealand, Auckland, New Zealand

Towards the end of the 20th century, we were successfully beginning to understand part of the genetic basis of some human diseases. Up to that time, progress had been relatively slow, largely depending upon establishing familial associations, and somewhat laboriously measured variations in candidate genes. This was usually in the form of single nucleotide polymorphisms (SNPs), measured one at a time with labor-intensive methods such as restriction fragment length polymorphism [1]. However, since the initial publication of work on the human genome [2], major advances in genotyping capability and reductions in cost, coupled with large collaborative population groups are enabling exponential advances in our understanding of human genetic variation. Genome-wide association studies (GWAS) are greatly increasing our understanding of the genetic basis of human disease, especially complex disease. Perhaps more importantly, they are more generally enhancing our knowledge of far more subtle differences between individuals, including behavioral characteristics, health, 'wellness' and performance. An analysis of GWAS publications since their first appearance in 2003 (fig. 1) emphasizes why Pennisi [3] described such studies as the breakthrough of the year in enabling knowledge of what makes each of us unique.

Since the earliest GWAS papers, there have been a number of commentaries in high-impact scientific journals, including a supplement in *Nature* (October 8), described as 'Human Genetics 2009'. The editorial points to the enhanced flow of human genetic information and the way that high density gene chip information is being utilized by online direct-to-consumer companies who claim to be predicting human health at the individual level. What is not being considered, however, is the key information that may be necessary to enable genetic data to predict human health or, more importantly, to develop strategies to modify the genetic predictions. That is, a parallel and integrated assessment of diet and environmental factors. In 2005, we commented on the need for international collaborative efforts in nutrigenomics to enable better understanding of the basis of human disease and 'wellness' characteristics that differ among individuals [4]. However, while there has been a proliferation

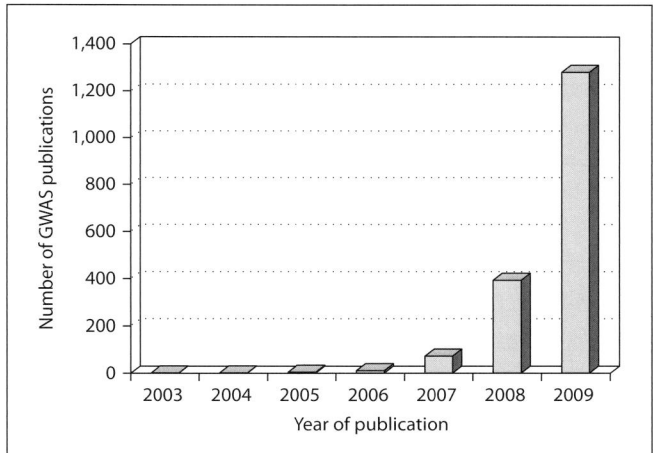

Fig. 1. Number of genome-wide association studies reported each year since 2003 in a PubMed literature search.

of studies on the genetic basis of disease (fig. 1), for the most part these have not been accompanied by stringent dietary and environmental data. It is suggested that this should become an essential input to such studies in the future.

Monogenic Disorders and Complex Disease

For much of the 20th century, knowledge of the genetic basis of human disease was limited to single-gene or Mendelian disease, where familial association is somewhat obvious. Most of these mutations are in the form of SNPs involving either missense or nonsense mutations [5]. Once the disease was accurately phenotyped and familial associations identified, it became relatively clear which gene was important. However, such diseases are relatively rare, and most of the common diseases are more complex, involving multiple genes and interactions with environment, including diet.

With complex disease, association studies are the only realistic approach, using large numbers of unrelated cases and controls, or family groupings such as trios involving 2 parents and an affected child [6]. Large numbers of markers that cover the genome are required to identify genes in complex disease. Perhaps more importantly, the presence or absence of a single gene variant is not usually sufficient to explain the disease phenotype. There is good reason to believe that genetic predisposition to complex disease is due to minor variations in a large number of genes, and their ability to interact with specific environmental factors. While these complex diseases are much more difficult to study, this knowledge may become increasingly important, since they are the most common cause of death in humans [7, 8]. There are, of course, even more technical challenges in gaining an effective understanding of the human diet than of genes [9].

Enabling Technologies in GWAS

Although the first GWAS appeared in the literature in 2003, the initial tools did not cover a representative area of the human genome. In 2004, Ishkanian et al. [10] described a tiling resolution DNA microarray that they described as showing 'complete coverage' of the human genome. Such tools are essential starting blocks for GWAS studies, which are based on enabling genotype-phenotype correlations, using the same principles as candidate gene studies. However, such studies are hypothesis free, since the variants measured span the entire human genome. The international HapMap project recognized the need for studies of this sort, and sought to characterize the major SNPs across the genome, and in different human population groups [11]. The notion was that these would provide an idea of population structure on all 'common' SNPs (>5% frequency), in 2 phases of increasing density across the genome. This would be supplemented by deep re-sequencing as appropriate. This resource has provided the enabling technology for genetic variant assays using gene chips, now able to cover more than 1 million SNPs across the genome. The 2 main genotyping providers are Affymetrix, whose variants are randomly distributed, and Illumina, who have utilized more highly selected tagging SNPs. Either or both of these gene chips are ideal to measure a large number of SNPs and also copy number variants [12]. Deep re-sequencing techniques are also available for interrogating specific areas of the genome. Large collaborative databases are essential for providing the necessary statistical power for confidence in data interpretation.

GWAS: Why Are They Important?

GWAS provide an important mechanism for moving away from candidate gene studies, which select genes for study based on known or suspected disease mechanisms. Instead, GWAS permit a comprehensive scan of the genome in an unbiased fashion. By this means they have drawn out associations with genes not previously suspected of being related to the disease. They permit examination of inherited genetic variability at unprecedented levels of resolution, and have even picked up some associations in regions not even known to harbor genes. The methods continue to be refined. In their 2009 review, Ioannidis et al. [13] recommend large-scale exact replication across both similar and diverse populations, fine mapping and resequencing, determination of the most informative markers and multiple independent informative loci, incorporation of functional information, and improved phenotype mapping of the implicated genetic effects. Even where replication proves that an effect exists, definitive identification of the causal variant is often elusive. While these are all important points, it is of concern that even the excellent Ioannidis et al. review fails to consider diet as one of the missing variables.

Crohn's disease provides a good example of the power of this methodology. Candidate gene studies very slowly uncovered some of the genetic basis for this disease, with an initial report on the first disease gene, Nucleotide oligomerisation domain 2 *(NOD2)* in 2001 [14]. Other genes were slowly and sometimes unconvincingly revealed, including other immune recognition genes such as Toll-like receptor 4 *(TLR4)* [15]. However, the first publications of GWAS on this disease [16, 17] revealed the importance of SNPs in hitherto unsuspected genes, including the interleukin 23 receptor, *IL23R*, and the autophagy gene, *ATG16L1*. These genes both involve response to environmental factors, especially bacteria and diet. GWAS methodology continues to yield important findings on the genetic basis of this disease [18]. However, studies on dietary interactions are substantially lagging behind the genetic evidence.

Use of Gene Chips and GWAS Datasets in Personalized Health Predictions

The publication of this burgeoning number of datasets has led to a proliferation of online genetic testing companies, which purport to provide a measure of genetic risk to an individual, who has provided saliva or buccal swab samples for DNA isolation and genotyping. Inevitably, there has been concern expressed about their relevance. For example, Ng et al. [19], compared data provided by 2 different direct-to-consumer genetics-testing companies on a small number of individuals, to find quite significant differences in the predictions claimed. For their 5 test individuals, in predictions of 7 diseases only 50% or fewer of the predictions agreed between the 2 companies. Their information showed that the accuracy of the raw data was high. However, they questioned whether the predicted disease risks had clinical validity, and how well a genetic variant correlates with a specific disease or condition. They found that the companies showed very similar predictions for diseases where the genetic risk was convincing, and they concluded that companies should communicate high risks better than they are currently doing. They also suggested that test data would become more relevant to human health if the companies tested for drug response markers. They pointed to differences between the genetic basis of disease in different ethnicities, and suggested that the information gathered should include consideration of behavior. Surprisingly, however, they failed to highlight the potential importance of diet and/or environment. Their 9 recommendations are reproduced in table 1.

Celiac disease provides an example where Ng et al. [19] showed good agreement between direct-to-consumer testing companies. Celiac disease represents a major food intolerance, with a current prevalence rate of approximately 1 per 100 individuals in the population [20]. This disease is characterized by a lifelong intolerance to gluten, which is found in wheat, barley and rye, and products derived from them. The most effective treatment for celiac disease is nutritional [21] and remission of symptoms can be well maintained in the absence of gluten. At present, this disease is usually diagnosed phenotypically, once symptoms have developed, and requires an invasive

Table 1. Recommendations for improvement of direct-to-consumer genetic testing, as identified by Ng et al. [19].

Addressed to	Recommendation
Industry	Report the genetic contribution for the markers tested
	Focus on high-risk predictions
	Directly genotype risk markers
	Test pharmacogenomic markers
	Agree on strong-effect markers
Community	Monitor behavioral outcomes
	Carry out prospective studies
	Replicate associated markers in other ethnicities
	Sequence rather than genotype

small intestinal biopsy for diagnosis. However, twin studies provide good evidence for a genetic basis of the disease, with 10% of first-degree relatives being affected, and 75% concordance between monozygotic twins [22]. Several genes are clearly involved, but the most consistent genetic component depends on the variants in HLA-DQ (DQ2 and/or DQ8) genes [23]. The main genes in celiac disease lead to a 7-fold increased disease risk, and can be diagnosed fairly consistently, either on a phenotype or genotype level. More recent GWAS also give insight into the other relevant genes for this disease [24]. There would seem to be a case for earlier genetic diagnosis in susceptible families, avoiding the inevitable suffering associated with the presence of symptoms.

Where slightly different interpretations occurred was where one company had kept up with the very latest literature but other companies had not. Crohn's disease provided an example where there were inconsistencies in diagnosis. Even though this disease has proved remarkably tractable in GWAS studies, with very strong probabilities of accurate diagnosis of genes [25], individually these have very low relative risks. This may suggest the importance of environmental interactions.

Gene-Diet Interactions: Crohn's Disease

The genetic basis of Crohn's disease has not been as easy to characterize as celiac disease. The genetic basis of the disease is, as with celiac disease, supported by twin studies. For example, Tysk et al. [26] have shown strong familial associations and around 44% concordance between monozygotic twins. Although key genes have been revealed by GWAS and other approaches, the odds ratios associated with individual risk alleles are not spectacular [25]. Furthermore, although key dietary items have been revealed, unlike celiac disease, there is no 'one size fits all' solution. For example, in our own studies, wheat products, dairy foods, red wine, corn, mushrooms, soy milk and yoghurt are all examples of foods for which a number of individuals with the disease report an exacerbation of risk. However, there are also a proportion of individuals who consistently report that they appear to benefit from regularly eating one or more of these foods. We have been able to demonstrate that at least some of these apparently inconsistent data, for example with mushrooms, are a result of gene-diet interactions [27]. In this example, a genetic variant in a solute transporter molecule, OCTN1, appeared important for Crohn's disease risk in some overseas populations; it did not show statistically significant association with disease risk in a New Zealand population. However, when the ability to tolerate mushrooms was factored in, those individuals with strong mushroom intolerance showed significantly enhanced levels of the OCTN1 variant as compared with the control population.

The experience with Crohn's disease leads to caution in interpreting dietary information in such a complex disease. There is a considerable effort to increase the sensitivity and accuracy of dietary information [9]. However, more accurate dietary questionnaires reveal a typical eating pattern for the individual. From an analysis of such data for an individual with Crohn's disease, one might conclude that a deficiency of wheat products, dairy foods, red wine, corn, mushrooms, soy milk and yoghurt has led to the development of the disease. However, the actual picture is likely to be the complete converse of this. The observation is that, when he or she actually eats these dietary items, disease symptoms develop, and thus the individuals learn to avoid foods that trigger symptoms. This means that it is the presence rather than the absence of these items that actually led to the establishment of symptoms of the disease. This is the complete converse of traditional dietary interpretation, and may lead the way to different thinking about dietary studies in association with GWAS. Certainly, effective methods are increasingly becoming available [28]. However such studies are performed, it is essential that they are done if we are to uncover the true role of genetic variants, and the interplay with diet and environment, in the etiology of complex disease.

Acknowledgments

Nutrigenomics New Zealand is a collaboration between AgResearch Ltd., Plant & Food Research and the University of Auckland, with funding through the Foundation for Research Science and Technology.

References

1 Breen G, Harold D, Ralston S, Shaw D, St Clair D: Determining SNP allele frequencies in DNA pools. Biotechniques 2000;28:464–466.
2 Venter JC, Adams MD, Myers EW, et al: The sequence of the human genome. Science 2001; 291:1304–1351. Erratum: Science 2001;292: 1838.
3 Pennisi E: Breakthrough of the year: Human genetic variation. Science 2007;318:1842–1843.
4 Kaput J, Ordovas JM, Ferguson L, et al: The case for strategic international alliances to harness nutritional genomics for public and personal health. Br J Nutr 2005;94:623–632.

5 Stenson PD, Ball EV, Mort M, et al: Human Gene Mutation Database (HGMD): 2003 update. Hum Mutat 2003;21:577–581.
6 Nowotny P, Kwon JM, Goate AM: SNP analysis to dissect human traits. Curr Opin Neurobiol 2001;11:637–641.
7 Bell J: Predicting disease using genomics. Nature 2004;429:453-456.
8 Frazer KA, Murray SS, Schork NJ, Topol EJ: Human genetic variation and its contribution to complex traits. Nat Rev Genet 2009;10: 241–251.
9 Poslusna K, Ruprich J, de Vries JH, Jakubikova M, van't Veer P: Misreporting of energy and micronutrient intake estimated by food records and 24 hour recalls, control and adjustment methods in practice. Br J Nutr 2009;101(suppl 2):S73–S85.
10 Ishkanian AS, Malloff CA, Watson SK, et al: A tiling resolution DNA microarray with complete coverage of the human genome. Nat Genet 2004;36:299–303.
11 Couzin J: Human genome: HapMap launched with pledges of $100 million. Science 2002;298:941–942.
12 Shelling AN, Ferguson LR: Genetic variation in human disease and a new role for copy number variants. Mutat Res 2007;622:33–41.
13 Ioannidis JP, Thomas G, Daly MJ: Validating, augmenting and refining genome-wide association signals. Nat Rev Genet 2009;10:318–329.
14 Ogura Y, Bonen DK, Inohara N, et al: A frameshift mutation in NOD2 associated with susceptibility to Crohn's disease. Nature 2001;411:603–606.
15 Browning BL, Huebner C, Petermann I, et al: Has Toll-like receptor 4 been prematurely dismissed as an inflammatory bowel disease gene? Association study combined with meta-analysis shows strong evidence for association. Am J Gastroenterol 2007;102:2504–2512.
16 Duerr RH, Taylor KD, Brant SR, et al: A genome-wide association study identifies IL23R as an inflammatory bowel disease gene. Science 2006;314:1461–1463.
17 Cummings JRF, Cooney R, Pathan S, et al: Confirmation of the role of ATG16L1 as a Crohn's disease susceptibility gene. Inflamm Bowel Dis 2007;13:941–946.
18 Marquez A, Cenit MC, Nunez C, et al: Effect of BSN-MST1 locus on inflammatory bowel disease and multiple sclerosis susceptibility. Genes Immun 2009;10:631–635.
19 Ng PC, Murray SS, Levy S, Venter JC: An agenda for personalized medicine. Nature 2009;461:724–726.
20 McGough N, Cummings JH: Coeliac disease: a diverse clinical syndrome caused by intolerance of wheat, barley and rye. Proc Nutr Soc 2005;64:434–450.
21 Greco L, Romino R, Coto I, et al: The first large population based twin study of coeliac disease. Gut 2002;50:624–628.
22 Di Gilio A, Fusco M, Mazzacca G: Grown-up coeliac children: the effects of only a few years on a gluten-free diet in childhood. Aliment Pharmacol Ther 2005;21:421–429.
23 Romanos J, van Diemen CC, Nolte IM, et al: Analysis of HLA and non-HLA alleles can identify individuals at high risk for celiac disease. Gastroenterology 2009;137:834–840.
24 Garner CP, Murray JA, Ding YC, et al: Replication of celiac disease UK genome-wide association study results in a US population. Hum Mol Genet 2009;18:4219–4225.
25 Wellcome Trust Case Control Consortium: Genome-wide association study of 14,000 cases of seven common diseases and 3,000 shared controls. Nature 2007;447:661–678.
26 Tysk C, Lindberg E, Järnerot G, Flodérus-Myrhed B: Ulcerative colitis and Crohn's disease in an unselected population of monozygotic and dizygotic twins: a study of heritability and the influence of smoking. Gut 1988;29:990–996.
27 Petermann I, Triggs CM, Huebner C, et al: Mushroom intolerance: a novel diet-gene interaction in Crohn's disease. Br J Nutr 2009;102:506–508.
28 Bureau A, Diallo MS, Ordovas JM, Cupples LA: Estimating interaction between genetic and environmental risk factors: efficiency of sampling designs within a cohort. Epidemiology 2008;19:83–93.

Lynnette R. Ferguson
Discipline of Nutrition, FM&HS, University of Auckland,
Auckland (New Zealand)
Tel. +64 9 373 7599, Fax +64 9 303 5963, E-Mail l.ferguson@auckland.ac.nz

Copy Number Variation, Eicosapentaenoic Acid and Neurological Disorders

With Particular Reference to Huntington's Disease and Associated CAG Repeats, and to Myalgic Encephalomyelitis and Viral Infection

Basant K. Puri[a] · Mehar S. Manku[b]

[a]MRI Unit, Imaging Sciences Department, MRC Clinical Sciences Centre, Imperial College London, Hammersmith Hospital, London, and [b]Amarin Neuroscience, Oxford, UK

It has been suggested that nutrigenomics, the study of the effects of nutrients on molecular level biological processes and the variable effects of nutrients on individuals, represents the new frontier of nutrition science [1]. One particular nutrient, eicosapentaenoic acid (EPA), is an important $n-3$ long-chain polyunsaturated fatty acid which has multiple important functions. The use of the semi-synthetic derivative ethyl-eicosapentaenoic acid (ethyl-EPA) in the treatment and prevention of certain neurological and cardiovascular disorders is becoming increasingly well known. In this paper, we discuss the early evidence that individual response to ethyl-EPA might be a function of copy number variation. To this end, the research carried out in Huntington's disease is germane, given that the genetic cause (increased CAG repeats) of this neurological disorder are well characterized, and that differences in the number of CAG repeats in Huntington's disease can be measured. Similarly, given the recent finding of retroviral infection being common in myalgic encephalomyelitis, the response of patients with the latter neurological disorder to ethyl-EPA might also be expected to show differences related to copy number variation.

Ethyl-EPA

EPA (C20:5$n-3$) is a long-chain $n-3$ polyunsaturated fatty acid that is a natural metabolite of the short-chain essential fatty acid α-linolenic acid. It is labile and can degrade rapidly. Ethyl-EPA is a semi-synthetic, highly purified EPA derivative which is more stable. Following oral administration and absorption, ethyl-EPA is acted on by esterases, particularly pancreatic lipase, to release EPA, so that ethyl-EPA acts as a pro-drug [2]. The EPA cyclo-oxygenase and the lipoxygenase metabolites include biologically active eicosanoids such as 3-series prostaglandins and resolvins [3]. EPA also down-regulates IL-1β-induced prostaglandin H synthase 2 expression in human microvascular endothelial cells, probably through its 5-lipoxygenase-dependent metabolites (EPA suppresses p38 mitogen-activated protein kinase phosphorylation in stimulated pulmonary microvascular endothelial cells) [4]. In respect of neurological disorders associated with cerebral atrophy, it is important to note that since prostaglandin biosynthesis can directly induce apoptosis in mammalian neuronal cells [5, 6], down-regulation of the prostaglandin synthesizing enzyme cascade might be associated with a protective effect of EPA against apoptotic changes in the brain [2].

Huntington's Disease

Huntington's disease is an autosomal dominant disease caused by an unstable expansion of CAG trinucleotide triplet repeats in the *huntingtin* gene at 4p16.3. The CAG repeats are transcribed and translated into polyglutamine expansion (polyQ) stretches, and the length of the repeats has been shown to correlate inversely with the age of onset of the disease [7, 8]. It is characterized by motor dysfunction; chorea and incoordination occur relatively early and dystonia, rigidity, and bradykinesia become more prominent with time. Death usually occurs within 15–25 years of onset of motor symptomatology [9, 10]. In terms of characteristic neuropathological changes, central, particularly striatal, neuronal degeneration takes place, to which mitochondrial dysfunction might contribute [11, 12]. The mechanism of such mitochondrial damage is not known at the time of writing, but there is evidence for an involvement of the c-Jun amino-terminal kinase (JNK) pathway induced by stress-signal kinase 1 (SEK1), for a specific role of p53 in the mitochondria-associated cellular dysfunction and behavioral abnormalities, and for possible mediation by nuclear factor-κB (NF-κB) [2].

It is noteworthy that EPA targets mitochondrial function and affects gene expression by acting on transcription factors such as peroxisome proliferator-activated receptors and also acts on the JNK and NF-κB pathways [13–15]. EPA inhibits phorbol 12-tetradecanoate 13-acetate-induced JNK-AP-1 transactivation and subsequent cellular transformation [16], deoxynivalenol-induced JNK activation in macrophages [17], lipopolysaccharide (LPS)-induced JNK activation in macrophages [18], LPS-induced JNK activation in microglia [19], and amyloid-β-induced JNK activation in the hippocampus [20, 21]. EPA has also been shown to inhibit tumor necrosis factor mRNA expression in LPS-stimulated macrophages and LPS-stimulated monocytes, possibly by reducing NF-κB activation by reducing the P65/P50 NF-κB dimers [22] or by inhibiting phosphorylation of the inhibitory subunit IκB, thereby keeping it in the non-phosphorylated form that in turn keeps NF-κB in an inactive form [19, 23]. In patients with bipolar disorder, ethyl-EPA treatment is associated with increased cerebral N-acetylaspartate, a putative marker of neuronal integrity [24].

A small 6-month randomized double-blind placebo-controlled trial of pure ethyl-EPA in stage III Huntington's disease showed that the fatty acid intervention was associated with improvement on the orofacial component of the Unified Huntington's Disease Rating Scale, while all the patients on placebo deteriorated on this scale [25]. Following subvoxel sinc-interpolation-based registration of follow-up 3D MRI brain scans with baseline scans [26], subtraction images showed that while the placebo was associated with progressive cerebral atrophy, the ethyl-EPA was associated with a reverse process [25]. A subsequent multi-center large-scale randomized placebo-controlled trial of ethyl-EPA was carried out. A pre hoc hypothesis was put forward by one of the authors, the late Prof. David Horrobin, suggesting that a genetic influence was likely in respect of the response to ethyl-EPA; he therefore suggested (before the study took place) that the results should be dichotomized around the median CAG repeat number. Indeed, the study went on to show that patients in the per protocol group as well as those with a lower CAG repeat number showed clinical improvement with ethyl-EPA compared with placebo [27], thus confirming Prof. Horrobin's hypothesis regarding the importance of considering pharmacogenetic factors in using EPA in this disease. Treatment with ethyl-EPA was again found to be associated with improved cerebral structure on MRI brain scans carried out in the patients attending the lead research center [2].

Myalgic Encephalomyelitis

Myalgic encephalomyelitis is a devastating disease which, according to the Revised CDC (Centers for Disease Control and Prevention) Criteria, include the following symptoms and signs (in addition to chronic fatigue): impaired memory or concentration; sore throat; tender cervical or axillary lymph nodes; myalgia; multi-joint pains; new headaches; unrefreshing sleep, and post-exertion malaise [28].

Three proton neurospectroscopy studies of myalgic encephalomyelitis, 2 systematic [29, 30] and 1 non-systematic [31], have reported an increased level of free choline-containing compounds in the brain [32]. It has been hypothesized that this may be the result of reduced incorporation of the choline polar head group in phospholipid molecules at the Sn3 position in both outer cell membranes and intracellular organelle membranes in neurons and glial cells in this disease, which may, in turn, result from impaired biosynthesis of membrane phospholipid molecules in the brain, as a result of reduced biosynthesis of long-chain polyunsaturated fatty acids (required at the Sn2 position of phospholipids) owing to putative viral infectious inhibition of the first long-chain polyunsaturated fatty acid biosynthetic step catalyzed by delta-6-desaturase [33, 34].

DNA from a human gammaretrovirus, xenotropic murine leukemia virus-related virus (XMRV), has recently been identified in peripheral blood mononuclear cells in 67% of patients compared with fewer than 4% of healthy controls [35]. Within a month of that publication, the same group announced that the proportion of patients showing evidence of XMRV infection was 95%. Cell culture experiments revealed that patient-derived XMRV is infectious and that both cell-associated and cell-free transmission of the virus are possible. Secondary viral infections were established in uninfected primary lymphocytes and indicator cell lines following exposure to activated peripheral blood mononuclear cells, B cells, T cells, or plasma derived from patients [35].

Interestingly, 2 placebo-controlled double-blind trials of the use of fatty acids, including EPA, in myalgic encephalomyelitis patients have given contrasting results. The earlier one, by Behan et al. [36], demonstrated significant benefit, while the second, by Peet and coworkers [37], was negative. Structural neuroimaging in a case report of treatment with high EPA-containing fatty acid supplementation has shown that clinical improvement in myalgic encephalomyelitis appears to be associated with marked reduction in the ventricle-to-brain ratio [38].

Retroviruses possess the ability to insert DNA copies (proviruses) of a viral genome into the chromosome of the host cell [39]. In respect of XMRV, which has also been associated with a subset of patients with prostate cancer, different retrovirus strains have been found in patients with myalgic encephalomyelitis and prostate cancer, although in all XMRV-positive myalgic encephalomyelitis cases the XMRV *gag* (736 nt) and *env* (352 nt) sequences were more than 99% similar to those previously reported for 3 prostate tumor-associated XMRV strains in a recent study [35]. Thus, if a retrovirus does have an etiological role in myalgic encephalomyelitis, copy number variation may be expected, and this in turn might partly account for variation in response to the virucidal properties of ethyl-EPA [40].

Conclusions

In this paper we have seen how the differential response of neurological disorders to treatment with ethyl-EPA may be a function of copy number variation. Future clinical studies involving ethyl-EPA should, when practicable, include genetic data from patients so that such a differential response may be better elucidated. This genetic influence may also account for the differential response to ethyl-EPA of patients suffering from psychiatric disorders such as depression and schizophrenia.

References

1 Peregrin T: The new frontier of nutrition science: nutrigenomics. J Am Diet Assoc 2001;101:1306.
2 Puri BK, Bydder GM, Manku MS, et al: Reduction in cerebral atrophy associated with ethyl-eicosapentaenoic acid treatment in patients with Huntington's disease. J Int Med Res 2008;36:896–905.
3 Serhan CN, Chiang N: Endogenous pro-resolving and anti-inflammatory lipid mediators: A new pharmacologic genus. Br J Pharmacol 2008;153 (suppl 1):S200–215.
4 Ait-Said F, Elalamy I, Werts C, et al: Inhibition by eicosapentaenoic acid of IL-1beta-induced PGHS-2 expression in human microvascular endothelial cells: involvement of lipoxygenase-derived metabolites and p38 MAPK pathway. Biochim Biophys Acta 2003;1631:77–84.

5 Takadera T, Shiraishi Y, Ohyashiki T: Prostaglandin E2 induced caspase-dependent apoptosis possibly through activation of EP2 receptors in cultured hippocampal neurons. Neurochem Int 2004;45:713–719.

6 Takadera T, Yumoto H, Tozuka Y, Ohyashiki T: Prostaglandin E(2) induces caspase-dependent apoptosis in rat cortical cells. Neurosci Lett 2002; 317:61–64.

7 Huntington's Disease Collaborative Research Group: A novel gene containing a trinucleotide repeat that is expanded and unstable on Huntington's disease chromosomes. The Huntington's Disease Collaborative Research Group. Cell 1993;72:971–983.

8 Kieburtz K, MacDonald M, Shih C, et al.: Trinucleotide repeat length and progression of illness in Huntington's disease. J Med Genet 1994;31: 872–874.

9 Kirkwood SC, Su JL, Conneally P, Foroud T: Progression of symptoms in the early and middle stages of Huntington disease. Arch Neurol 2001;58: 273–278.

10 Marder K, Zhao H, Myers RH, et al: Rate of functional decline in Huntington's disease. Huntington study group. Neurology 2000;54:452–458.

11 Panov AV, Gutekunst CA, Leavitt BR, et al: Early mitochondrial calcium defects in Huntington's disease are a direct effect of polyglutamines. Nat Neurosci 2002;5:731–736.

12 Sawa A, Wiegand GW, Cooper J, et al: Increased apoptosis of Huntington disease lymphoblasts associated with repeat length-dependent mitochondrial depolarization. Nat Med 1999;5:1194–1198.

13 Jump DB: Dietary polyunsaturated fatty acids and regulation of gene transcription. Curr Opin Lipidol 2002;13:155–164.

14 Jump DB: The biochemistry of n–3 polyunsaturated fatty acids. J Biol Chem 2002;277:8755–8758.

15 Murck H, Manku M: Ethyl-EPA in Huntington disease: potentially relevant mechanism of action. Brain Res Bull 2007;72:159–164.

16 Liu G, Bibus DM, Bode AM, et al: Omega 3 but not omega 6 fatty acids inhibit AP-1 activity and cell transformation in JB6 cells. Proc Natl Acad Sci USA 2001;98:7510–7515.

17 Moon Y, Pestka JJ: Deoxynivalenol-induced mitogen-activated protein kinase phosphorylation and IL-6 expression in mice suppressed by fish oil. J Nutr Biochem 2003;14:717–726.

18 Lo CJ, Chiu KC, Fu M, Chu A, Helton S: Fish oil modulates macrophage P44/P42 mitogen-activated protein kinase activity induced by lipopolysaccharide. J Parenter Enteral Nutr 2000;24:159–163.

19 Moon DO, Kim KC, Jin CY, et al: Inhibitory effects of eicosapentaenoic acid on lipopolysaccharide-induced activation in BV2 microglia. Int Immunopharmacol 2007;7:222–229.

20 Lynch AM, Loane DJ, Minogue AM, et al: Eicosapentaenoic acid confers neuroprotection in the amyloid-beta challenged aged hippocampus. Neurobiol Aging 2007;28:845–855.

21 Minogue AM, Lynch AM, Loane DJ, Herron CE, Lynch MA: Modulation of amyloid-beta-induced and age-associated changes in rat hippocampus by eicosapentaenoic acid. J Neurochem 2007;103:914–926.

22 Lo CJ, Chiu KC, Fu M, Lo R, Helton S: Fish oil decreases macrophage tumor necrosis factor gene transcription by altering the NF kappa B activity. J Surg Res 1999;82:216–221.

23 Zhao Y, Joshi-Barve S, Barve S, Chen LH: Eicosapentaenoic acid prevents LPS-induced TNF-alpha expression by preventing NF-kappaB activation. J Am Coll Nutr 2004;23:71–78.

24 Frangou S, Lewis M, Wollard J, Simmons A: Preliminary in vivo evidence of increased N-acetyl-aspartate following eicosapentaenoic acid treatment in patients with bipolar disorder. J Psychopharmacol 2007;21:435–439.

25 Puri BK, Bydder GM, Counsell SJ, et al: MRI and neuropsychological improvement in Huntington disease following ethyl-EPA treatment. Neuroreport 2002;13:123–126.

26 Puri BK: Monomodal rigid-body registration and applications to the investigation of the effects of eicosapentaenoic acid intervention in neuropsychiatric disorders. Prostaglandins Leukot Essent Fatty Acids 2004;71:177–179.

27 Puri BK, Leavitt BR, Hayden MR, et al: Ethyl-EPA in Huntington disease: a double-blind, randomized, placebo-controlled trial. Neurology 2005;65:286–292.

28 Fukuda K, Straus SE, Hickie I et al: The chronic fatigue syndrome: a comprehensive approach to its definition and study. International Chronic Fatigue Syndrome Study Group. Ann Intern Med 1994;121: 953–959.

29 Puri BK, Counsell SJ, Zaman R, et al: Relative increase in choline in the occipital cortex in chronic fatigue syndrome. Acta Psychiatr Scand 2002;106: 224–226.

30 Chaudhuri A, Condon BR, Gow JW, Brennan D, Hadley DM: Proton magnetic resonance spectroscopy of basal ganglia in chronic fatigue syndrome. Neuroreport 2003;14:225–228.

31 Tomoda A, Miike T, Yamada E, et al: Chronic fatigue syndrome in childhood. Brain Dev 2000;22:60–64.

32 Cox IJ, Puri BK: In vivo MR spectroscopy in diagnosis and research of neuropsychiatric disorders. Prostaglandins Leukot Essent Fatty Acids 2004;70:357–360.
33 Puri BK: Long-chain polyunsaturated fatty acids and the pathophysiology of myalgic encephalomyelitis (chronic fatigue syndrome). J Clin Pathol 2007;60:122–124.
34 Puri BK, Tsaluchidu S, Treasaden IH: Serial structural MRI analysis and proton and 31PMR spectroscopy in the investigation of cerebral fatty acids in major depressive disorder, Huntington's disease, myalgic encephalomyelitis and in forensic schizophrenic patients. World Rev Nutr Diet 2009;99:31–45.
35 Lombardi VC, Ruscetti FW, Das Gupta J, et al: Detection of an infectious retrovirus, XMRV, in blood cells of patients with chronic fatigue syndrome. Science 2009;326:585–589.
36 Behan PO, Behan WM, Horrobin D: Effect of high doses of essential fatty acids on the postviral fatigue syndrome. Acta Neurol Scand 1990;82:209–216.
37 Warren G, McKendrick M, Peet M: The role of essential fatty acids in chronic fatigue syndrome: a case-controlled study of red-cell membrane essential fatty acids (EFA) and a placebo-controlled treatment study with high dose of EFA. Acta Neurol Scand 1999;99:112–116.
38 Puri BK, Holmes J, Hamilton G: Eicosapentaenoic acid-rich essential fatty acid supplementation in chronic fatigue syndrome associated with symptom remission and structural brain changes. Int J Clin Pract 2004;58:297–299.
39 Lewin B: Genes IX, Sudbury, MA, Jones and Bartlett, 2008.
40 Puri BK: The use of eicosapentaenoic acid in the treatment of chronic fatigue syndrome. Prostaglandins Leukot Essent Fatty Acids 2004;70:399–401.

Prof. Mehar S. Manku
Amarin Neuroscience Ltd.
Oxford OX4 4GA (UK)
Tel. +44 1865 7785921034, E-Mail mehar.manku@amarincorp.com

Nutrigenetics: A Tool to Provide Personalized Nutritional Therapy to the Obese

Amelia Marti · Estibaliz Goyenechea · J. Alfredo Martínez

Institute of Nutrition and Food Sciences, University of Navarra, Pamplona, Spain

Obesity is a multifactorial disorder in which excessive body fat deposition arises when energy intake is higher than energy expenditure [1]. The growing prevalence of obesity around the world is mainly attributed to changes in lifestyle (e.g. increased consumption of high energy-yielding foods enriched with carbohydrates and fats, or reduced physical activity) that may impact genetic susceptibility [2]. More than 1 billion people are currently overweight or obese [3]. This health burden is worsened because an excess in body adipose tissue is associated with clinical complications such as diabetes, hypertension, dyslipemia, impaired immune competence, hormonal disturbances, some types of cancer and higher mortality rates [4].

Many theories have been proposed to explain the origin of this epidemic, such as the thrifty gene or genetically based hypotheses, the fetal programming hypothesis, the environmental (unbalanced diets and sedentary lifestyles) hypothesis, the ethnic shift hypothesis or the assortative mating hypothesis, all of which underline the complex theory that suggests that there is not a single cause of obesity but it is a consequence of an interaction between genetic and lifestyle influences [5].The mutual interactions between the genetic profile and the environment undoubtedly complicate the understanding of the specific roles of genes and external influences in obesity [6].

Current obesity treatments are based on [7]:
- dietary strategies to reduce energy intake or manipulate macronutrient distribution;
- exercise programs to increase physical activity;
- behavioral or psychological approaches;
- pharmacological prescriptions to increase thermogenesis or reduce appetite or food utilization;
- surgical procedures to control nutrient absorption.

In this context, identification of additional candidate genes may allow for the provision of more individualized recommendations (dietary advice, physical activity and/or drug therapy) to prevent excessive weight gain and achieve effective weight loss and successful long-term maintenance of weight reduction on the basis of an identified genetic predisposition [4]. Therefore, the interactions between the most relevant gene polymorphisms affecting the amount and composition of weight loss as well as the changes in obesity-associated risk factors depending on the characteristics of the nutritional strategy (energy deficit and dietary macronutrient distribution) are under investigation [8]. In the future, the advances in molecular and genetic biotechnology will pave the way to combine research for new candidate genes, the identification of novel polymorphisms and the profiling of gene expression patterns putatively involved in gene-nutrient interactions concerning weight homeostasis [9].

Indeed, linkage studies, candidate gene association investigations and genome-wide association studies (GWAS) will contribute to substantial advances in nutrigenetic-based personalized therapies, which will also benefit from advances in phenotype measurements including photonic scanners, air displacement pletismography, CT and MRI, US and validated dietary intake measurements [5]. Also, scientific progress on omics technologies will extend beyond common single nucleotide polymorphism (SNPs) and screen the role of copy number variation, siRNA and miRNA involvement, as well as epigenetic changes affecting DNA methylation, chromatin folding, covalent histone modifications and polycombs affecting gene-environment interactions and obesity [10].

Observational Studies Evidencing Gene-Nutrient Interactions on Weight Gain

Gene-environment interactions can be assessed through cross-sectional and retrospective case-control designs when information on dietary patterns and lifestyles as well as on genotyping is available [11]. These research approaches have been successfully focused on candidate genes related to appetite control (e.g. LEP, MC4R, FTO), energy and lipid utilization (e.g. ADBRs, UCPs, APOA5), adipocyte metabolism and signaling [e.g. peroxisome proliferator-activated receptor (PPAR), interleukin-6 (IL6)], where the outcome variables were obesity risk, BMI, body composition or appetite/satiety measurements (table 1).

Genes Regulating Food/Energy Intake

The assessment of several polymorphisms in candidate obesity genes and their interactions with the dietary intake of $n-6$ polyunsaturated fatty acids in a subsample of the EPIC-Heidelberg cohort revealed an increased obesity risk for variants of the leptin gene, which encodes a protein participating in food intake regulation and body weight homeostasis [12]. Also, the highly polymorphic melanocortin receptor 4 gene (MC4R), which is involved in appetite control at the central nervous system level, may show an interaction with dietary intake in obese subjects since carriers of the 103I allele had significantly higher daily energy and carbohydrate intakes than did

Table 1. Selected observational studies concerning gene × nutritional intake interactions on obesity/adiposity markers

Gene(s)	Ref.	Controlled nutritional factor	Main variable	Effect modification/outcome depending on gene polymorphism
PPARG	Luan, 2001 [20]	Total fat P/S ratio	BMI	BMI was greater among Ala allele carriers only when the P/S ratio was low, and in Pro homozygotes when this ratio is high.
PPARG	Marti, 2002 [23]	CHO	BMI/ obesity risk	Pro 12 Ala carriers were associated with increased risk of obesity in those subjects in which >49% energy came from CHO.
11 genes (15 SNPs)	Nieters, 2002 [12]	n–6 PUFA	Obesity risk	A substantial elevation of obesity risk with increasing intake of n–6 fatty acids in carriers (1 or 2 alleles) of TNFα, leptin and PPARG variants.
ADBR2	Martinez, 2003 [15]	CHO CHO/fat ratio	BMI/ obesity risk	Women with a high CHO intake (>49% VET) had greater risk of obesity in Gln27Gln heterozygotes.
PPARG	Memisoglu, 2003 [21]	Total fat MUFA	BMI	Intake of monounsaturated fat was inversely associated with BMI among 12 Ala variant carriers.
PPARA	Robitaille, 2004 [24]	Total fat MUFA	WC	Saturated fat intake was related to WC only in Leu162Leu homozygotes.
PPARG	Nelson, 2007 [22]	PUFA	BMI	Polyunsaturated fat consumption induced higher BMI values in Ala carriers of the Pro12 Ala variant.
UCP3	Dancott, 2004 [18]	Energy intake	Body composition	No evidence of interaction between UCP3-5 and UCP3-55 in regard to dietary intake.
ADBR3	Miyaki, 2005 [16]	Total energy	Obesity risk	Arg 64 allele carriers were associated with higher obesity risk than Trp64Trp homozygotes only in the highest energy consumers.
APOA5	Corella, 2007 [17]	Energy and fat intake	BMI	Carriers of the Apo45-1131C allele had lower obesity risk only when in the high fat intake group, but higher obesity risk with low fat intake.
IL6R	Song, 2007 [25]	Total energy	BMI/WC	Association between higher energy intake and abdominal obesity in T allele carriers of the Asp358 Ala polymorphism.
FTO	Timpson, 2008 [14]	Macronutrient intake	Appetite/ satiety	Children carrying the A variant allele (rs9939609AT) showed higher calorie and total fat intake.

Table 1. Continued

Gene(s)	Ref.	Controlled nutritional factor	Main variable	Effect modification/outcome depending on gene polymorphism
MC4R	Pichler, 2008 [13]	Macronutrient intake	BMI	High CHO consumption was associated with BMI in those V103I risk allele carriers.

ADBR = Adrenoreceptor; APO = apoenzyme; CHO = carbohydrate; FTO = fat mass and obesity associated gene; IL6 = interleukin-6 receptor; MC4R = melanocortin receptor; MUFA = monounsaturated fatty acid; PPAR = peroxisome proliferator-activated receptor; P/S ratio = ratio of polyunsaturated to saturated fatty acids; PUFA = polyunsaturated fatty acid; WC = waist circumference

non-carriers [13]. Another gene that has been found to be related to appetite in children and that may show a diet × gene interaction is the fat mass and obesity associated locus (FTO), since the rs 9939609 AT polymorphism may stimulate energy and fat intake [14].

Genes Regulating Energy and Lipid Utilization
The gene encoding for the adrenergic receptor 2 protein (ADBR2), which is involved in lipolysis and other metabolic functions, has been found to participate in a gene-environment interaction since women carrying the Gln variant had 2.56 times greater risk of obesity with a high carbohydrate intake (>45% energy). Similarly, a higher carbohydrate/fat ratio (>1.77) was significantly associated with being obese as affected by the Glu allele [15]. Moreover, a high energy intake interacted with the Trp64Arg polymorphism of ADBR3, another gene participating in lipid utilization which led to a significant increase in the risk of obesity of Japanese men [16].

Interestingly, the apolipoprotein A5 (APOA5) –1131T>C SNP, which is involved in triglyceride metabolism, appears to modulate the effect of fat intake on BMI and obesity risk in both men and women [17]. On the other hand, the –5 and –55 genetic variants of the uncoupling protein UCP3 gene, which participates in thermogenesis, showed no modulation of body composition induced by the energy intake [18].

Genes Regulating Adipogenesis and Adipokines
The importance of the nuclear peroxisome proliferator-activated receptor gamma (PPARG) regulating adipogenesis and adipocyte differentiation has been demonstrated in families with loss-of-function mutations, whose gene expression in sensitive to fatty acids [19]. An interaction between the Pro12Ala polymorphism PPARG and total fat intake or the P/S ratio (unsaturated score) was found on BMI, Ala allele carriers had greater BMI when the P/S ratio was low [20]. Some of these findings were only partly confirmed in another study, which showed that polyunsaturated fat consumption induced higher BMI values in Ala carriers of the Pro12Ala polymorphism [21].

Moreover, another trial concerning this PPARG gene variant revealed that associations between total fat monounsaturated fatty acid intake with BMI were different in PPARG 12Ala variant allele-carriers compared with non-carriers [22]. Thus, the intake of monounsaturated fatty acid was not associated with BMI among homozygous wild-type women, but was inversely associated with this adiposity marker among 12Ala variant allele carriers. Furthermore, a case-control study with 313 subjects, reported that Ala carriers were associated with an increased risk of obesity in those subjects consuming >49% total energy from carbohydrates [23], while the Pro12Ala genotype showed the opposite trend. On the other hand, an association between the PPAR alfa-L162V polymorphism and waist circumference was only identified for saturated fat intake in Leu162Leu homozygotes [24]. Functions of the IL6 receptor may be affected by an interaction between the GG vs. TT+GT genotypes: Asp358Ala gene variant and dietary energy, which modifies the risk for abdominal obesity waist circumference [25].

Intervention Studies Concerning Genetic Modification Effects on Weight Loss and Maintenance

Nutritional intervention trials provide more reliable evidence concerning the assessment of interactions between the genetic make-up and dietary factors than observational studies, since various sources of biase are minimized [4]. In this context, a number of studies have focused on genes regulating energy intake [e.g. MC3R, pro-opiomelanocortin (POMC), LEP, LEPLR, FTO], lipid metabolism and adipogenesis [e.g. PLIN, APOA5, LIPC, fatty acid binding protein 2 (FABP2), PPARG], thermogenesis (e.g. ADBRs, UCPs) and adipokine synthesis (e.g. ADIPOQ, IL6), whose functions may be influenced by the dietary intake and, therefore, have an impact on body weight gain and composition (table 2).

Genes Regulating Food/Energy Intake
Mutations in genes encoding neuropeptides such as MC4R or POMC, which participate in the hypothalamic axis controlling appetite and satiety, may specifically modify the response to weight-lowering treatments [5]. This outcome has been demonstrated for 2 variants concerning the MC3R gene (CI7A and 6241A), which interacted in childhood obesity affecting weight loss after following a well-designed energy-restricted program [26], but not for the R236G substitution in the POMC gene [27]. A lifestyle adaptation produced no effect in weight loss or fat distribution depending on the recently described FTO gene [28]. However, a modification in the effect produced by a hypocaloric diet plus exercise on the gene make-up concerning the LEPR gene was found for the AA genotype (Lys656Lys), which showed a higher fat mass loss compared to minor allele carriers [29]. Furthermore, the A-2549 allele for the LEP gene was associated with lower BMI and leptinemia in women following a hypocaloric diet [30].

Table 2. Selected genes and nutritional interactions concerning weight loss and maintenance after different nutritional interventions

Gene(s)	Ref.	Nutritional intervention	Main variable	Effect modification/outcome depending on gene polymorphism
LEP	Mammes, 1998 [30]	Low calorie diet	Leptin levels	The A^{-2549} allele was associated with lower BMI reduction in women.
ADRB3	Nakamura, 2000 [41]	3-month weight reduction program	Visceral/subcutaneous fat area	After 3 months, changes in visceral fat areas in 64 Arg/64 Arg subjects were smaller than those in 64 Trp/64 Trp subjects.
UCP3 × ADBR3	Kim, 2004 [40]	12-week low calorie diet	BMI and fat distribution	After 12 weeks, wild-type group showed the highest decreases in total and visceral fat areas, followed by 'only UPC3 variant' group.
APOA5	Aberle, 2005 [33]	Short-term fat restriction	BMI change (kg/m^2)	Weight reduction was higher in C allele carriers of the 1131T>C polymorphism
PLIN	Corella, 2005 [32]	Low calorie diet	Weight loss (kg)	GG homozygotes lost more weight than A allele carriers
IL6 × PPARG	Goyenechea, 2006 [43]	Energy restricted diet	Weight regain (kg)	The C allele: IL6 partially protected against weight regain, while the 2 variants improved the ability for weight maintenance.
LIPC	Santos, 2006 [34]	Different CHO content in hypocaloric diet	Weight loss (kg)	Lower obesity risk linked to the 514C>T polymorphism and high intake of fiber.
PLIN (7 SNPs)	Jang, 2006 [31]	12-week calorie restriction	Abdominal fat area (cm)	Subjects with nGA/nGA haplotype at SNPs 11482G>A/14995A>T had increased FFA levels with a rapid loss in abdominal fat, whereas GA/GA haplotype carriers reduced FFA levels.
POMC	Santoro, 2006 [27]	Hypocaloric balanced diet	Weight loss (kg)	The R236G substitution does not preclude the possibility to lose weight in obese children.
UCP3	Cha, 2006 [38]	1-month very low calorie diet	Weight loss (kg)	Haplotype ht1 [CGTACC] was significantly associated with an increased reduction in body weight.
UCP2-3	Yoon, 2007 [39]	1-month very low calorie diet	Fat loss (%)	Common haplotype, UCP2-UCP3-ht1 (GGCdelCGTACC), and a promoter SNP of UCP2, UCP2–866G>A, were associated with VLCD-induced fat mass reduction.
ADBR3	Shiwaku, 2007 [37]	Low calorie diet and exercise	Weight loss (kg)	Arg64 allele carriers lost less weight than Trp64Trp homozygotes

Table 2. Continued

Gene(s)	Ref.	Nutritional intervention	Main variable	Effect modification/outcome depending on gene polymorphism
MC3R	Santoro, 2007 [26]	Weight loss program	BMI change (kg/m^2)	After 12-month follow-up carriers of C17A and 6241A variants showed a significantly higher BMI z score.
FABP2	De Luis, 2008 [35]	Low calorie diet and exercise	Fat loss (%)	The allele carriers had greater decrease in fat mass than Ala54Ala homozygotes.
FABP2	De Luis, 2008 [29]	Hypocaloric diets (low carb/low fat)	BMI, fat loss and WC	Similar weight loss is achieved depending on the Ala54Thr polymorphism with both diets.
FTO	Haupt, 2008 [28]	Lifestyle modification	Weight loss (kg) and fat distribution (%)	No effect of the intervention on assessed variables.
ADIPOQ	Goyenechea, 2009 [42]	Energy restricted diet	Weight (re)gain (kg)	The A allele on the –11391G/A polymorphism provides protection against weight regain.
LEPR	Abete, 2009 [45]	Energy restriction	Fat mass loss (%)	The AA genotype group (Lys109Arg) showed a higher fat carrier loss compared to minor allele carriers.
PPARG	Razquin, 2009 [36]	Mediterranean diet	Waist circumference	The 12 Ala allele carriers reduce more waist circumference compared with wild-type subjects that followed a Mediterranean dietary pattern.

ADBR = Adrenoreceptor; ADIPOQ = adiponectin; APO = apoenzyme; FABP = fatty acid binding protein; FTO = fat mass and obesity associated gene; IL6 = interleukin 6; LEP = leptin; LEPR = leptin receptor; MC3R = melanocortin receptor; PLIN = perilipin; POMC = pro-opiomelanocortin; PPAR = peroxisome proliferator-activated receptor; UCP-3 = uncoupling protein 3; WC = waist circumference.

Genes Affecting Lipid Metabolism and Adipogenesis

The function of some gene polymorphisms related to lipid metabolism such as PLIN (Perilipin), APOA5 (apoprotein A5), LIPC (hepatic lipase) or FABP (fatty acid binding protein) may be differentially affected by the slimming program depending on the variant. Thus, the genetic variation at the perilipin locus has been associated with changes in abdominal fat reduction following a hypocaloric diet prescribed to mildly lose weight [31]. Also, PLIN11482A carriers are apparently resistant to weight loss [32]. In addition, weight reduction was higher in C allele carriers of the APOA5 1131T>C polymorphism [33] when submitted to short-term fat restriction. Other gene variants that have been found to interact with the weight-lowering process following an energy-restriction approach are those of the LIPC 514CT polymorphism, in which fiber intake may produce a multiplicative effect [34]. A mutation in the gene encoding for FABP interacted with the fat-loss process, since Thr allele carriers had a greater decrease in adipose tissue mass than Ala54Ala homozygotes [35]. Finally, it has been reported that a Mediterranean diet pattern within the PREDIMED trial protects against waist circumference enlargement in 12Ala carriers for the PPARG gene [36].

Genes Involving Proteins Related to Thermogenesis Processes
At least 2 genes involved in energy yielding processes have been implicated in weight-loss interactions between genes and dietary intake: ADBR3 and UCP3. Thus, the Arg64 allele carriers lost less weight than Trp64Trp homozygotes for the ADBR3 gene when submitted to a very low calorie diet combined with exercise [37], while the UCP2 –866G>A and the major haplotype [CGCdelCGTACC] had a differentially significant reduction in fat mass in the obese following a very restricted energy diet [38]. One of the effects of UCP3 haplotypes on obesity phenotypes was dependent on very low calorie diets [39]. Interestingly, a combined action of 2 different polymorphisms concerning the UCP3 promoter and ADBR3 genes was evidenced since an effect was only found on fat distribution for homozygotes under the same low calorie diet [40]. Interestingly, the Trp64Arg polymorphism on the ADBR3 gene may affect regional distribution of fat loss [41].

Genes Encoding Adipokines and Proteins Related to Adipocyte Metabolism
Additional evidence about gene × nutrient interactions on weight homeostasis after following a hypocaloric diet was described for an adipokine gene: adiponectin (ADIPOQ). The A allele on the –11391G/A gene polymorphism provides protection against weight regain [42]. Also, a synergetic outcome was demonstrated for obese subjects carrying the IL6 174 C>G and Pro12Ala polymorphisms, who were protected against weight regain [43].

Nutritional Studies Concerning Gene-Dependent Effects on Obesity-Related Manifestations

Obesity is often accompanied by a number of clinical complications, some of which can substantially improve after following adequate nutritional advice. Obesity is dependent on the individual genetic make-up, which has been shown by some SNPs affecting genes that are involved in lipid metabolism and on weight homeostasis (table 3).

Changes in insulin resistance or dyslipemia showing an effect modification induced by an energy-restricted diet have been described for some genes affecting a single nucleotide CD36 (–22674T/C) promoter SNP [44], LEPR (Lys109Arg) variant [45], PGC1α (Gly482Ser) missense mutation [46]. Also, *n*–3 fatty acid supplementation may modify the TG response depending on the Pro12Ala polymorphism [47].

Table 3. Selected nutritionally slimming intervention studies concerning gene-nutrition interactions with favorable effects on metabolic markers accompanying obesity

Gene(s)	Ref.	Nutritional intervention	Main variable	Effect modification/outcome depending on gene polymorphism
FABP2	Georgopoulos, 2000 [50]	Saturated fat overload	Triacylglycerol	Saturated fat load produces higher hypertriglyceridemia in allele T carriers (A54T).
PPARG	Lindi, 2003 [47]	n–3 fatty acid supplementation	Serum triglycerides	Carriers of the Ala12 allele had lower triglycerides in response to n–3 fatty acid supplementation compared to ProPro subjects.
APOE	Moreno, 2005 [49]	PUFA/SFA intake	Insulin sensitivity	Carriers of the G variant allele (–219G→T) specifically reduced insulin resistance when fed on diet rich in monounsaturated fat.
PPARG × ADRB2	Rosado, 2007 [51]	Hypocaloric diet	Satiety	Carriers of the Ala12 allele (PPARG) had higher satiety and fat oxidation than ProPro subjects.
ADIPO Q	Perez-Martinez, 2008 [48]	CHO/fat intake	Insulin resistance	Homozygote CC men (–11377 C/G) improved insulin sensitivity when fed on diets low in saturated fat.
CD 36 promoter	Goyenechea, 2008 [44]	Low calorie diet	Total cholesterol	Allele –22674C is associated with improved lipid profile during weight loss maintenance.
LEPR	De Luis, 2008 [29]	Low fat/low CHO hypocaloric diets	Leptin	Lys65Lys homozygote carriers under a low-fat diet reduced more leptin levels plasma.
PGC1α	Goyenechea, 2008 [46]	Low calorie diet	Insulin sensitivity	Enhanced short-term improvement on insulin response in carriers of the gly482Ser variant.

ADBR = Adrenoreceptor; ADIPOQ = adiponectin; APO = apoenzyme; FABP = fatty acid binding protein; LEPR = leptin receptor; PCG1α = peroxisome proliferator-activated receptor gamma coactivator α; PPAR = peroxisome proliferator-activated receptor; PPARG = peroxisome proliferator-activated receptor gamma coactivator; PUFA = polyunsaturated fatty acid; SFA = saturated fatty acid.

Another trial investigating the role of macronutrient intake within hypocaloric diets demonstrated that under a low fat diet Lys65Lys homozygote carriers of the LEPR polymorphism showed a greater reduction in plasma leptin [29]. The participation of fat intake on insulin resistance depending on the genotype was evidenced in an experiment in which homozygous CC men carrying the –11377C/G polymorphism for the ADIPOQ gene improved insulin sensitivity when fed on diets low in saturated fat [48]. This study complemented other research that found that carriers of the G variant allele (–219G→T) of the APOE gene specifically reduced insulin resistance when fed a diet rich in monounsaturated fatty acids [49]. Another study observed that a saturated fat load was associated with a greater elevation in postprandial triglycerides in the Thr54/Thr54 polymorphism of the FABP2 gene [50]. On the other hand, an interaction between variants in PPARG and ADBR2 genes affecting eating behavior and body composition was found when a hypocaloric diet was prescribed [51].

Conclusions

Genotype-environment interactions arise when the response of a phenotype (e.g. body weight) to environmental changes (e.g. overfeeding) depends on the individual's genetic background [4]. Most of the genetic studies on human obesity have assumed the absence of genotype-environment interactions simply because of the difficulties in assessing such interactive effects in quantitative genetic models.

There are several plausible scenarios for the interaction between genetic and environmental factors. A higher obesity risk (represented by a quantitative trait BMI) will arise from the presence of obesity-related gene variants and environmental influences (i.e. high consumption of carbohydrates, low levels of physical activity) for a population carrying a given polymorphism. Indeed, individuals inherit a number of gene variants in key loci, but they also make specific lifestyle choices (e.g. low-fat vs. high-fat diets, high vs. low levels of physical activity) that affect weight gain or loss. Thus, while environmental factors may be changed in the short term, genetic factors can not, but they might interplay [52].

The gene-environment relationship is a key issue not only in understanding the pathogenesis of multifactorial diseases, but also in designing appropriate treatments, such as 'personalized nutrition' [53]. Indeed, the large-scale European intervention trial NUGENOB concerning the comparison of the impact of more than 40 genetic polymorphisms on weight loss with hypocaloric diets containing different macronutrient distributions showed that much work is required in this area and that gene expression profiling is involved in body weight and composition control [54–56].

References

1 Marti A, Moreno–Aliaga MJ, Hebebrand J, Martinez JA: Genes, lifestyles and obesity. Int J Obes 2004; 28:S29–S36.
2 Marti A, Martinez-González MA, Martinez JA: Interaction between genes and lifestyle factors on obesity. Proc Nutr Soc 2008;67:1–8.
3 Kelly T, Yang W, Chen CS, Reynolds K, He J: Global burden of obesity in 2005 and projections to 2030. Int J Obes 2008;32:1431–1437.
4 Moreno-Aliaga MJ, Santos JL, Marti A, Martínez JA: Does weight loss prognosis depend on genetic make-up? Obes Rev 2005;6:155–168.

5 Walley AJ, Asher JE, Froguel P: The genetic contribution to non-syndromic human obesity. Nat Rev Genet. 2009;10:431–442.
6 Newell A, Zlot A, Silvey K, Arail K: Addressing the obesity epidemic: a genomics perspective. Prev Chronic Dis 2007;4:1–6
7 Abete I, Parra MD, Zulet MA, Martínez JA: Different dietary strategies for weight loss in obesity: role of energy and macronutrient content. Nutr Res Rev 2006;19:5–17.
8 Martinez JA, Parra MD, Santos JL, et al: Genotype-dependent response to energy-restricted diets in obese subjects: towards personalized nutrition. Asia Pac J Clin Nutr 2008;17:S119–S122.
9 Ochoa MC, Moreno-Aliaga MJ, Martínez-González MA, et al: Predictor factors for childhood obesity in a Spanish case-control study. Nutrition 2007;23:379–384.
10 Campión J, Milagro FI, Martínez JA: Individuality and epigenetics in obesity. Obes Rev 2009;10:383–392.
11 Qi L, Cho YA: Gene-environment interaction and obesity. Nutr Rev 2008;66:684–694.
12 Nieters A, Becker N, Linseisen J: Polymorphisms in candidate obesity genes and their interaction with dietary intake of n–6 polyunsaturated fatty acids affect obesity risk in a sub-sample of the EPIC-Heidelberg cohort. Eur J Nutr 2002;41:210–221.
13 Pichler M, Kollerits B, Heid IM, et al: Association of the melanocortin-4 receptor V103I polymorphism with dietary intake in severely obese persons. Am J Clin Nutr 2008;88:797–800.
14 Timpson NJ, Emmett PM, Frayling TM, et al: The fat mass- and obesity-associated locus and dietary intake in children. Am J Clin Nutr 2008;88:971–978.
15 Martínez JA, Corbalán MS, Sánchez-Villegas A, et al: Obesity risk is associated with carbohydrate intake in women carrying the Gln27Glu beta2-adrenoceptor polymorphism. J Nutr 2003;133:2549–2554.
16 Miyaki K, Sutani S, Kikuchi H, et al: Increased risk of obesity resulting from the interaction between high energy intake and the Trp64Arg polymorphism of the beta3-adrenergic receptor gene in healthy Japanese men. J Epidemiol 2005;15:203–210.
17 Corella D, Lai CQ, Demissie S, et al: APOA5 gene variation modulates the effects of dietary fat intake on body mass index and obesity risk in the Framingham Heart Study. J Mol Med 2007;85:119–128.
18 Damcott CM, Feingold E, Moffett SP, et al: Genetic variation in uncoupling protein 3 is associated with dietary intake and body composition in females. Metabolism 2004;53:458–464.
19 Steemburgo T, Azevedo MJ, Martinez JA: Interação entre gene e nutriente e sua associação à obesidade e ao diabetes melito. Arq Bras Endocrinol Metab 2009;53:485–496.
20 Luan J, Browne PO, Harding AH, et al: Evidence for gene-nutrient interaction at the PPARgamma locus. Diabetes 2001;50:686–689.
21 Memisoglu A, Hu FB, Hankinson SE, et al: Interaction between a peroxisome proliferator-activated receptor gamma gene polymorphism and dietary fat intake in relation to body mass. Hum Mol Genet 2003;12:2923–2929.
22 Nelson TL, Fingerlin TE, Moss L, et al: The PPARgamma Pro12Ala polymorphism is not associated with body mass index or waist circumference among Hispanics from Colorado. Ann Nutr Metab 2007;51:252–257.
23 Marti A, Corbalán MS, Martínez-González MA, Forga L, Martínez JA: CHO intake alters obesity risk associated with Pro12Ala polymorphism of PPARgamma gene. J Physiol Biochem 2002;58:219–220.
24 Robitaille J, Brouillette C, Houde A, et al: Association between the PPARalpha-L162V polymorphism and components of the metabolic syndrome. J Hum Genet 2004;49:482–489.
25 Song Y, Miyaki K, Araki J, et al: The interaction between the interleukin-6 receptor gene genotype and dietary energy intake on abdominal obesity in Japanese men. Metabolism 2007;56:925–930.
26 Santoro N, Perrone L, Cirillo G, et al: Effect of the melanocortin-3 receptor C17A and G241A variants on weight loss in childhood obesity. Am J Clin Nutr 2007;85:950–953.
27 Santoro N, Perrone L, Cirillo G, et al: Weight loss in obese children carrying the proopiomelanocortin R236G variant. J Endocrinol Invest 2006;29:226–230.
28 Haupt A, Thamer C, Staiger H, et al: Variation in the FTO gene influences food intake but not energy expenditure. Exp Clin Endocrinol Diabetes 2009;117:194–197.
29 de Luis DA, Aller R, Izaola O, Sagrado MG, Conde R: Influence of Lys656Asn polymorphism of leptin receptor gene on leptin response secondary to two hypocaloric diets: a randomized clinical trial. Ann Nutr Metab 2008;52:209–214.
30 Mammès O, Betoulle D, Aubert R, et al: Novel polymorphisms in the 5′ region of the LEP gene: association with leptin levels and response to low-calorie diet in human obesity. Diabetes 1998;47:487–489.
31 Jang Y, Kim OY, Lee JH, et al: Genetic variation at the perilipin locus is associated with changes in serum free fatty acids and abdominal fat following mild weight loss. Int J Obes 2006;30:1601–1608

32 Corella D, Qi L, Sorlí JV, et al: Obese subjects carrying the 11482G>A polymorphism at the perilipin locus are resistant to weight loss after dietary energy restriction. J Clin Endocrinol Metab 2005;90:5121–5126.

33 Aberle J, Evans D, Beil FU, Seedorf U: A polymorphism in the apolipoprotein A5 gene is associated with weight loss after short-term diet. Clin Genet 2005;68:152–154.

34 Santos JL, Boutin P, Verdich C, et al: Genotype-by-nutrient interactions assessed in European obese women: a case-only study. Eur J Nutr 2006;45:454–462.

35 de Luis DA, Aller R, Izaola O, Sagrado MG, Conde R: Influence of Ala54Thr polymorphism of fatty acid-binding protein 2 on weight loss and insulin levels secondary to two hypocaloric diets: a randomized clinical trial. Diabetes Res Clin Pract 2008;82:113–118.

36 Razquin C, Alfredo Martinez J, Martinez-Gonzalez MA, et al: The Mediterranean diet protects against waist circumference enlargement in 12Ala carriers for the PPARgamma gene: 2 years' follow-up of 774 subjects at high cardiovascular risk. Br J Nutr 2009; 9:1–8.

37 Shiwaku K, Nogi A, Anuurad E, et al: Difficulty in losing weight by behavioral intervention for women with Trp64Arg polymorphism of the beta3-adrenergic receptor gene. Int J Obes Relat Metab Disord 2003;27:1028–1036.

38 Cha MH, Shin HD, Kim KS, Lee BH, Yoon Y: The effects of uncoupling protein 3 haplotypes on obesity phenotypes and very low-energy diet-induced changes among overweight Korean female subjects. Metabolism 2006;55:578–586.

39 Yoon Y, Park BL, Cha MH, et al: The effects of uncoupling protein 3 haplotypes on obesity phenotypes and very low-energy diet-induced changes among overweight Korean female subjects. Effects of genetic polymorphisms of UCP2 and UCP3 on very low calorie diet-induced body fat reduction in Korean female subjects. Biochem Biophys Res Commun 2007;359:451–456.

40 Kim OY, Cho EY, Park HY, Jang Y, Lee JH: Additive effect of the mutations in the beta3-adrenoceptor gene and UCP3 gene promoter on body fat distribution and glycemic control after weight reduction in overweight subjects with CAD or metabolic syndrome. Int J Obes Relat Metab Disord 2004;28:434–441.

41 Nakamura M, Tanaka M, Abe S, et al: Association between beta 3-adrenergic receptor polymorphism and a lower reduction in the ratio of visceral fat to subcutaneous fat area during weight loss in Japanese obese women. Nutr Res 2000;20:25–34.

42 Goyenechea E, Collins LJ, Parra D, et al: The –11391 G/A polymorphism of the adiponectin gene promoter is associated with metabolic syndrome traits and the outcome of an energy-restricted diet in obese subjects. Horm Metab Res 2009;41:55–61.

43 Goyenechea E, Parra D, Martínez JA: Weight regain after slimming induced by an energy-restricted diet depends on interleukin-6 and peroxisome-proliferator-activated-receptor-gamma2 gene polymorphisms. Br J Nutr 2006;96:965–972.

44 Goyenechea E, Collins LJ, Parra D, et al: CD36 gene promoter polymorphisms are associated with low density lipoprotein-cholesterol in normal twins and after a low-calorie diet in obese subjects. Twin Res Hum Genet 2008;11:621–628.

45 Abete I, Goyenechea E, Crujeiras AB, Martínez JA: Inflammatory state and stress condition in weight-lowering Lys109Arg LEPR gene polymorphism carriers. Arch Med Res 2009;40:306–310.

46 Goyenechea E, Crujeiras AB, Abete I, Parra D, Martínez JA: Enhanced short-term improvement of insulin response to a low-caloric diet in obese carriers the Gly482Ser variant of the PGC-1alpha gene. Diabetes Res Clin Pract 2008;82:190–196.

47 Lindi V, Schwab U, Louheranta A, et al: Impact of the Pro12Ala polymorphism of the PPAR-gamma2 gene on serum triacylglycerol response to n–3 fatty acid supplementation. Mol Genet Metab 2003;79:52–60.

48 Pérez-Martínez P, López-Miranda J, Cruz-Teno C, et al: Adiponectin gene variants are associated with insulin sensitivity in response to dietary fat consumption in Caucasian men. J Nutr 2008;138:1609–1614.

49 Moreno JA, Pérez-Jiménez F, Marín C, et al: The apolipoprotein E gene promoter (–219G/T) polymorphism determines insulin sensitivity in response to dietary fat in healthy young adults. J Nutr 2005;135:2535–2540.

50 Georgopoulos A, Aras O, Tsai MY: Codon-54 polymorphism of the fatty acid-binding protein 2 gene is associated with elevation of fasting and postprandial triglyceride in type 2 diabetes. J Clin Endocrinol Metab 2000;85:3155–3160.

51 Rosado E, Bressan J, Martins M, Cecon P, Martínez JA: Polymorphism in the PPARgama2 and beta2-adrenergic genes and diet lipids effects on body composition, energy expenditure and eating behaviour of obese women. Appetite 2007;49:635–643.

52 Martínez JA, Enríquez L, Moreno MJ, Martí A: Genetics of obesity. Public Health Nutr 2007;10:1138–1144.

53 Martínez JA: Genomic and personalized medicine; in Willard FH, Ginsburg GS (eds): San Diego Academic Press. Barcelona, Elsevier, 2008, vol 2, pp 1170–1186.
54 Sørensen TI, Boutin P, Taylor MA, et al: Genetic polymorphisms and weight loss in obesity: a randomised trial of hypo-energetic high- versus low-fat diets. PLoS Clin Trials 2006;1:e12.
55 Goossens GH, Petersen L, Blaak EE, et al: Several obesity- and nutrient-related gene polymorphisms but not FTO and UCP variants modulate postabsorptive resting energy expenditure and fat-induced thermogenesis in obese individuals: the NUGENOB study. Int J Obes 2009;33:669–679.
56 Viguerie N, Vidal H, Arner P, et al: Adipose tissue gene expression in obese subjects during low-fat and high-fat hypocaloric diets. Diabetologia 2005; 48:123–131.

J. Alfredo Martinez
Institute of Nutrition and Food Sciences, University of Navarra
ES–31008 Pamplona (Spain)
Tel. +34 948425600, Fax +34 948425649, E-Mail jalfmtz@unav.es

Xenobiotic Metabolizing Genes, Meat-Related Exposures, and Risk of Advanced Colorectal Adenoma

Leah M. Ferrucci[a,b] · Amanda J. Cross[a] · Marc J. Gunter[c] · Jiyoung Ahn[d] · Susan T. Mayne[b] · Xiaomei Ma[b] · Stephen J. Chanock[a] · Meredith Yeager[a] · Barry I. Graubard[a] · Sonja I. Berndt[a] · Wen-Yi Huang[a] · Richard B. Hayes[d] · Rashmi Sinha[a]

[a]Division of Cancer Epidemiology and Genetics, National Cancer Institute, National Institutes of Health, Bethesda, Md., [b]Yale School of Public Health, New Haven, Conn., [c]Department of Epidemiology and Population Health, Albert Einstein College of Medicine, and [d]Division of Epidemiology, Department of Environmental Medicine, New York University School of Medicine, New York, N.Y., USA

The potential for carcinogenic action of meat-related exposures, such as heterocyclic amines (HCAs), polycyclic aromatic hydrocarbons (PAHs), and *N*-nitroso compounds (NOCs) [1, 2], might explain positive associations between red and processed meat intake and colorectal neoplasia [3]. HCAs and PAHs are formed in meats cooked well-done at high temperatures [4] and produce intestinal tumors in rodents [5–7]. NOCs are some of the strongest known chemical carcinogens [2] and induce tumors in both the colon and rectum of numerous animal species [8]. Nitrate and nitrite, which are added to processed meats, can form NOCs [9]. NOCs can also form endogenously in the colon through the conversion of nitrate and nitrite [10], a reaction which is thought to be catalyzed by heme iron from red meat [11, 12].

HCAs, PAHs, and some NOCs are considered procarcinogens, as they require metabolic activation to attain full potential. Phase I and phase II xenobiotic metabolizing enzymes (XMEs) are involved in the activation and detoxification of these substrates [13–17]. Single nucleotide polymorphisms (SNPs) in genes that encode XMEs are hypothesized to alter enzyme expression and function [14], resulting in differential metabolism of xenobiotics between individuals [18]. A number of colorectal adenoma studies have evaluated interactions between XME genes and meat consumption with inconsistent results [19–30], but the majority of these investigated a limited number of genes. In addition, HCAs and PAHs from meat were estimated in just 2 studies [21, 22], while only 1 prior analysis evaluated nitrate/nitrite from processed meat [28].

Utilizing detailed meat-cooking data, we investigated the interaction of HCAs, PAHs, and nitrate/nitrite from meat with several XME gene variants in relation to advanced colorectal adenoma. Examining these interactions with asymptomatic colorectal adenomas, precursors to colorectal cancer [31–33], is valuable as diet should not have been altered by disease. Our analysis expands on findings of increased risk of prevalent colorectal adenoma with well-done red meat and cooking-related mutagens in the Prostate, Lung, Colorectal, and Ovarian (PLCO) Cancer Screening Trial [34].

Materials and Methods

Study Population
The PLCO Cancer Screening Trial is a randomized, multi-center clinical trial investigating the efficacy of screening for prostate, lung, colorectal and ovarian cancer [35, 36]. Participants aged 55–74 were recruited from 10 centers in the United States. Participants completed a self-administered baseline risk factor questionnaire, a food frequency questionnaire (FFQ), and provided biological samples. The study was approved by the institutional review boards at the National Cancer Institute and the 10 study centers. All participants provided written informed consent.

Cases and controls for this study were selected from participants enrolled in the screening arm of the PLCO Cancer Screening Trial between 1993 and 1999 (n = 77,483). At baseline, participants in the screening arm underwent flexible sigmoidoscopy of the distal colorectum (60 cm). Those with neoplastic lesions were referred for full colonoscopic examination and diagnostic work-up by the participant's personal physician. Trained abstractors obtained medical records and pathology reports pertaining to removed lesions, and lesions were coded according to location, size and morphology.

Participants were eligible for this study if they had: (1) undergone a successful sigmoidoscopy with insertion to at least 50 cm with > 90% of mucosa visible or a suspect lesion identified; (2) completed the baseline risk factor questionnaire, and (3) provided a blood sample for use in etiologic studies. Of the 42,037 participants meeting these criteria, 4,834 were further excluded due to self-reported history of Crohn's disease, ulcerative colitis, familial polyposis, Gardner's syndrome, colorectal polyps, or cancer (other than non-melanoma skin cancer). We randomly selected 772 of the 1,234 cases with at least 1 distal (descending colon and sigmoid or rectum) advanced colorectal adenoma for genotyping. Advanced adenomas were those with at least 1 of the following 3 characteristics: (1) size of ≥ 1 cm; (2) high-grade dysplasia, or (3) villous components, including tubulovillous. Of the 26,651 controls with a negative sigmoidoscopy (no polyps or other suspect lesion detected), we selected 777 controls frequency-matched to cases by gender and ethnicity (non-Hispanic white, non-Hispanic black, and other). Participants with insufficient dietary data (missed 7 or more food items on the FFQ, n = 83) were further excluded, leaving a total of 720 advanced colorectal adenoma cases and 746 controls.

Gene Selection and Genotyping
All genes and SNPs were selected a priori based on known or suggested functional relevance and a minor allele frequency of ≥ 5% in Caucasians (Appendix 1). DNA was extracted from stored buffy coat or whole blood samples using Qiagen standard protocols (QIAamp DNA Blood Midi or Maxi kit; www1.qiagen.com). All genotyping was conducted at the Core Genotyping Facility of the Division of Cancer Epidemiology and Genetics, National Cancer Institute, using TaqMan (Applied Biosystems, Foster City, Calif., USA; www.appliedbiosystems.com). All of the assays were validated and optimized and methods specific to *GSTM1*, *GSTT1* and *GSTP1* have been reported elsewhere

[37]. Internal laboratory quality controls were Coriell DNA samples consisting of homozygous major allele, heterozygous and homozygous minor allele genotypes for each polymorphism under investigation. In every 384 samples, there were 4 of each control type and 4 no template controls. External blinded quality controls from 40 individuals were also interspersed and showed > 99% interassay concordance. Genotyping data were obtained for > 90% of subjects, with data missing for the following reasons: insufficient DNA, genotyping failures, or fingerprint profile review showing subject-specific ambiguities.

Dietary Data

Participants completed a 137-item FFQ with a detailed meat-cooking module on their usual diet during the previous year. Most (89%) participants in the trial completed the FFQ prior to or the same day as the sigmoidoscopy. Using the Computerized Heterocyclic Amines Resource for Research in Epidemiology of Disease (CHARRED; www.charred.cancer.gov) software application [4], we generated intake estimates of 2 HCAs (ng/day): 2-amino-3,8-dimethylimidazo[4,5-*f*]quinoxaline (MeIQx), and 2-amino-1-methyl-6-phenyl-imidazo[4,5-*b*]pyridine (PhIP), as well as benzo[*a*]pyrene (B[*a*]P). We estimated nitrate and nitrite from processed meats using a nitrate/nitrite database based on laboratory measured values of these compounds from 10 types of processed meat samples that represented 90% of the processed meat consumed in the United States [4].

Statistical Analysis

We evaluated departure from Hardy-Weinberg equilibrium among the controls using Pearson's χ^2 tests. ORs and 95% CIs for the association between genotypes and advanced colorectal adenoma were calculated using unconditional logistic regression, adjusting for gender, ethnicity (non-Hispanic white, non-Hispanic black, other), and age (continuous). To evaluate the association between hypothesized gene pathways and colorectal adenoma, we included all the SNPs for genes potentially involved in the metabolism of each substrate in a model and compared it to a null model. We also conducted gene-specific global tests of association by including all of the SNPs in a given gene in a model and compared that to a null model that included none of the SNPs [38]. SNPs were coded with 2 dummy variables corresponding to the variant genotypes. The likelihood-ratio test for the gene-specific global test had 2k degrees of freedom (k representing the number of SNPs for the gene). Tests for linear trend were based on assigning ordinal values (0, 1 and 2) to the most prevalent genotypes in order of homozygous for the common allele, heterozygous and homozygous for the rare allele.

We evaluated effect modification of the associations between the meat-related exposure and colorectal adenoma by each of the XME genotype variants. We compared models with all of the cross product terms (diet on the continuous scale by genotype) to null models that included only the main effects. If this likelihood ratio test was statistically significant at the 0.05 level, we examined the effect of the dietary variable as a continuous measure stratified by genotype. Finally, to account for multiple comparisons, we corrected the p values for interactions using the False Discovery Rate [39].

Results

Cases and controls were similar with respect to the matching factors of gender and ethnicity (table 1). Cases tended to be older and were more likely to be current smokers and to have a first-degree relative with colorectal cancer. Cases also had fewer years of education and lower levels of physical activity compared to controls.

Table 1. Baseline characteristics of subjects in a nested case-control study of advanced colorectal adenoma in the PLCO Cancer Screening Trial (n = 1,466).

Characteristics	Cases (n = 720)[a]	Controls (n = 746)[a]	p value[b]
Age, years	63.1 ± 5.2	61.9 ± 5.2	<0.01
Gender, n (%)			0.74
Male	501 (69.6)	513 (68.8)	
Female	219 (30.4)	233 (31.2)	
Ethnicity, n (%)			0.81
Non-Hispanic white	681 (94.6)	704 (94.4)	
Non-Hispanic black	15 (2.1)	19 (2.6)	
Other	24 (3.3)	23 (3.1)	
Study center, n (%)			<0.01
Colorado	65 (9.0)	84 (11.3)	
Georgetown	36 (5.0)	43 (5.8)	
Hawaii	14 (1.9)	13 (1.7)	
Henry Ford Health System	61 (8.5)	90 (12.1)	
Minnesota	136 (18.9)	173 (23.2)	
Washington	77 (10.7)	75 (10.1)	
Pittsburg	112 (15.6)	58 (7.8)	
Utah	62 (8.6)	38 (5.1)	
Marshfield	130 (18.1)	156 (20.9)	
Alabama	27 (3.8)	16 (2.1)	
First degree family history of colorectal cancer, n (%)	90 (12.5)	67 (9.0)	0.03
Education, n (%)			0.04
12 years or less	245 (34.0)	217 (29.1)	
At least some college	475 (66.0)	528 (70.9)	
Body mass index (kg/m^2)	27.9 ± 4.8	27.5 ± 4.6	0.09
Physical activity (h/week)	2.5 ± 1.8	2.8 ± 1.8	<0.01
Regular use of NSAIDs, n (%)	418 (58.1)	449 (60.2)	0.42
Smoking status, n (%)			<0.01
Never	243 (33.8)	300 (40.2)	
Former cigarette smoker	344 (47.8)	353 (47.3)	
Current cigarette smoker	98 (13.6)	50 (6.7)	
Never cigarettes, but pipe and cigar	34 (4.7)	43 (5.8)	
Alcohol (g/day)	14.5 ± 25.1	12.6 ± 24.0	0.27
Total caloric intake (kcal/day)	2,114 ± 834	2,168 ± 827	0.17
Red meat (g/day)	86.8 ± 64.3	87.7 ± 67.6	0.88
MeIQx (ng/day)	37.0 ± 51.8	35.8 ± 43.7	0.86
PhIP (ng/day)	203.1 ± 461.4	205.8 ± 458.6	0.83
B[a]P (ng/day)	30.7 ± 57.1	31.5 ± 53.3	0.92

Data are means ± standard deviations unless otherwise indicated.
NSAIDs = non-steroidal anti-inflammatory drugs.
[a] Numbers may not sum to total due to missing values
[b] p values are for χ^2 test for categorical variables and Wilcoxon rank sum test for continuous variables.

Table 2. Meat exposure XME gene pathways in relation to advanced colorectal adenoma

Meat exposure	Genes	p value[a]
HCAs	CYP1A1, NAT1, NAT2, SULT1A1, SULT1A2	0.312
PAHs	CYP1A1, CYP1B1, CYP3A4, EPHX1, GSTM1, GSTP1, GSTT1, NQO1, SULT1A1, SULT1A2	0.172
NOCs	CYP2A6, CYP2C9, CYP2E1, GSTM1, GSTT1, GSTP1, NAT1, NAT2, NQO1	0.225

[a] Global pathway test based on inclusion of all SNPs for a given pathway compared to a model without any SNPs.

Our investigation of XME pathways, in which we identified the multiple genes hypothesized to be involved in the metabolism of HCAs, PAHs and NOCs, yielded no statistically significant findings in relation to colorectal adenoma (table 2). Our results for *EPHX1, GSTM1, GSTM2, GSTT1, NAT1* and *NAT2* were similar to previously published results in the larger advanced colorectal adenoma PLCO case-control subset [37, 40–42] (data not shown). Expanding upon these earlier analyses, in our gene-specific global tests, we found associations for *GSTM1* (p value for global test = 0.03) and *NAT1* (p value for global test = 0.05) with advanced colorectal adenoma (data not shown). For individual genes and SNPs, we did not find any statistically significant associations between *CYP1A1, CYP1B1, CYP2A6, CYP2C9, CYP2E1, CYP3A4, NQO1, SULT1A1,* or *SULT1A2,* and advanced colorectal adenoma in this population (data not shown).

We found a suggestive interaction between intake of PhIP and variation in *CYP1B1* (rs10012 p for interaction = 0.019; rs1056836 p for interaction = 0.019) and *NQO1* (p for interaction = 0.007) with advanced colorectal adenoma (table 3). We also found evidence of interaction with intake of B[*a*]P for variation in *CYP1B1* (p for interaction = 0.005) and *CYP3A4* (p for interaction = 0.021). In addition, there was a possible interaction with intake of nitrate/nitrite and *CYP1A1* (p for interaction = 0.022). However, when we corrected for multiple comparisons, none of the resulting p values for interaction fell below a False Discovery Rate threshold of 0.20. When stratified by genotype, for *CYP1B1* rs10012, there was a statistically significant increased risk of colorectal adenoma with increasing intake of PhIP for participants with either the CG/GG genotypes (OR = 1.53; 95%CI = 1.02–2.30) and risk was also elevated among those with the CC genotype for *CYP1B1* rs1056836 (OR = 1.86; 95%CI = 1.07–3.22).

Discussion

Overall, we observed evidence of possible interactions between intake of meat-related HCAs, PAHs, and nitrate/nitrite and genetic variants in *CYP1A1, CYP1B1, CYP3A4,*

Table 3. ORs and 95% CIs for the association between dietary variables and advanced colorectal adenoma stratified by genotype.

Dietary intake	Gene	Locus	Genotype	Cases/controls	OR[a]	$p_{interaction}$[b]	Corrected[c] $p_{interaction}$
PhIP per 1,000 ng/day	CYP1B1	rs10012	CC	344/375	0.81 (0.58–1.12)	0.019	0.384
			CG	293/296	1.47 (0.93–2.30)		
			GG	71/59	1.76 (0.60–5.21)		
			CG/GG	364/355	1.53 (1.02–2.30)		
	CYP1B1	rs1056836	CC	232/250	1.86 (1.07–3.22)	0.019	0.384
			CG	337/344	0.86 (0.64–1.15)		
			GG	137/137	0.82 (0.33–2.08)		
			CG/GG	474/481	0.85 (0.64–1.13)		
	NQO1	rs1800566	CC	416/474	1.03 (0.76–1.40)	0.007	0.340
			CT	244/225	0.99 (0.60–1.61)		
			TT	25/17	–		
			CT/TT	269/242	0.80 (0.52–1.24)		
B[a]P per 100 ng/day	CYP1B1	rs10012	CC	344/375	0.74 (0.55–1.00)	0.005	0.340
			CG	293/296	1.25 (0.94–1.68)		
			GG	71/59	1.66 (0.73–3.81)		
			CG/GG	364/355	1.29 (0.99–1.68)		
	CYP3A4	rs2242480	GG	558/579	1.02 (0.83–1.21)	0.021	0.384
			GA	126/131	1.13 (0.69–1.85)		
			AA	12/14	–		
			GA/AA	138/145	0.89 (0.56–1.42)		
Nitrate + Nitrite per 0.5 mg/day	CYP1A1	rs1048943	AA	646/684	1.03 (0.92–1.15)	0.022	0.384
			AG	44/38	1.11 (0.75–1.59)		
			GG	2/3	–		
			AG/GG	46/41	1.14 (0.79–1.64)		

Data are limited to SNPs with statistically significant tests for interaction before correction.
[a]Adjusted for age, gender and ethnicity.
[b]Likelihood ratio test for model with cross-product terms of dietary variables (coded as continuous) with the genotype variables (coded as dummy variables) compared to null model with only main effects for dietary variables and genotypes.
[c]Based on false discovery rate.

and *NQO1* with risk of advanced colorectal adenoma in the PLCO Cancer Screening Trial. Yet, when stratified by genotype, strong variation in risk of colorectal adenoma with increasing intake of the meat-related exposures was not obvious and correction for multiple comparisons indicated our findings may be due to chance. We did not observe any statistically significant main effects for *CYP1A1, CYP1B1, CYP2A6, CYP2C9, CYP2E1, CYP3A4, NQO1, SULT1A1* or *SULT1A2* on risk of advanced colorectal adenoma. Our gene-based analyses for *GSTM1* and *NAT1* support previously reported SNP based analyses in PLCO [37, 41].

A strength of this analysis was our substrate-oriented pathway-based approach, in which we assessed a range of XME genes involved in the activation and detoxification of xenobiotics, and comprehensively examined interactions with meat-related intake of HCAs, PAHs and nitrate/nitrite. Our study was further strengthened by the inclusion of advanced colorectal adenoma cases, an outcome clinically relevant for progression to colorectal cancer. Importantly, since adenomas are largely asymptomatic, it is unlikely that cases would have changed their dietary habits. In addition, the majority of participants completed the FFQ prior to diagnosis, reducing the potential for recall bias. Our sample size is larger than many prior XME gene-meat interaction studies of colorectal adenoma and few have quantitatively estimated intake of the specific potentially carcinogenic meat-related exposures, instead relying on meat cooking method or doneness level as proxies.

A limitation of our analysis, like other studies of gene-environment interactions, is limited power to observe small associations and the potential for chance findings due to multiple comparisons. To gain power, we used a method for testing gene-environment interactions that assumes independence of the gene and the environmental factor [43], but in general, we did not observe smaller p values (data not shown). Future research of XME gene-meat interactions should assess both activating and detoxifying XME genes and evaluate the more specific meat-related exposures, rather than overall meat intake or meat cooking method/doneness. Yet these analyses can become complex, as there is a certain amount of error associated with the measurement of dietary exposures and their associated exposures. Finally, our measure of nitrate/nitrite is a proxy for processed meat-related exposure to NOCs and the nitrate/nitrite database does not contain data on the levels of these compounds in other foods.

In our interaction analyses, there was variation in the association between the meat-related variables and advanced colorectal adenoma across the *CYP1B1* genotypes. *CYP1B1* is involved in the metabolism of PAHs [14, 15, 44] and in fact, we did see a suggestive interaction with B[*a*]P, a known marker of PAHs [4]. Other studies have also found similar effect modification of the association between well-done red meat or total meat on colorectal cancer risk by combined *CYP1B1* variants [45, 46]. However, specific functional data for this variant and PAH metabolism are lacking and further work is required to characterize the biological mechanism underlying this potential interaction.

We found increased risk of colorectal adenoma with increasing PhIP intake among participants with the less common allele of *CYP1B1* rs10012 compared to the common allele and participants with the *CYP1B1* rs1056836 common allele (CC). Functionality of these variants in relation to PhIP is not well-characterized and, thus far, has been studied only in combination with other SNPs for this gene [47]. Another possible reason for an interaction between PhIP and the *CYP1B1* rs10012 variant is the relatively high correlation between PhIP and B[*a*]P (0.58) in our population.

Variation in the association between our dietary variables and risk of colorectal adenoma by *CYP1A1*, *CYP3A4*, and *NQO1* was not straightforward. As hypothesized [48, 49], we did observe a suggestive interaction between *CYP3A4* variants and B[*a*]P intake on risk of advanced colorectal adenoma, but there have been no other studies of interaction with meat intake to verify this observation. *CYP3A4* is more common than other CYP3A isoforms in the intestine [50] and there is also wide range in expression levels of this enzyme across individuals [51], but little evidence as to which genetic variants control this variation [52]. One study of *CYP1A1* noted increased risk of colorectal adenoma among those with high meat intake [27]; however, 3 studies of colorectal cancer did not observe effect modification by meat [45, 53] or HCA intake [54]. One other study of colorectal cancer observed a possible interaction between *NQO1* phenotypes and red meat intake [55].

In general, there is little consensus in the literature for XME gene-meat interactions in relation to colorectal neoplasia for *CYP2A6* phenotypes [28, 56], *CYP2E1* [46, 57, 58], *EPHX1* [19, 25–27, 30, 55, 59], or *SULT1A1* [20, 27, 45, 60–62]. In addition, there are limited data on *CYP2C9* [46] and *SULT1A2* [27]. Although we did not find evidence of effect modification by *NAT1* or *NAT2*, studies of these genotypes or phenotypes point toward an increased risk of colorectal neoplasia for rapid acetylators with high intake of meat, HCAs or PAHs [21, 22, 63–65]. Overall, these varied results could be due to several reasons, including differences in study populations and the study of adenomas versus cancer.

Our approach focused on a wide range of genes involved in the metabolism of 3 groups of potentially carcinogenic meat-related exposures: HCAs, PAHs, and nitrate/nitrite. Given our sample size, these analyses were largely exploratory. The substrate-focused pathway-based approach encompasses the multiple levels at which these potentially carcinogenic meat-related exposures are activated or detoxified in the body. With future consortial efforts, studies will have the opportunity to investigate potential effect modification of the association between meat-related exposures and colorectal adenoma by XME gene variants in greater detail.

Acknowledgments

This research was supported (in part) by the Intramural Research Program of the National Institutes of Health, National Cancer Institute, by grant TU2 CA105666 from the National Cancer Institute, and by contracts from the Division of Cancer Prevention, National Cancer Institute, National Institutes of Health, Department of Health and Human Services.

The authors thank Drs. Christine Berg and Philip Prorok, Division of Cancer Prevention, National Cancer Institute, the Screening Center investigators and staff of the Prostate, Lung, Colorectal, and Ovarian (PLCO) Cancer Screening Trial, and Mr. Tom Riley and staff, Information Management Services, Inc.

Appendix 1. XME genes included in main effect (pathway, gene and SNP) and/or interaction analyses

Gene	Locus
CYP1A1	Ex7+129C>A (T461N; rs1799814)
	Ex7+131A>G (I462V; rs1048943)[a]
CYP1B1	Ex2+143C>G (R48G; rs10012)
	Ex3+251G>C (V432L; rs1056836)
CYP2A6	Ex3-15T>A (L160H; rs1801272)
CYP2C9	Ex3-52C>T (R144C; rs1799853)
CYP2E1	-332T>A (rs2070673)
	IVS4+23T>C (rs6413421)
CYP3A4	IVS10+12G>A (rs2242480)
EPHX1[b]	Ex3-28T>C (Y113H; rs1051740)
	Ex4+52A>G (H139R; rs2234922)
GSTM1[c]	Ex4+10+>- (rs1065411)
GSTP1[c]	Ex5-24A>G (I105V; rs1695)
	Ex17-4C>T (H1085H; rs1799817)
GSTT1[c]	Ex5-49+>- (rs4630)
NAT1[a]	Ex3-177A>T (T1088A; rs1057126)
	Ex3-170A>C (C1095A; rs15561)
	IVS2-338C>T (C-334T; rs4986988)
	IVS2-34A>T (A-40T; rs4986989)
NAT2[a]	Ex2-367G>A (R268K; rs1208)
	Ex2-313G>A (G286E; rs1799931)
	Ex2+288C>T (Y94Y; rs1041983)
	Ex2+347T>C (I114T; rs1801280)
	Ex2+487C>T (L161L; rs1799929)
	Ex2-580G>A (R197Q; rs1799930)
NQO1	Ex4-3C>T (R139W; rs4986998)
	Ex6+40C>T (P187S; rs1800566)[a]
SULT1A1	Ex10+127A>G (G212G; rs6839)
SULT1A2	336bp 3' of STP (rs3194168)

[a] SNP main effects previously published for advanced colorectal adenoma in the PLCO Cancer Screening Trial.
[b] SNP main effects and interactions with red meat and dietary B[a]P previously published for advanced colorectal adenoma in the PLCO Cancer Screening Trial.
[c] SNP main effects and interactions with red meat, HCAs and B[a]P previously published for advanced colorectal adenoma in the PLCO Cancer Screening Trial.

References

1 Sinha R, Norat T: Meat cooking and cancer risk. IARC Sci Publ 2002;156:181–186.
2 Cross AJ, Sinha R: Meat-related mutagens/carcinogens in the etiology of colorectal cancer. Environ Mol Mutagen 2004;44:44–55.
3 World Cancer Research Fund/American Institute for Cancer Research: Food, Nutrition, Physical Activity, and the Prevention of Cancer: A Global Perspective. Washington DC, AICR, 2007.
4 Sinha R, Cross A, Curtin J, et al: Development of a food frequency questionnaire module and databases for compounds in cooked and processed meats. Mol Nutr Food Res 2005;49:648–655.
5 Ito N, Hasegawa R, Sano M, et al: A new colon and mammary carcinogen in cooked food, 2-amino-1-methyl-6-phenylimidazo[4,5-b]pyridine (PhIP). Carcinogenesis 1991;121503–1506.
6 Ochiai M, Imai H, Sugimura T, Nagao M, Nakagama H: Induction of intestinal tumors and lymphomas in C57BL/6N mice by a food-borne carcinogen, 2-amino-1-methyl-6-phenylimidazo[4,5-b]pyridine. Jpn J Cancer Res 2002;93:478–483.
7 Ohgaki H, Takayama S, Sugimura T: Carcinogenicities of heterocyclic amines in cooked food. Mut Res 1991;259:399–410.
8 Bogovski P, Bogovski S: Animal Species in which N-nitroso compounds induce cancer. Int J Cancer 1981;27:471–474.
9 Mirvish SS: Role of N-nitroso compounds (NOC) and N-nitrosation in etiology of gastric, esophageal, nasopharyngeal and bladder cancer and contribution to cancer of known exposures to NOC. Cancer Lett 1995;93:17–48.
10 Mirvish SS, Haorah J, Zhou L, et al: Total N-nitroso compounds and their precursors in hot dogs and in the gastrointestinal tract and feces of rats and mice: possible etiologic agents for colon cancer. J Nutr 2002;132(suppl 11):3526S–3529S.
11 Cross AJ, Pollock JR, Bingham SA: Haem, not protein or inorganic iron, is responsible for endogenous intestinal N-nitrosation arising from red meat. Cancer Res 2003;63:2358–2360.
12 Hughes R, Cross AJ, Pollock JR, Bingham S: Dose-dependent effect of dietary meat on endogenous colonic N-nitrosation. Carcinogenesis 2001;22:199–202.
13 Xue W, Warshawsky D: Metabolic activation of polycyclic and heterocyclic aromatic hydrocarbons and DNA damage: a review. Toxicol Appl Pharmacol 2005;206:73–93.
14 Shimada T: Xenobiotic-metabolizing enzymes involved in activation and detoxification of carcinogenic polycyclic aromatic hydrocarbons. Drug Metab Pharmacokinet 2006;21:257–276.
15 Nebert DW, Dalton TP: The role of cytochrome P450 enzymes in endogenous signalling pathways and environmental carcinogenesis. Nat Rev Cancer 2006;6:947–960.
16 Glatt H, Pabel U, Meinl W, et al: Bioactivation of the heterocyclic aromatic amine 2-amino-3-methyl-9H-pyrido [2,3-b]indole (MeAalphaC) in recombinant test systems expressing human xenobiotic- metabolizing enzymes. Carcinogenesis 2004;25:801–807.
17 Muckel E, Frandsen H, Glatt HR: Heterologous expression of human N-acetyltransferases 1 and 2 and sulfotransferase 1A1 in Salmonella typhimurium for mutagenicity testing of heterocyclic amines. Food Chem Toxicol 2002;40:1063–1068.
18 Turesky RJ: Interspecies metabolism of heterocyclic aromatic amines and the uncertainties in extrapolation of animal toxicity data for human risk assessment. Mol Nutr Food Res 2005;49:101–117.
19 Tranah GJ, Giovannucci E, Ma J, et al: Epoxide hydrolase polymorphisms, cigarette smoking and risk of colorectal adenoma in the Nurses' Health Study and the Health Professionals Follow-up Study. Carcinogenesis 2004;25:1211–1218.
20 Tiemersma EW, Voskuil DW, Bunschoten A, et al: Risk of colorectal adenomas in relation to meat consumption, meat preparation, and genetic susceptibility in a Dutch population. Cancer Causes Control 2004;15:225–236.
21 Shin A, Shrubsole MJ, Rice JM, et al: Meat intake, heterocyclic amine exposure, and metabolizing enzyme polymorphisms in relation to colorectal polyp risk. Cancer Epidemiol Biomarkers Prev 2008;17:320–329.
22 Ishibe N, Sinha R, Hein DW, et al: Genetic polymorphisms in heterocyclic amine metabolism and risk of colorectal adenomas. Pharmacogenetics 2002;12:145–150.
23 Roberts-Thomson IC, Ryan P, Khoo KK, et al: Diet, acetylator phenotype, and risk of colorectal neoplasia. Lancet 1996;347:1372–1374.
24 Tiemersma EW, Kloosterman J, Bunschoten A, Kok FJ, Kampman E: Role of EPHX genotype in the associations of smoking and diet with colorectal adenomas. IARC Sci Publ 2002;156:491–493.
25 Ulrich CM, Bigler J, Whitton JA, et al: Epoxide hydrolase Tyr113His polymorphism is associated with elevated risk of colorectal polyps in the presence of smoking and high meat intake. Cancer Epidemiol Biomarkers Prev 2001;10:875–882.

26 Cortessis V, Siegmund K, Chen Q, et al: A case-control study of microsomal epoxide hydrolase, smoking, meat consumption, glutathione S-transferase M3, and risk of colorectal adenomas. Cancer Res 2001;61:2381–2385.

27 Goode EL, Potter JD, Bamlet WR, Rider DN, Bigler J: Inherited variation in carcinogen-metabolizing enzymes and risk of colorectal polyps. Carcinogenesis 2007;28:328–341.

28 Ward MH, Cross AJ, Divan H, et al: Processed meat intake, CYP2A6 activity and risk of colorectal adenoma. Carcinogenesis 2007;28:1210–1216.

29 Saebo M, Skjelbred CF, Brekke Li K, et al: CYP1A2 164 A→C polymorphism, cigarette smoking, consumption of well-done red meat and risk of developing colorectal adenomas and carcinomas. Anticancer Res 2008;28:2289–2295.

30 Skjelbred CF, Saebo M, Hjartaker A, et al: Meat, vegetables and genetic polymorphisms and the risk of colorectal carcinomas and adenomas. BMC Cancer 2007;7:228.

31 Winawer SJ, Zauber AG, Ho MN, et al:. Prevention of colorectal cancer by colonoscopic polypectomy. The National Polyp Study Workgroup. N Engl J Med 1993;329:1977–1981.

32 Anderson WF, Guyton KZ, Hiatt RA, et al: Colorectal cancer screening for persons at average risk. J Natl Cancer Inst 2002;94:1126–1133.

33 Stryker SJ, Wolff BG, Culp CE, et al: Natural history of untreated colonic polyps. Gastroenterology 1987;93:1009–1013.

34 Sinha R, Peters U, Cross AJ, et al: Meat, meat cooking methods and preservation, and risk for colorectal adenoma. Cancer Res 2005;65:8034–8041.

35 Prorok PC, Andriole GL, Bresalier RS, et al: Design of the Prostate, Lung, Colorectal and Ovarian (PLCO) Cancer Screening Trial. Control Clin Trials 2000;21(suppl 6):273S–309S.

36 Gohagan JK, Prorok PC, Hayes RB, Kramer BS: The Prostate, Lung, Colorectal and Ovarian (PLCO) Cancer Screening Trial of the National Cancer Institute: history, organization, and status. Control Clin Trials 2000;21(suppl 6):251S–272S.

37 Moore LE, Huang WY, Chatterjee N, et al : GSTM1, GSTT1, and GSTP1 polymorphisms and risk of advanced colorectal adenoma. Cancer Epidemiol Biomarkers Prev 2005;14:1823–1827.

38 Chapman JM, Cooper JD, Todd JA, Clayton DG: Detecting disease associations due to linkage disequilibrium using haplotype tags: a class of tests and the determinants of statistical power. Hum Hered 2003;56:18–31.

39 Benjamini Y, Drai D, Elmer G, Kafkafi N, Golani I: Controlling the false discovery rate in behavior genetics research. Behav Brain Res 2001;125:279–284.

40 Huang WY, Chatterjee N, Chanock S, et al: Microsomal epoxide hydrolase polymorphisms and risk for advanced colorectal adenoma. Cancer Epidemiol Biomarkers Prev 2005;14:152–157.

41 Moslehi R, Chatterjee N, Church TR, et al: Cigarette smoking, N-acetyltransferase genes and the risk of advanced colorectal adenoma. Pharmacogenomics 2006;7:819–829.

42 Hou L, Chatterjee N, Huang WY, et al: CYP1A1 Val462 and NQO1 Ser187 polymorphisms, cigarette use, and risk for colorectal adenoma. Carcinogenesis 2005;26:1122–1128.

43 Mukherjee B, Chatterjee N: Exploiting gene-environment independence for analysis of case-control studies: an empirical bayes-type shrinkage estimator to trade-off between bias and efficiency. Biometrics 2008;64:685–694.

44 Shimada T, Fujii-Kuriyama Y: Metabolic activation of polycyclic aromatic hydrocarbons to carcinogens by cytochromes P450 1A1 and 1B1. Cancer Sci 2004;95:1–6.

45 Cotterchio M, Boucher BA, Manno M, et al: Red meat intake, doneness, polymorphisms in genes that encode carcinogen-metabolizing enzymes, and colorectal cancer risk. Cancer Epidemiol Biomarkers Prev 2008;17:3098–3107.

46 Kury S, Buecher B, Robiou-du-Pont S, et al: Combinations of cytochrome P450 gene polymorphisms enhancing the risk for sporadic colorectal cancer related to red meat consumption. Cancer Epidemiol Biomarkers Prev 2007;16:1460–1467.

47 Han JF, He XY, Herrington JS, et al: Metabolism of 2-amino-1-methyl-6-phenylimidazo[4,5-b]pyridine (PhIP) by human CYP1B1 genetic variants. Drug Metab Dispos 2008;36:745–752.

48 Rihs HP, Pesch B, Kappler M, et al: Occupational exposure to polycyclic aromatic hydrocarbons in German industries: association between exogenous exposure and urinary metabolites and its modulation by enzyme polymorphisms. Toxicol Lett 2005;157:241–255.

49 Lamba JK, Lin YS, Schuetz EG, Thummel KE: Genetic contribution to variable human CYP3A-mediated metabolism. Adv Drug Deliv Rev 2002;54:1271–1294.

50 Canaparo R, Finnstrom N, Serpe L, et al: Expression of CYP3A isoforms and P-glycoprotein in human stomach, jejunum and ileum. Clin Exp Pharmacol Physiol 2007;34:1138–1144.

51 Shimada T, Yamazaki H, Mimura M, Inui Y, Guengerich FP: Interindividual variations in human liver cytochrome P-450 enzymes involved in the oxidation of drugs, carcinogens and toxic chemicals: studies with liver microsomes of 30 Japanese and 30 Caucasians. J Pharmacol Exp Ther 1994;270:414–423.

52 Wojnowski L, Kamdem LK: Clinical implications of CYP3A polymorphisms. Expert Opin Drug Metab Toxicol 2006;2:171–182.
53 Murtaugh MA, Sweeney C, Ma KN, Caan BJ, Slattery ML: The CYP1A1 genotype may alter the association of meat consumption patterns and preparation with the risk of colorectal cancer in men and women. J Nutr 2005;135:179–186.
54 Kobayashi M, Otani T, Iwasaki M, et al. Association between dietary heterocyclic amine levels, genetic polymorphisms of NAT2, CYP1A1, and CYP1A2 and risk of colorectal cancer: a hospital-based case-control study in Japan. Scand J Gastroenterol 2009: 1–8.
55 Turner F, Smith G, Sachse C, et al: Vegetable, fruit and meat consumption and potential risk modifying genes in relation to colorectal cancer. Int J Cancer 2004;112:259–264.
56 Nowell S, Sweeney C, Hammons G, Kadlubar FF, Lang NP: CYP2A6 activity determined by caffeine phenotyping: association with colorectal cancer risk. Cancer Epidemiol Biomarkers Prev 2002;11: 377–383.
57 Le Marchand L, Donlon T, Seifried A, Wilkens LR: Red meat intake, CYP2E1 genetic polymorphisms, and colorectal cancer risk. Cancer Epidemiol Biomarkers Prev 2002;11:1019–1024.
58 Morita M, Le Marchand L, Kono S, et al: Genetic polymorphisms of CYP2E1 and risk of colorectal cancer: the Fukuoka Colorectal Cancer Study. Cancer Epidemiol Biomarkers Prev 2009;18:235–241.
59 Robien K, Curtin K, Ulrich CM, et al: Microsomal epoxide hydrolase polymorphisms are not associated with colon cancer risk. Cancer Epidemiol Biomarkers Prev 2005;14:1350–1352.
60 Lilla C, Risch A, Verla-Tebit E, et al: SULT1A1 genotype and susceptibility to colorectal cancer. Int J Cancer 2007;120:201–206.
61 Tiemersma EW, Kampman E, Bueno de Mesquita HB, et al: Meat consumption, cigarette smoking, and genetic susceptibility in the etiology of colorectal cancer: results from a Dutch prospective study. Cancer Causes Control 2002;13:383–393.
62 Moreno V, Glatt H, Guino E, et al: Polymorphisms in sulfotransferases SULT1A1 and SULT1A2 are not related to colorectal cancer. Int J Cancer 2005; 113:683–686.
63 Lilla C, Verla-Tebit E, Risch A, et al: Effect of NAT1 and NAT2 genetic polymorphisms on colorectal cancer risk associated with exposure to tobacco smoke and meat consumption. Cancer Epidemiol Biomarkers Prev 2006;15:99–107.
64 Nothlings U, Yamamoto JF, Wilkens LR, et al: Meat and heterocyclic amine intake, smoking, NAT1 and NAT2 polymorphisms, and colorectal cancer risk in the multiethnic cohort study. Cancer Epidemiol Biomarkers Prev 2009;18:2098–2106.
65 Yeh CC, Sung FC, Tang R, Chang-Chieh CR, Hsieh LL: Polymorphisms of cytochrome P450 1A2 and N-acetyltransferase genes, meat consumption, and risk of colorectal cancer. Dis Colon Rectum 2009; 52:104–111.

Rashmi Sinha
Division of Cancer Epidemiology and Genetics, National Cancer Institute, National Institutes of Health, Department of Health and Human Services
Bethesda, MD 20892 (USA)
Tel. +1 301-496-6426, Fax +1 301-496-6829, E-Mail sinhar@mail.nih.gov

Strategies to Improve Detection of Hypertension Genes

Steven C. Hunt

Cardiovascular Genetics Division, Department of Internal Medicine, University of Utah, Salt Lake City, Utah, USA

The identification of genes that are associated with hypertension has been a slower process than for other diseases, despite a similar heritability in many cases. This is, in part, likely to be a result of a great number of genes being involved with the blood pressure control pathways and their accompanying small effects on the phenotypes that are being measured.

With blood pressure fluctuating so acutely with changes in posture, stress, activity level, and even while talking, strong responses to these fluctuations are required to keep blood pressure appropriate for tissue perfusion and cellular function. Because of the importance of blood pressure control, there are redundant compensatory pathways for this pressure normalization. Therefore, a gene that may compromise one pathway may not be found to be associated with hypertension because other pathways can adequately compensate and normalize the phenotypes being studied. What might be detected in these situations are associations of a gene with the compensating factors that change to normalize a causal pathway. The altered levels of the compensating factors will likely be smaller than the causal phenotype levels if there were no compensation, and are probably more difficult to detect. Both initiating genes and compensating genes are involved in eventual hypertension development, in line with the strong polygenic nature of hypertension.

Recent genome-wide association studies (GWAS) have begun to suggest genes related to hypertension and blood pressure levels [1–9]. Comparing the results of each GWAS as a whole, there is little overlap of the significant gene associations. When targeted in silico look-ups of association regions are done in other GWAS, a few genes are then replicated because the penalty for multiple corrections is decreased. These few genes, such as SH2B3 or CACNB2, show very small influences on blood pressure in accordance with the theory of large numbers of genes working together in pathways for fine blood pressure control. Interestingly, few of the physiological candidate genes that have been found associated with hypertension over the last 20 years of research have been replicated by GWAS.

In light of these difficulties, elucidation of a few concepts suggested by the literature may increase the ability to detect more genes and to verify the genes already suggested for their involvement with hypertension. These include: (1) selecting of subjects with strong family histories of hypertension; (2) identifying age ranges that show the highest heritability of blood pressure in the target population; (3) measuring local tissue-specific electrolyte or hormone concentrations in addition to systemic concentrations; (4) using acute interventions to investigate genetic interactions with environmental factors such as diet, activity and stress; (5) determining the appropriate time window after intervention to identify initiators versus compensators of blood pressure elevation; (6) genotyping subjects involved in large clinical trials to detect intervention interactions with genotype, and (7) increasing the density of SNPs in and around candidate genes for hypertension in genome-wide or candidate gene association studies.

Subject Selection

Persons with strong family histories of hypertension, still the strongest genetic risk factor we have to predict future hypertension [10, 11], are more likely to have multiple genes predisposing to blood pressure elevation. Not only are these persons likely to have more hypertension genes, the genes shared among family members are sufficiently expressed to lead to hypertension in multiple family members – in genetic terms they are penetrant genes. Unaffected relatives in families with strong histories of hypertension have significantly higher risks of developing hypertension compared to the general population [10, 12]. Relative risks above 2 are almost always seen in a positive family history of hypertension compared to relative risks for a specific gene in large hypertension genome-wide association studies in the 1.1–1.5 range. From birth to young adulthood, the combined effects of these genes seem to be adequately compensated, as hypertension does not generally develop until ages 40 or older. Aging is an extremely strong risk factor for hypertension, with the lifetime risk of hypertension approaching 90%, as reported in the Framingham Heart Study [13]. This result suggests that compensating mechanisms may lose their effectiveness with age allowing the effects of initiating hypertension genes to be detected.

While a proportion of the non-genetic variance in blood pressure is due to measurement errors and random variation, a significant part is the result of environmental factors. Selection of hypertensive subjects who have more environmental risk factors as opposed to stronger genetic predispositions may lead to difficulties in detecting genes with small effects even though the combination of genetic and environmental risk factors may increase the risk of hypertension. On the other hand, selection of high-risk subjects and modulation of environmental risk factors should allow detailed investigation of gene and environment interactions and will likely improve the ability to detect hypertension genes.

Selecting an Intervention

In the detection of initiating factors, one must correctly choose an intervention that affects the initiating genes by increasing or decreasing expression. One obvious choice would be dietary salt manipulation or saline infusions. Since 40–50% of the population appear to have blood pressures that are quite responsive to salt, this has been the most frequent intervention. It is still unclear whether sodium changes from low to high or high to low are best to unmask sodium excretion abnormalities. A feeding study in Japan showed differences in sodium excretion between salt-sensitive and salt-resistant subjects when changed from a low to high salt diet, but not vice versa [14]. However, an earlier study found that compared to salt-resistant patients, salt-sensitive patients had blunted renal responses when sodium intake was reduced rather than increased [15]. Saline infusions have been effective in validating the association of the alpha adducin gene with hypertension [16]. Weight loss interventions would be expected to affect the salt sensitivity pathways, as obese subjects are more likely to be salt sensitive, and salt sensitivity is decreased following weight loss [17]. Other interventions include potassium supplementation, angiotensin II infusions, antihypertensive medication institution, and stressed blood pressure procedures such as posture change, isometric handgrip procedures, exercise and mental challenges.

Study Time Windows

Animal models suggest that when the blood pressure system is stressed with high salt intake, an initial genetic response may be only transiently expressed. Compensatory mechanisms quickly counteract the abnormal genetic response to the initial stressor, reducing the blood pressure back to normal or near-normal levels. The Japanese salt study referenced above [14], showed that the sodium excretion differences were maintained between salt-sensitive and salt-resistant subjects only for a few days after the intervention, after which the excretion curves became similar again. Investigating the causes of the delayed sodium excretion would be effective during that window but not before or after.

Figure 1 shows a genetic cause of hypertension, the knockout of the microsomal prostaglandin E synthase-1 gene in the mouse [18]. Chronic salt loading acts as an initiator of sodium retention in the knockout mouse during days 1–3. This sodium retention is subsequently hidden or normalized after compensating mechanisms increasing sodium excretion are activated, even when sodium loading continues. Measuring sodium balance after day 3 in the 2 mouse strains would not identify this gene as being associated with sodium balance. The compensatory factors that are invoked to normalize the sodium retention are blood pressure increases that lead to premature death in these mice. In this case, the blood pressure difference would be detected as a compensating factor or the result of a compensating factor, but in other

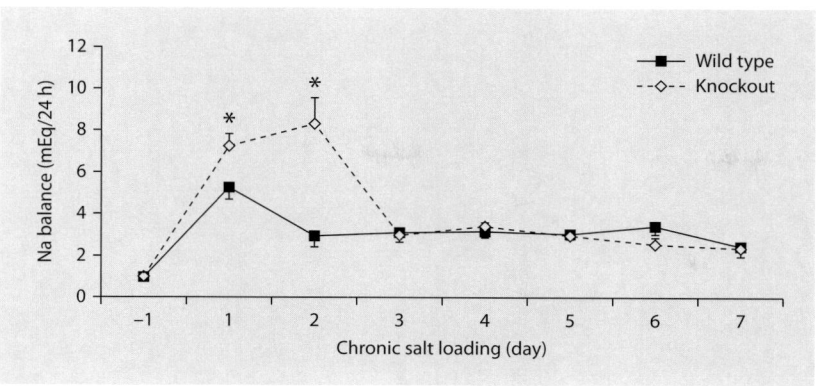

Fig. 1. Transient acute but not chronic sodium retention in the microsomal prostaglandin E synthase-1 knockout (KO) mouse. From Jia et al. [18]. * p < 0.05.

examples, the compensating factor might not be measured in the experiment, and it may not lead to elevated blood pressure. It seems likely that there may be time windows throughout life when specific genetic factors have greater expression and contribute to the development of hypertension.

The existence of these time windows is further suggested by the low infant twin blood pressure heritability [19]. Adult twin blood pressure heritability is much larger [20–22] and suggests that heritability is not constant over age [23–26]. Results from the HyperGEN study, fitting both the traditional constant heritability model and a model that allows heritability to change with age (fig. 2), suggests that blood pressure heritability is much larger in particular age ranges [26]. The maximum heritability also differs by racial group, suggesting that different populations may have different heritability patterns. For systolic blood pressure, blacks had an estimated peak heritability of 0.68 at age 59 compared to an average heritability of 0.29; whites had an estimated peak heritability of 0.69 at age 74 compared to an average heritability of 0.24. The differences between the peak and average heritability were highly significant ($p < 10^{-12}$). If these results are verified in other populations, they suggest that in order to maximize the ability to detect hypertension genes, the population-specific age-dependent heritability should first be estimated and subjects selected within the maximum range.

Tissue versus Central Phenotype Measurement

The importance of the kidney in blood pressure control and hypertension development and tissue-specific gene expression was shown in elegant experiments in which the AT1R gene was knocked out either systemically or just in the kidney [27]. In mice

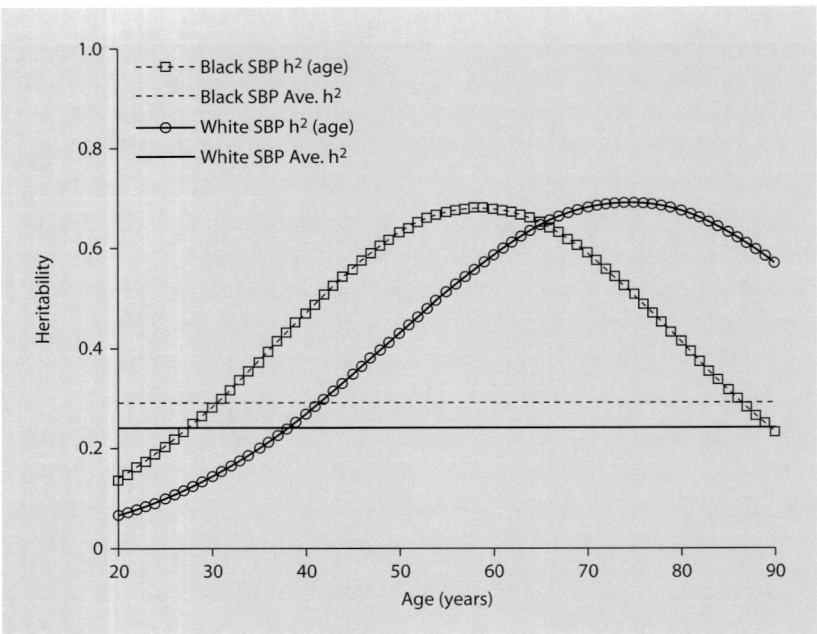

Fig. 2. Systolic blood pressure (SBP) average and age-specific heritabilities in white and black participants in the HyperGEN study. From Shi et al. [26].

where the AT1R gene was systemically knocked out but which then received a transplant of a normal kidney with functioning AT1 receptors, blood pressure increased and hypertension eventually developed during chronic angiotensin II infusion. When the AT1R gene was functional systemically and a kidney with the AT1R gene knocked out was transplanted into the mouse, hypertension did not develop during angiotensin II infusion. The study concluded that both central and kidney AT1 receptors help control blood pressure, but that the kidney receptors were required for the development of hypertension. These experiments also confirmed the earlier transplant experiments that showed that hypertension follows the kidney [28]. Kidneys transplanted from normotensive rats into hypertensive rats removed the hypertension and kidneys transplanted from hypertensive rats into normotensive rats caused hypertension. These experiments suggest that if polymorphims in kidney expressed genes such as the AT1R gene are associated with hypertension, one should measure the intermediate phenotypes in the kidney rather than systemically.

An example of such an intermediate phenotype is plasma angiotensinogen. Experiments on the relevance of circulating angiotensinogen versus angiotensinogen acting locally in the renal tubules show that kidney-specific angiotensinogen and the resulting angiotensin II produced play important roles in sodium excretion somewhat independently of circulating angiotensin II [29–31]. This reinforces the concept

Table 1. Systolic and diastolic blood pressure reductions by angiotensinogen (AGT) genotypes after intervention in 3 clinical trials. From Hunt [40]

	AGT G-6A			
	AA	GA	GG	AA-GG difference
TOHP Na reduction	−2.7/−2.2	−1.3/−0.7	−0.2/1.1	−2.5/−1.5
TOHP weight loss	−3.5/−2.4	−0.9/−1	−1.1/0.3	−2.6/−1.4
SAGA salt diet	−8.6/−3.9	−9.0/−5.2	−5.3/−1.0	−3.3/−2.9
DASH fruit/vegetable diet	−5.2/−3.0	−2.3/−1.2	−1.3/0.3	−3.9/−3.3
DASH diet	−6.9/−3.5	−5.6/−3.2	−2.8/0.2	−4.1/−3.7

All blood pressure data are in mm Hg. TOHP = Trials of Hypertension Prevention II [33]; SAGA = Dutch clinical trial using SAGA salt [32]; DASH = Dietary Approaches to Stop Hypertension [34].

that the tissue in which hypertension risk factors are measured may be critical for detecting gene associations.

Intervention Studies

Some genes have been consistently related to elevated blood pressure and hypertension but the observed effects of these genes are small and therefore hard to replicate in all studies. The majority of the associated genes have been related to renal electrolyte handling, similar to mechanisms of the rarer monogenic hypertension disorders, possibly because this class of genes have been studied to a greater extent than genes not acting primarily in the kidney. The greater number of positive findings in the kidney-related genes may also be a result of the kidney genes having slightly larger effect sizes. The GWAS are beginning to find associations for a number of genes that are not specifically kidney related. Because there are many causes of hypertension, it would be expected that any one gene would only have a small effect when averaged across large numbers of people.

Intervention studies are one strategy that appear to magnify the baseline effects of genes so that they are more easily detected. Multiple interventions including reduced dietary salt, increased dietary potassium, increased fruits and vegetables, lower fat intake, weight loss, and drug treatment appear to help reduce blood pressure to a greater extent in subjects genetically susceptible to hypertension than in those not as susceptible. The results support the concept that those at highest genetic risk of hypertension compared to those at low risk show a greater improvement in blood pressure for interventions that target the defective genetic pathways.

Table 1 summarizes 3 clinical trials in which individuals at a greater risk of hypertension due to the -6A polymorphism in the AGT gene had the greatest reductions in blood pressure after intervention [32–34]. The Trials of Hypertension Prevention

II enrolled subjects with borderline hypertension, the Dietary Approaches to Stop Hypertension (DASH) trial enrolled borderline or stage 1 hypertensive subjects, and the Dutch SAGA salt trial enrolled never-treated hypertensive subjects. All 3 trials showed a significant difference across AGT genotypes for change in blood pressure with the intervention. While sodium reduction was involved in 2 of the trials, similar results could be seen for weight loss [33], potassium supplementation [32] and the DASH diet even when sodium was held constant [34]. All interventions that target the genetically compromised pathway are likely to be effective in controlling blood pressure. Therefore, the -6A subjects on average appear to be salt sensitive and respond well to appropriate interventions despite their higher baseline risk for hypertension. Subjects with the AGT -6G alleles would not be expected to respond as well and other interventions may be more effective.

The genetic effects of the -6A AGT allele on blood pressure can probably be easily confounded by other mechanisms. Obesity and the associated increase in adipocytes, which are an important source of circulating angiotensinogen, may have larger effects on blood pressure than the AGT gene in normal-weight subjects [35]. The combination of obesity with AGT should magnify the risks of hypertension beyond the additive effects of either one alone, even though it would be difficult to differentiate between the 2 risk factors. Higher LDL-C levels increase blood pressure responses to infused angiotensin II, making blood pressure more sensitive to angiotensin II even though the baseline blood pressure levels may not be elevated [36, 37]. Greater blood pressure reactivity in the presence of high LDL-C may interact with stress and other environmental factors to eventually result in hypertension. Polymorphisms at the AT1 receptor also may affect the renin-angiotensin physiological pathway, with CC homozygotes at position A1166C of the AT1R gene showing smaller blood pressure responses to infused angiotensin II than A allele carriers [36].

Improving Genome-Wide Association Results

Genomic-wide association analyses of many common disease traits have been very successful at finding new genes [38]. Hypertension and blood pressure traits had had fewer genes suggested from these studies until very large meta analyses were performed that were powered sufficiently to detect very small genetic effects [5, 7]. While these genes need further validation, it is noteworthy that few of the physiological candidate genes found to be associated with hypertension have been detected in the genome-wide scans. This suggests that other unknown but important genes for hypertension are also being missed. An important reason appears to be that the density of the SNPs on the arrays are not sufficient around these candidate genes [39]. Only 52% of the HAPMAP SNPs in 160 hypertension candidate genes were captured by the Affymetrix 500k array. The greater the density of SNPs in a candidate gene, the greater the likelihood that an association can be found. More dense arrays are now available, but additional efforts should be made to target known candidate genes in these large studies. In addition, the less common SNPs should not be routinely excluded, as the sample size in these meta analyses may be sufficient to detect associations with SNPs with allele frequencies in the 0.5–5% range. Validated results from the genome-wide studies should be analyzed in existing clinical trials to test for intervention interactions, as has been done for AGT.

Summary

Multiple factors contribute to the development of hypertension, including genetic factors and environmental exposures. Various pathophysiological mechanisms are at play in the pathogenesis of hypertension and this pathogenesis, by necessity, exhibits substantial variation at the level of the individual, as it depends on the relative contribution of inherited genes and individual lifetime environmental exposures. Over time, long-term compensatory mechanisms, including responses to either chronic hypertension or to therapeutic intervention, can only obscure the initiating mechanisms of disease. Acute compensating mechanisms can also mask initiating gene effects during or after an intervention, so that early phenotype assessments during the intervention may be more likely to detect the genetic initiators. Compensatory mechanisms, working over days, weeks or even years, will likely be variably effective in minimizing the expected blood pressure rise, making it difficult to detect genetic initiating mechanisms in cross-sectional, 'steady state', or 'in balance' studies. If the lifetime risk of hypertension indeed approaches 90% [13], the power to identify genetic factors can only decrease with duration of disease and treatment, and prediction of hypertension becomes of vanishing significance. With multiple factors at play, we cannot expect that all causes are mutually exclusive, but it is reasonable to assume that one of these mechanisms is predominant in the initiation of the disease in any one individual. Given the heterogeneity of essential hypertension argued above, it becomes evident that the chance of identifying genetic factors that contribute to disease development will be greatest if study subjects at highest genetic predisposition are observed during age ranges when heritability is at a maximum, using the correct phenotypes, measured in the correct tissues, during the correct time window. Genes found to be significant in such studies should be densely typed in clinical trials and large population studies to assess public health and clinical applications of the findings.

Acknowledgments

This work was supported by NIH grants AG18734 and HL090668.

References

1. Wellcome Trust Case Control Consortium: Genome-wide association study of 14,000 cases of seven common diseases and 3,000 shared controls. Nature 2007; 447:661–678.
2. Levy D, Larson MG, Benjamin EJ, et al: Framingham Heart Study 100K Project: genome-wide associations for blood pressure and arterial stiffness. BMC Med Genet 2007;8(suppl 1):S3.
3. Sabatti C, Service SK, Hartikainen AL, et al: Genome-wide association analysis of metabolic traits in a birth cohort from a founder population. Nat Genet 2009;41:35–46.
4. Wang Y, O'Connell JR, McArdle PF, et al: Whole-genome association study identifies STK39 as a hypertension susceptibility gene. Proc Natl Acad Sci USA 2009;106:226–231.
5. Newton-Cheh C, Johnson T, Gateva V, et al: Genome-wide association study identifies eight loci associated with blood pressure. Nat Genet 2009;41:666–676.
6. Org E, Eyheramendy S, Juhanson P, et al: Genome-wide scan identifies CDH13 as a novel susceptibility locus contributing to blood pressure determination in two European populations. Hum Mol Genet 2009;18:2288–2296.
7. Levy D, Ehret GB, Rice K, et al: Genome-wide association study of blood pressure and hypertension. Nat Genet 2009;41:677–687.
8. Yang HC, Liang YJ, Wu YL, et al: Genome-wide association study of young-onset hypertension in the Han Chinese population of Taiwan. PLoS One 2009;4:e5459.
9. Adeyemo A, Gerry N, Chen G, et al: A genome-wide association study of hypertension and blood pressure in African Americans. PLoS Genet 2009;5:e1000564.
10. Hunt SC, Williams RR, Barlow GK: A comparison of positive family history definitions for defining risk of future disease. J Chron Dis 1986;39:809–821.
11. Hunt SC, Gwinn M, Adams TD: Family history assessment: strategies for prevention of cardiovascular disease. Am J Prev Med 2003;24:136–142.
12. Williams RR, Hunt SC, Heiss G, et al: Usefulness of cardiovascular family history data for population-based preventive medicine and medical research (the Health Family Tree Study and the NHLBI Family Heart Study). Am J Cardiol 2001;87:129–135.
13. Vasan RS, Beiser A, Seshadri S, et al. Residual lifetime risk for developing hypertension in middle-aged women and men: The Framingham Heart Study. Jama. 2002 Feb 27;287(8):1003–10.
14. Sanada H, Yatabe J, Midorikawa S, et al: Single-nucleotide polymorphisms for diagnosis of salt-sensitive hypertension. Clin Chem 2006;52:352–360.
15. Weinberger MH, Stegner JE, Fineberg NS: A comparison of two tests for the assessment of blood pressure responses to sodium. Am J Hypertens 1993;6:179–184.
16. Manunta P, Cusi D, Barlassina C, et al: Alpha-adducin polymorphisms and renal sodium handling in essential hypertensive patients. Kidney Int 1998;53:1471–1478.
17. Rocchini AP, Key J, Bordie D, et al: The effect of weight loss on the sensitivity of blood pressure to sodium in obese adolescents. N Engl J Med 1989;321:580–585.
18. Jia Z, Zhang A, Zhang H, Dong Z, Yang T: Deletion of microsomal prostaglandin E synthase-1 increases sensitivity to salt loading and angiotensin II infusion. Circ Res 2006;99:1243–1251.
19. Levine RS, Hennekens CH, Perry A, et al: Genetic variance of blood pressure levels in infant twins. Am J Epidemiol 1982;116:759–764.
20. Feinleib M, Garrison RJ, Fabsitz R, et al: The NHLBI twin study of cardiovascular disease risk factors: methodology and summary of results. Am J Epidemiol 1977;106:284–295.
21. Miller JZ, Weinberger MH, Christian JC, Daugherty SA: Familial resemblance in the blood pressure response to sodium restriction. Am J Epidemiol 1987;126:822–830.
22. Hunt SC, Hasstedt SJ, Kuida H, et al: Genetic heritability and common environmental components of resting and stressed blood pressures, lipids, and body mass index in Utah pedigrees and twins. Am J Epidemiol 1989;129:625–638.
23. Vaughn TT, Pletscher LS, Peripato A, et al: Mapping quantitative trait loci for murine growth: a closer look at genetic architecture. Genet Res 1999;74:313–322.
24. Pérusse L, Moll PP, Sing CF: Evidence that a single gene with gender- and age-dependent effects influences systolic blood pressure determination in a population-based sample. Am J Hum Genet 1991;49:94–105.
25. Cheng LS-C, Carmelli D, Hunt SC, Williams RR: Evidence for a major gene influencing 7-year increases in diastolic blood pressure with age. Am J Hum Genet 1995;57:1169–1177.
26. Shi G, Gu CC, Kraja AT, et al: Genetic effect on blood pressure is modulated by age: the Hypertension Genetic Epidemiology Network Study. Hypertension 2009;53:35–41.

27 Crowley SD, Gurley SB, Oliverio MI, et al: Distinct roles for the kidney and systemic tissues in blood pressure regulation by the renin-angiotensin system. J Clin Invest 2005;115:1092–1099.
28 Dahl LK, Heine M, Thompson K: Genetic influence of the kidneys on blood pressure: evidence from chronic renal homografts in rats with opposite predispositions to hypertension. Circ Res 1974;40:94–101.
29 Rohrwasser A, Morgan T, Dillon HF, et al: Elements of a paracrine tubular renin-angiotensin system along the entire nephron. Hypertension 1999;34:265–1274.
30 Navar LG, Nishiyama A: Why are angiotensin concentrations so high in the kidney? Curr Opin Nephrol Hypertens 2004;13:107–115.
31 Kobori H, Alper AB Jr, Shenava R, et al: Urinary angiotensinogen as a novel biomarker of the intrarenal renin-angiotensin system status in hypertensive patients. Hypertension 2009;53:344–350.
32 Hunt SC, Geleijnse JM, Wu LL, et al: Enhanced blood pressure response to mild sodium reduction in subjects with the 235T variant of the angiotensinogen gene. Am J Hypertens 1999;12:460–466.
33 Hunt SC, Cook NR, Oberman A, et al: Angiotensinogen genotype, sodium reduction, weight loss, and prevention of hypertension: trials of hypertension prevention, phase II. Hypertension 1998;32:393–401.
34 Svetkey LP, Moore TJ, Simons-Morton DG, et al: Angiotensinogen genotype and blood pressure response in the Dietary Approaches to Stop Hypertension (DASH) study. J Hypertens 2001;19:1949–1956.
35 Janke J, Engeli S, Gorzelniak K, Luft FC, Sharma AM: Mature adipocytes inhibit in vitro differentiation of human preadipocytes via angiotensin type 1 receptors. Diabetes 2002;51:1699–1707.
36 Vuagnat A, Giacche M, Hopkins PN, et al: Blood pressure response to angiotensin II, low-density lipoprotein cholesterol and polymorphisms of the angiotensin II type 1 receptor gene in hypertensive sibling pairs. J Mol Med 2001;79:175–183.
37 Nickenig G, Sachinidis A, Michaelsen F, et al: Upregulation of vascular angiotensin II receptor gene expression by low-density lipoprotein in vascular smooth muscle cells. Circulation 1997;95:473–478.
38 Manolio TA, Collins FS: The HapMap and genome-wide association studies in diagnosis and therapy. Annu Rev Med 2009;60:443–456.
39 Sober S, Org E, Kepp K, et al: Targeting 160 candidate genes for blood pressure regulation with a genome-wide genotyping array. PLoS One 2009;4:e6034.
40 Hunt SC: Genetic architecture of complex traits predisposing to nephropathy: hypertension. Semin Nephrol, in press.

Steven C. Hunt, PhD
Cardiovascular Genetics Division, University of Utah
420 Chipeta Way, Room 1160
Salt Lake City, Utah 84108 (USA)
Tel. +1 801 581 3888, ext. 234, Fax +1 801 581 6862, E-Mail steve.hunt@utah.edu

Diet, Nutrition and Modulation of Genomic Expression in Fetal Origins of Adult Disease

Alan A. Jackson[a,b] · Graham C. Burdge[a] · Karen A. Lillycrop[b,c]

[a]Institute of Human Nutrition, University of Southampton School of Medicine, Southampton General Hospital, [b]National Institutes of Health Research, Nutrition Biomedical Research Unit, Southampton Universities NHS Trust, Southampton General Hospital, [c]Developmental and Cell Biology, University of Southampton School of Biological Sciences, Southampton, UK

The greatest burden of ill-health for adults in most societies relates to disorders of the cardiovascular system and to cancers [1]. These diseases are caused by lifestyle choices in which poor diet and relatively low levels of activity play a major role [1]. There is a large body of literature which shows that environmental exposures, including nutrition, play a significant role in the etiology of the disease, but there is variable susceptibility amongst individuals exposed to seemingly similar risk factors or environments. Cancer is a condition which results from a derangement in the cellular processes which regulate cell division, terminal differentiation and apoptosis, with damage to the genetic material of the cell being central. Exposures which lead to these derangements usually precede the appearance of the clinical disease by a prolonged period of time, often several decades [2]. While gene mutation has a role in the etiology of cancer, there is increasing evidence showing that epigenetic processes such as DNA methylation and covalent modification to histones are also involved [3]. Epigenetic changes of this kind represent potential for altered gene activity, and hence cellular dysregulation. However, the underlying propensity may only be manifest when the gene is exposed to an appropriate environmental signal with the direction of the response and nature of the cellular dysregulation a function of the specific epigenetic change [4, 5].

It has been known for many years that exposure of the individual to nutritional and other environmental challenges during critical periods of early development can markedly affect later size, shape, structure, function and behavior. However, Barker et al. [6] were the first to provide clear evidence that there might also be a direct link between early nutritional exposure and risk of chronic disease, building the evidence that is supportive of a causal association [6, 7]. In this they have refined a new conceptual approach to the way in which we consider the evolution of this group of diseases based upon a new developmental model, the so called 'fetal origins hypothesis'. Based initially on ecological observations and later on retrospective cohort studies, there is now a considerable body of epidemiological and experimental data that supports the hypothesis. In the earlier observations, the size and shape of the baby at birth was shown to be related to the risk during adult life of coronary heart disease, hypertension, stroke, type 2 diabetes, obesity and some cancers [6]. These relations were shown to be graded across the usual range of birth weights seen in the population and not a special feature of very high or very low birth weight, indicating that they might be a consequence of the usual range of exposure found within a population [4, 7]. The results have been reproduced across a number of populations, and although there may be some debate around the details, the general principal appears to apply widely [4, 6, 7].

Epidemiology

Methodologically, the major advance was to be able to identify groups of adults in whom size at birth had been recorded with reliability and could be related on an individual basis to current health, risk of chronic disease, morbidity or mortality from specific disease conditions [8]. By identifying such populations it has been possible to carry out a range of elegant retrospective cohort investigations providing clear evidence that the pace and pathway of early growth is a major risk factor for this particular group of chronic diseases [6, 8]. The first studies were carried out in Hertfordshire (England), where it was shown that for both men and women as birth weight increased, the risk of death from coronary heart disease decreased. Based on observations of this kind, the 'fetal origins hypothesis' proposes that poor nutritional exposure during early development of the fertilized ovum, embryo, fetus, infant or child permanently determines the structure and function of the body through the process of programming [7–9]. This translation of genotype into a defined phenotype from a very early stage of development, sets the basis upon which all later exposures, nutritional and those of the wider environment, build. It defines the opportunity and limit for future structure and function [8–10]. More refined exploration of other data sets in which more detailed data are available for later growth during childhood and adolescence, such as the Helsinki Birth Cohort, provide the opportunity to identify particular pathways of growth that may be associated with particular disease outcomes [6]. Together these explorations provide a rich description of how the structural phenotype captured simply as measures of size, shape and body composition mark differences in the functional phenotype which in themselves presage variable vulnerability to a wider range of environmental challenges, which can ultimately lead to ill-health [6, 7]. These findings from these observational studies are supported by evidence derived from 'natural' experiments.

Experiments of Nature

The most well explored human model of a defined intervention for a specific period of time is given by the experience provided as a result of the Dutch famine during 1944–1945. This was a sharply defined period of severe food shortage for a population which previously had enjoyed reasonable nutritional health. During this period the food ration fell below 1,000 kcal/day and even the extra rations allowed for pregnant and lactating women and young children could not be provided [11, 12]. The change in food availability had a disastrous effect on the population, but although fertility decreased women continued to become pregnant and deliver babies and health records continued to be kept. It has been possible to time the relative exposure of the famine in relation to the time of conception and the progress of the pregnancies. Women who were exposed early in pregnancy, around the time of embryonic growth and the elaboration of the early fetal form had babies which were of relatively good size, but later in life suffered the more extensive and severe manifestations of ill health for a range of systems. Those exposed during later pregnancy, at a time when many of the structures and functions of the fetus have been established, but when the weight gained is greatest, had babies who were most obviously affected by having a lower birth weight. They still carried an increased risk for later ill health, but this was less marked than those exposed during the earlier stages of development. Those fetuses exposed to famine during late gestation were more likely to demonstrate impaired glucose tolerance during adult life. Those exposed in mid-gestation had an increased likelihood of impaired glucose tolerance, but also were more likely to display microalbuminuria indicative of altered renal function or obstructive airways disease indicative of altered respiratory function. Exposure early in gestation was associated with later glucose intolerance, an atherogenic lipid profile, altered blood coagulation, obesity, stress sensitivity, coronary heart disease and breast cancer [11, 12].

These observations demonstrate an effect on a wide range of functions and systems, variability in outcome in relation to the timing of the exposure indicative of special tissue vulnerability at sensitive periods of development, disjunction between the specific functional effects and the size of the baby at birth. In addition to the specific time-related effects from one tissue or system to another, there is also evidence that for those conceived during the famine there was an increased risk of schizophrenia, anti-social personality disorder, and congenital neural defects, demonstrating a wide range of effects on the central nervous system [11, 12]. The vulnerability implied by increased sensitivity and stress responsiveness increases the potential susceptibility to all stressors and associated metabolic consequences. Importantly, stressors interact with and impact upon nutritional state and wellbeing through a range of effects that include altered appetite, modification in the delivery of nutrients to tissues, altered tissue demands for nutrients and increased nutrient losses. The effects found on liver function (coagulation changes and lipid profiles) and renal health (micralbuminuria) imply the likelihood of altered responsiveness to potential or actual environmental toxins, including carcinogens, altered excretion, modified inter-organ co-operativity and integration of function [11, 12]. Not all of the effects should be construed as being necessarily negative. Those women who were exposed to the famine during their own fetal life later showed increased reproductive success [13]. Importantly it has been shown the effects can be passed on to the third generation, arguing strongly for non-genomic transmission of information or memory [14].

Thus, birth size provides some useful information, but has to be seen as a relatively crude indicator of the intrauterine nutritional exposure and experience, patterns of exposure during fetal life set structure and functionality that have long-term impact on the capacity of individual tissues to function and their integration as components of a whole body system, growth and development after birth may be modulated by experience before birth, but how current environmental exposure builds on that experience is itself of importance for later health or disease risk.

Cancer Risk and Early Life

The fundamental lesion in cancer is damage to DNA, which can be brought about by a range of physical, chemical or microbiological factors. Because the cell usually has mechanisms to protect itself, sustained damage to DNA must take place against a background of a cellular capability that is inadequate to cope by protecting or effectively repairing the damaged DNA. The capability of the cell to achieve effective prevention or repair depends upon the cellular microenvironment, in particular the nutrient microenvironment of the cell. This microenvironment reflects the overall nutritional wellbeing of the individual, a balance between nutrient intake and the specific nutrient demands for usual activity and coping with the rigors imposed by the wider external environment [4]. Cells that contain critically damaged DNA but do not undergo apoptosis are potentially neoplastic. Dysregulation of the life cycle of individual cells is, therefore a fundamental feature of cancer causation. This is in part determined by the immediate nutrient environment, but also by the nutrient environment experienced during very early development [4, 5].

The studies from the women who experienced the Dutch hunger winter during early life showed that there was a 5 times increase in risk of developing cancer of the breast in women exposed to famine while in utero [15]. Birth size has been related to increased risk of breast cancer in a number of studies and, in general, larger size at birth is associated with an increased risk of cancer of the breast [2, 5]. In 2007 the World Cancer Research Fund and American Institute of Cancer Research [2] produced the most comprehensive review of any aspect of the medical literature ever conducted. This global effort by some of the world's leading nutrition and cancer scientists identified major factors related to the foods eaten, nutritional status achieved and physical activity undertaken as causal factors for major cancers. This analysis was comprehensive, detailed and rigorous, using sound, validated methods and hence its conclusions are the most authoritative statement there is currently on the causes of cancer. It is estimated that on average at least 30% of cancers could be prevented with appropriate modifications to diet and lifestyle, and in some situations as much as 70% [16]. There is convincing evidence that abdominal fatness causes colorectal cancer, and probably causes cancer of the pancreas and endometrium and pre-menopausal breast cancer. There is also convincing evidence that achieved height 'causes' colorectal and postmenopausal breast cancer, and probably 'causes' cancer of the pancreas and ovary and premenopausal breast cancer. This very strong relationship between achieved height itself and specific cancer cannot be a direct effect of height on the risk of cancer, but must be a reflection that the complex of factors that contribute to the achievement of height, must also relate strongly, and probably directly to the factors which increase the risk of cancer. Other aspects of development of the bony skeleton have been related to cancer in women in the Helsinki Birth Cohort, where 300 women were diagnosed with breast cancer [6]. Growth of bony skeleton is important for reproductive health in many ways, but most critically during child birth where small pelvic bones increase the risk of obstructed labor. Small pelvic bones are often a persistent consequence of poor nutrition during infancy and childhood. In Helsinki, the dimensions of the mothers' bony pelvis were measured routinely in order to assess the likelihood of an obstructed labor. A higher risk of either breast cancer or ovarian cancer in the daughter was associated with the shape and pattern of the mother's pelvis, itself a marker of the mother's sex hormone status around the time her reproductive capability was being established [17, 18]. The stem cells for the breast form at around 6 weeks after conception and the authors postulated that higher concentrations of sex hormones in the mother around this time gave rise to genetic instability in the differentiating putative breast cells in their daughters [17]. Further, they found that broader hips in the mother were predictive of ovarian cancer in their daughters, leading to the suggestion that ovarian cancer may be initiated by exposure of the fetal ovary to maternal sex hormones [18].

Growth and Development

Growth is a complex process that takes place in both space and time. Early exposures can have lasting effects, both on structure and on function. The most obvious example of this is when a noxious exposure acts during a sensitive period of the development of a tissue or organ, impairing the development and leading to lifelong alterations of structure, for example with teratogens such as thalidomide or hypervitaminosis A [19, 20]. However, a limitation or lack of a specific nutrient can have an equally damaging structural effect, such as hypovitaminosis A, or poor folate status and neural tube defects [21, 22]. These obvious structural changes at the level of the whole body are extreme forms of less dramatic damage which can be inflicted at the cellular or subcellular levels.

An understanding of how early nutritional exposure enables normal growth and body proportions, measured indirectly as achieved height and weight, is an imperative if the relationships identified in epidemiological studies of populations are to be interpreted [7, 9, 10, 23, 24]. Growth is a structured process which includes increases in length and mass, changes in body composition and relative proportions and maturation of function. The elaboration of the processes that enable structure and function at every stage of growth and development result from a complex interaction amongst genetic endowment and the hormonal milieu with the availability of energy and nutrients to fuel and enable cellular elaboration [25]. In an article in the *Lancet* in 1970, Elsie Widdowson used the term 'harmony of growth' to capture the pace, proportions and partitioning of nutrients that are fundamental for the achievement of normal growth, appropriate body proportions and effective maturation of function [26]. Thus, growth and development are tightly organized and regulated processes with complex and subtle changes taking place in space and time, with each successive change being dependent upon and determined by having achieved the early stages with a measure of success. Any significant constraint at any particular stage of development may lead to alteration of structure and function, which may be difficult or impossible to repair or make good at later times. Any tissue or organ is particularly vulnerable at the time of rapid cellular replication, leading to sensitive periods during development which differ in their critical timing from tissue to tissue or from function to function. Throughout there is a close interdependent relationship between structure and function, thereby capturing a memory of differences in earlier exposure to an altered cellular or tissue, hormonal or nutritional milieu. For any complex organism, this variability in structure and function can obtain at any or every level of organization, extending from the molecular and subcellular, through the organization and regulation of cells, tissues and organs, up to whole body integration of responses to wider environmental challenge. Size at any age is a relatively crude summary statement of the extent to which the availability of energy and pattern of nutrients matches that required for that stage of development, and size at birth is a very crude summary of the nutrients that have been available to the fetus.

The size of newborn babies and their growth during infancy and childhood have changed over time [27, 28]. During approximately the last 100–150 years, children have been getting larger and growing to maturity more rapidly, known as the secular trend in growth with progressively greater final adult height in many developed countries. Thus, within the same population there has been a progressive increase in attained adult height for both males and females, a reflection of increased height at 5–7 years of age of 1–2 cm every 10 years [27, 28]. This has been associated with a decrease in the age of menarche from around 16 to around 13 years of age in the 100 years from 1860 [27]. For a number of countries in western Europe this attained adult height appears to have achieved a plateau of around 1.8 m, for example in Denmark, Sweden, Norway and the Netherlands. It has been suggested that the plateau is achieved around 18 years following post-neonatal mortality falling to around 4/1,000 deliveries [23, 24]. In many senses this increase in height is indicative of improvement in public health and much of the increase has been attributed to factors that contribute to improved nutrition from a very early age. Importantly if achieved height is a risk factor for some cancers and there has been a secular trend in height over many years, what are the common factors that underlie this important relationship?

Size and Body Composition at Birth

The new growth standards developed by WHO show how infants and children should grow when provided with the opportunity for a healthy environment [29]. Across the globe the pattern of growth of children from a wide range of backgrounds is similar. However, even within this similarity for all populations there is variability within the normal range. The suggestion posed by the 'fetal origins hypothesis' is that even within this observed 'normal' range of variability there is differential risk of later chronic disease.

There has been the general observation that infants who are smaller at birth tend to have a different body composition to those who are heavier, most notably that they are relatively more adipose. An extreme example of this difference has been noted in populations where size at birth is very low, for example in India. Yajnick et al. [30] have described the phenotype of the Indian baby as being fat/thin, a pattern that is carried through to adulthood and marks the phenotype which is closely associated with the cardio-metabolic syndrome. Although the baby may be small at birth the relative deficit of different body compartments is not equal. There are substantial deficits in length and lean tissue, but relative preservation of adipose tissue, especially centrally placed adipose. This population has substantially increased risk of type 2 diabetes, associated with relative adiposity throughout life, which may be directly associated with dietary limitations of vitamin B_{12} [31]. One important question is whether this is a peculiarly Indian phenotype and problem, or simply an extreme example of a more common phenotypic difference in size and shape, and also for wider aspects of metabolic function.

Kensara et al. [32, 33] compared the extent to which early life variability in size relates to differences in size, shape and whole body function later in life using the Hertfordshire cohort and comparing individuals from the lowest and highest fifths of birth size within the 'normal' range. These men were studied when they were around 70 years old. At this age the percentage body fat was about 5% greater for those of lower birth weight compared with those of higher birth weight. This meant that for the same weight or BMI at 70 years of age, those of lower birth weight had reduced lean mass, but greater fat mass, especially greater central fat [32]. Resting metabolic rate (RMR) was measured as a summary statement of metabolic activity and 38% of the variability in RMR could be explained by variation in current size (height and weight) and size at birth. Those in the lower birth weight category had lower resting expenditure, 32% of which was explained by differences in birth size, indicative of a reduced metabolic demand, a reduced metabolic capacity, and altered cellular environment. Size at birth uniquely explained 17% of the variability, more than current size which uniquely explained 6% of the variability, with 15% of the variability explained on a shared basis by size at birth and current height and weight [33]. The compositional changes meant that for any given BMI the men of lower birth weight had 5% more fat [32]. Therefore, the differences in body composition identified for the Indian baby with the fat/thin phenotype may represent a more general difference in phenotype associated with differences in size at birth, which in itself marks important variability in overall and specific metabolic function and efficiency [34]. Although differences in genotype may explain a part of this variability, the observation that the WHO growth standards apply globally [29] indicate that there are major environmental factors that impact on the variability, which include nutrition factors, either directly or indirectly.

Developmental Plasticity

The epidemiological and metabolic studies carried out in humans argue strongly that nutrient exposure from the earliest stages of life can exert an impact on functional capability at all later ages, indicating that a single genotype can give rise to a range of different phenotypes. This process, characterized as developmental plasticity, is a widespread biological phenomenon which is considered to enable survival in range of environments, and the ability to cope with the range of stresses or stressors experienced from one situation to another [35]. This variable phenotype may promote the ability to cope in the short term, but carries with it potential vulnerability in the longer term especially if the later environment exposes phenotypic susceptibility. Greater achieved height and central adiposity may confer advantages under some circumstances, but they are not necessarily an unalloyed benefit. It is very difficult to explore these relationships mechanistically in humans, given the long time between the exposure and the outcome, and animal models provide a valuable opportunity to determine possible mechanisms in some detail.

Animal Models

There are a wide range of studies on the reproductive performance in animals – conducted for the purpose of enhancing animal husbandry – which have explored the effects of general or specific nutritional interventions before or during pregnancy, during lactation and during the later life of the offspring. These generally have an interest in relatively short-term outcomes, determined by market considerations. It is clear that more extreme dietary manipulations lead to adverse outcomes in the short and longer term, with the specific consequence being determined by the timing, severity and duration of the insult [7, 19–22]. An important observation which arises from the epidemiological studies is that for chronic non-communicable disease the variability in risk is seen as a graded effect within the usual variability of birth size and growth within the population. For the diet or nutritional exposure to operate as an important factor in promoting or enabling the altered risk in outcome would require that the effects of importance should be demonstrable across the range of intakes usually seen and considered to be compatible with health within the population. Further, if the impact is cumulative during life it might be explained simply by sensitive periods during development leading to differences in structure and function which constrain the maximal capability of one or other function, or limit the ability to regulate and integrate [7, 25]. However the observation that these effects can be communicated between generations, and by embryo transfer, requires acquired genetic mechanisms of retained memory, considered most likely to be through epigenetic processes such as DNA methylation and covalent modification of histones [5]. This potentially implicates those processes through which 1-carbon moieties such as methyl groups are made available to metabolism and the mechanisms through which methylation of the promoter region of specific regulatory genes is enhanced or constrained from one situation to another [5].

The induction of changes to the phenotype of the offspring, in response to the prenatal environment, that persists throughout the lifespan implies stable changes to gene transcription resulting in altered activities of metabolic pathways and the set point homeostatic control processes and in differences in the structure of tissues. One important consideration in understanding the mechanism responsible for phenotype induction is the interaction between any process resulting in different phenotypes, environmental cues and gene polymorphisms, in particular those located in gene promoters. Studies on gene expression demonstrate stable effects on transcription [5]. Importantly, some of the genes which showed altered expression following prenatal undernutrition are transcription factors which affect multiple pathways in development and nutrient homeostasis: for example PPARα and the glucocorticoid receptor (GR) [36]. Modified regulation of expression of a few key transcription factors may alter the activities of a large number of metabolic and developmental pathways. The methylation of CpG dinucleotides which are clustered at the 5′ promoter regions of genes, confers stable silencing of transcription. Methylation patterns are largely established during embryogenesis or in early postnatal life [37]. DNA methylation also plays a key role in cell differentiation by silencing the expression of specific genes during development and differentiation of individual tissues, and thus the timing of gene methylation is tissue and gene-specific [38, 39]. Covalent modifications of histones influence chromatin structure and hence the ability of transcriptional machinery to gain access to DNA. DNA methylation can induce transcriptional silencing by blocking the binding of transcription factors and/or through promoting the binding of the methyl CpG binding protein (MeCP)-2. The latter binds to methylated cytosines and, in turn, recruits histone-modifying complexes composed of deacetylases and histone methyl transferases to the DNA, resulting in a closed chromatin structure and transcriptional silencing [40, 41].

Epigenetic regulation of gene promoters is established during development and is responsible for patterns of transcriptional expression and silencing in adults, perturbations to this process represent a candidate molecular mechanism for induction of persistent alterations in phenotype by the environment early in life. Perturbations as diverse as lack of maternal grooming, uterine artery ligation or embryo culture have been shown to lead to epigenetic modulation of transcription, structural and functional effects in the short and long term [5, 42–45].

Varying the maternal intake of nutrients involved in 1-carbon metabolism across a wide range can induce graded changes in DNA methylation and gene expression in the offspring, which persist into adulthood [45]. However, for this mechanism to operate in the induction of phenotypes associated with the 'fetal origins hypothesis' would require that it can operate within the range of dietary intakes typical for a population. Feeding a diet which is adequate but restricted in protein to pregnant rats is a well established model of phenotype induction. This is because feeding pregnant dams graded amounts of protein across a range of intakes not associated with any obvious pathology leads to graded increases in blood pressure in the offspring [46]. This modest change to maternal macronutrient intake during pregnancy induced hypomethylation of the PPARα and GR promoter and increased expression of PPARα and GR in the liver of the offspring. There was also an increase in the expression of PPARα and GR target genes such acyl-CoA oxidase and phosphoenolpyruvate carboxykinase, respectively, supporting the suggestion that altered epigenetic regulation of transcription factors modifies that activities of important metabolic pathways [36, 47]. Sequence analysis of the PPARα promoter showed that the methylation status of only a few CpG dinucleotides was altered by the reduced protein diet during pregnancy [48]. This suggests that the process of induced epigenetic change is targeted and that the resulting change in transcription may reflect changes in the interaction of the gene with relatively few transcription factors, thus inducing specific changes in the regulation of gene function and hence response to environmental differences. Methylation of the PPARα and GR promoters was also reduced in the heart of animals whose mothers had been exposed to a reduced protein diet during pregnancy [5]. Further, the PPARα promoter was hypomethylated in the whole umbilical cord offspring of rats fed a reduced protein diet during pregnancy [5], suggesting that hypomethylation of PPARα and GR promoters had already been established very early in pregnancy, before cell lineages had become definitively established. Hypomethylation of the GR promoter was associated with an increase in histone modifications which facilitate transcription while those that suppress gene expression were reduced or unchanged [47].

Induction of the altered phenotype (hypertension and endothelial function) in the offspring of rats fed the reduced protein diet during pregnancy was prevented by supplementation of this diet with glycine or folic acid [49–51]. Hypomethylation of the hepatic PPARα and GR promoters was also prevented by the addition of 5 times more folic acid than contained in the reduced protein diet [36]. Thus, 1-carbon metabolism plays a central role in the induction of an altered phenotype. In this model there is an important interaction between the metabolism of macronutrients and micronutrients, and further that these interactions operate through differential methylation of the promoter region of regulatory genes through seemingly epigenetic mechanisms. The regulatory genes themselves play a central role in metabolic integration in terms of responsiveness to stress (GR), and macronutrient partitioning and central fat deposition (PPARα). Feeding the reduced protein diet during pregnancy in the F0-generation results in elevated blood pressure, endothelial dysfunction, insulin resistance and adverse glucose homeostasis in the F1, F2 and even the F3 generations, despite no further unusual dietary exposure for subsequent generations [52–55]. This implies that transmission of a phenotype induced in the F1 generation to the F2 generation and further into the F3 generation may involve preservation of levels of DNA methylation of specific genes. As the female line appears sufficient for transmission of this epigenetic information between generations the level of methylation of the PPARα and GR promoters in gametes must be similar to that of somatic cells.

The de novo methylation of CpG dinucleotides is catalyzed by DNA methyltransferase (Dnmt) 3a and 3b. The pattern of methylation is maintained through mitosis by gene-specific methylation of hemimethylated DNA by Dnmt1 [37]. Changes in the activity of Dnmt as a result of altered 1-carbon metabolism represent one candidate mechanism for transmission of information regarding maternal 1-carbon metabolism status to the fetus for induction of modified epigenetic regulation of transcription and thus modified phenotype. Feeding the reduced protein diet to rats during pregnancy induced a reduction in Dnmt1 expression and in the binding of Dnmt1 at the GR promoter. [47]. However, the expression of Dnmt3a, Dnmt3b and methyl binding domain-2, and the binding of Dnmt3a at the GR promoter were unaltered [47]. This suggests that hypomethylation of the GR promoter in the liver of the offspring and probably other genes including PPARα, is induced by the maternal diet as a result of a lower capacity to maintain patterns of cytosine methylation during mitosis. Modulation of Dnmt1 expression by differences in 1-carbon metabolism provide a link between maternal diet and epigenetic regulation of gene expression in the fetus. This is supported by the finding that lower Dnmt1 expression induced by the reduced protein diet during pregnancy was prevented by increasing the folic acid content of the diet. [47] and is consistent with the a central role for Dnmt1 in the induction of an altered phenotype [49, 50].

We suggest 2 possible mechanisms by which feeding a reduced protein diet during pregnancy may alter 1-carbon metabolism. Firstly, it is possible that a decreased availability of glycine leads to an altered flux of methyl groups between different metabolic fates and a constraint on the remethylation of homocysteine to methionine [56, 57]. Second, increased maternal corticosteroid levels [58], possibly a result of the stress induced by constrained nutrient availability, may reduce folic acid availability [59]. The latter could explain how maternal corticosteroid blockade prevents the induction of hypertension in the offspring of mothers who had reduced protein diets during pregnancy [60], as well as prevention of altered phenotype by folic acid administration [36, 50].

Based upon current data, we have suggested a mechanism for the induction of an altered phenotype in the offspring as a consequence of nutrient constraint during pregnancy in which promoter methylation is lost in a gene-specific manner during mitosis due to decreased Dnmt1 expression and activity [5, 36, 61]. This is accompanied by reduced binding of the MeCP2-histone deacetylase-histone methyltransferase complex leading to persistence of histone modifications that permit transcription.

Epigenetics and Cancer

A change in the epigenetic regulation of genes has been implicated as a causal mechanism in specific cancers including lung, prostate, breast [62], colon [63] and hemopoietic cancers [64]. Specifically, increased cancer risk is associated with global hypomethylation of the genome with concurrent hypermethylation or hypomethylation of the promoter of specific genes. The mechanism by which global hypomethylation is induced is unclear, but may reflect the global decline in DNA methylation associated with increasing age [62]. The age-related decline in global hypomethylation is related to a reduction in Dnmt1 activity [65] which, in turn, may induce expression of oncogenes such as c-*Myc* and c-N-*ras*. [65]. Thus, it appears that modulation of Dnmt1 activity is a key regulatory step in both fetal programming and in the induction of tumorigenesis This may be accompanied by de novo methylation of tumor suppressor genes [66] by increased Dnmt3a activity, leading to aberrant activation of genes involved in cell proliferation and cell differentiation [67]. Together these changes represent a shift in the regulation of gene control which, in turn, may predispose the genome to further changes in methylation, which result ultimately in neoplasia.

Conclusion

The observation that nutrition in early life can induce both hypomethylation and hypermethylation of specific CpG dinucleotides suggests a mechanism for induction of different disease endpoints (e.g. metabolic disease of cancer) by variation in the same environmental exposure, which is marked by differences in the direction of association between birth weight and disease risk. One particular example of the role of epigenetics in modulating gene activity by shifting the balance between agonist and suppressor proteins is the induction tumorigenesis by activation of telomerase in differentiated cells. Telomerase activity is down-regulated in most cells during terminal differentiation in embryogenesis as a result of methylation of the CpG promoter region. It has been proposed that activation of telomerase in preneoplastic cells is due to a shift in the regulation between the activator c-*Myc* and the suppressor WT1, by changes in the methylation status of specific CpG within the binding domains of these transcription factors in the promoter of the catalytic sub-unit which confers RT activity (hTERT) [68]. One consequence of hTERT activation is to increase Dnmt1 activity [69], which leads to copying of aberrant patterns of cytosine methylation. This suggests a synergistic role for hTERT and Dnmt1 in controlling cell proliferation and the methylation status of the genome.

The addition of supplemental folic acid to the reduced protein diet provided during pregnancy reversed many of the effects of the low protein diet on blood pressure and vascular reactivity as well as on the methylation of the promoter region for PPARα and GR and their relative expression in the offspring. By contrast when the control protein diet was supplemented with folic acid the effects on the offspring were very different, with an increase in blood pressure and increases in the concentration of triacylglycerol and non-esterified fatty acids in the blood [70]. If the addition of supplemental folic acid to the reduced protein diet provided during pregnancy reversed many of the phenotypic and epigenetic effects of the low protein diet in the offspring would a similar effect be seen if the supplemental folic acid were provided to the offspring postnatally? Supplementation with folic acid postnatally induced increased weight gain, lower plasma β-hydroxybutyrate concentration and increased hepatic and plasma triacylglycerol concentration compared with offspring not given supplemental folic acid. In the liver of folic acid supplemented offspring there was an increased methylation of the promoter region for PPARα and the GR, and a decrease in the methylation of the promoter region for the insulin receptor, with reciprocal changes in mRNA expression. Hence increased intakes of supplemental folic acid intake during the juvenile period did not simply reverse the phenotype induced by the maternal diet, but produced distinct changes in both the phenotype and the epigenotype. This indicates that the effect of the increased intake of folic acid is contingent on the timing of the supplementation relative to the developmental stage of the organism and the overall nutrient pattern within the diet. Importantly, whereas during pregnancy the effect of the supplemental folic acid is buffered by maternal metabolism, the juvenile offspring were exposed directly to folic acid provided in the diet [71]. Bidirectional responses in relation to the previous nutritional exposure have also been shown for other systems, for example in rats the expression of 11β-hydroxysteroid dehydrogenase-2 in response to leptin administration from day 3 to 10 of life was increased in the offspring of well nourished mothers, but decreased in the offspring of undernourished mothers: by contrast leptin suppressed expression of PPARα in maternally well nourished offspring and enhanced expression in maternally undernourished offspring [72].

The observational evidence from epidemiological studies is substantial. Not surprisingly, not all of the evidence fits in a simple way, but there is a substantial weight of evidence that argues that patterns of growth and development during fetal life, infancy and childhood relate strongly to the risk of non-communicable disease during later adult life. The experience drawn from the Dutch winter famine, where there was limited exposure to a very low food intake for a defined period of time, is supportive. Moreover it provides evidence that the timing as well as the severity of the exposure lead to differences in the phenotypic outcome in terms of markers of risk for later ill-health as well as specific disease patterns. Taken together, the evidence argues that the variability in risk cannot be explained simply on the basis of genetic or genomic variability, but appears to be a complex interaction of nutrient exposure and the hormonal milieu at the critical time when tissues and systems are especially sensitive to environmental perturbations, which modifies the opportunity for genetic expression, most likely through epigenetic mechanisms. Animal studies show that modest manipulations of the maternal diet during pregnancy can lead to epigenetic changes in the promoter region of critical regulatory genes, which are carried through generations. These epigenetic changes lead directly to differential expression of the genes and a shift in the set point and responsiveness of regulatory systems. It appears that it is this shift that alters responsiveness of the organism to wider environmental or nutritional perturbations, lowering the threshold for adverse effects and increasing susceptibility to abnormal function. The evidence suggests that aspects of the regulation and control of 1-carbon metabolism are of particular importance in setting the extent of epigenetic modification and, our understanding of the critical factors that determine and control these interactions needs greater refinement. At each age the response to current nutritional exposure appears to be modified to an extent by previous nutritional experience. It appears that metabolic plasticity is directionally dependent on earlier nutritional status and we still do not know what might underlie this response. Population studies show that whereas higher birth weight within an acceptable range is related to better long-term outcome for many of the health issues of concern, such as cardiovascular disease and type 2 diabetes, the opposite is true for cancers such as those of the breast and prostate. If the objective is to move to interventions that will protect the population from ill-health there is an important and urgent need to understand the basis of these different relationships to ensure that the public health implications can be appreciated.

References

1 World Health Organization: Diet, nutrition and the prevention of chronic disease. Report of as joint WHO/FAO Expert Consultation. WHO Technical report series 916. Geneva, World Health Organization, 2003.
2 World Cancer Research Fund/American Institute for Cancer Research: Food, nutrition, physical activity and the prevention of cancer: a global perspective. Washington, American institute for Cancer Research, 2007.
3 Vucic EA, Brown CL, Lam WL: Epigenetics of cancer progression. Pharmacogenomics 2008;9:215–234.
4 Jackson AA: Integrating ideas of life course across cellular, individual and population in cancer causation. J Nutr 2005;135(suppl 12):2927S–2933S.
5 Burdge GC, Lillycrop KA, Jackson AA: Nutrition in early life, and risk of cancer and metabolic disease: alternative endings in an epigenetic tale? Br J Nutr 2009;101: 619–630.

6 Barker DJP, Osmond C, Kajantie E, Eriksson JG: Growth and chronic disease: findings in the Helsinki Birth Cohort. Ann Human Biol 2009;36:445–458.
7 Jackson AA: Nutrients, growth, and the development of programmed metabolic function. Adv Exp Med Biol 2000;478:41–55.
8 Barker DJP: Mothers, babies and health in later life, ed 2. Edinburgh, Churchill Livingstone, 1998.
9 Jackson AA: All that glitters. Br Nutr Foundation Nutr Bull 2001;25:11–24.
10 Wootton SA, Jackson AA: Influence of undernutrition in early life on growth, body composition and metabolic competence; in Henry CJ (ed): Early Environment and Later Outcomes. Society for the Study of Human Biology Symposium. Cambridge, Cambridge University Press, 1995.
11 Painter RC, Roseboom TJ, Bleker OP: Prenatal exposure to the Dutch famine and disease in later life: an overview. Reprod Toxicol 2005;20:345–352.
12 Roseboom T, de Rooij S, Painter R: The Dutch famine and its long-term consequence for adult health. Early Human Dev 2006;82:485–491.
13 Painter RC, Westendorp RG, de Rooij SR, et al: Increased reproductive success of women after prenatal undernutrition. Hum Reprod 2008;23:2591–2595.
14 Painter RC, Osmond C, Gluckman P, et al: Transgenerational effects of prenatal exposure to the Dutch famine on neonatal adiposity and health in later life. BJOG 2008;115:1243–1249.
15 Painter RC, De Rooij SR, Bossuyt PM, et al: A possible link between prenatal exposure to famine and breast cancer: a preliminary study. Am J Hum Biol 2006;18:853–856.
16 World Cancer Research Fund/American Institute for Cancer Research: Policy and action for cancer prevention. Food, nutrition, and physical activity: a global perspective. Washington, AICR, 2009.
17 Barker DJ, Osmond C, Thornburg KL, et al: A possible link between the pubertal growth of girls and breast cancer in their daughters. Am J Hum Biol 2008;20:127–131.
18 Barker DJ, Osmond C, Thornburg KL, Kajantie E, Eriksson JG: A possible link between the pubertal growth of girls and ovarian cancer in their daughters. Am J Hum Biol 2008;20:659–662.
19 Kalter H, Warkany J: Experimental production of congenital malformations in strains of inbred mice by maternal treatment with hypervitaminosis A. Am J Pathol 1961;38:1–21.
20 Woollam DH: Thalidomide disaster considered as an experiment in mammalian teratology. Br Med J 1962;2:236–237.
21 Wilson JG, Roth CB, Warkany J: An analysis of the syndrome of malformations induced by maternal vitamin A deficiency: effects of restoration of vitamin A at various times during gestation. Am J Anat 1953;92:189–217.
22 MRC Vitamin Study Research Group: Prevention of neural tube defects: results of the Medical Research Council Vitamin Study. Lancet 1991;338:131–137.
23 Schmidt IM, Jørgensen MH, Michaelsen KF: Height of conscripts in Europe: is postneonatal mortality a predictor? Ann Hum Biol 1995;22:57–67.
24 Larnkaer A, Attrup Schrøder S, et al: Secular change in adult stature has come to a halt in northern Europe and Italy. Acta Paediatr 2006;95:754–765.
25 Jackson AA: Perinatal nutrition: the impact on postnatal growth and development; in Gluckman PD, Heyman MA (eds): Pediatrics and perinatology, ed 2. London, Arnold, 1996, p 298–303.
26 Widdowson EM: Harmony of growth. Lancet 1970;1:902–905.
27 Tanner JM: Fetus into Man: Physical Growth from Conception to Maturity. Cambridge (Mass.), Harvard University Press, 1990.
28 Cole TJ: Secular trends in growth. Proc Nutr Soc 2000;59:317–324.
29 de Onis M, Garza C, Onyango AW, Borghi E: Comparison of the WHO Child Growth Standards and the CDC 2000 growth charts. J Nutr 2007;137:144–148.
30 Yajnik CS, Fall CH, Coyaji KJ, et al: Neonatal anthropometry: the thin-fat Indian baby. The Pune Maternal Nutrition Study. Int J Obes Relat Metab Disord 2003;27:173–180.
31 Yajnik CS, Deshpande SS, Jackson AA, et al: Vitamin B_{12} and folate concentrations during pregnancy and insulin resistance in the offspring: the Pune Maternal Nutrition Study. Diabetologia 2008;51:29–38.
32 Kensara OA, Wootton SA, Phillips DI, et al: Fetal programming of body composition: relation between birth weight and body composition measured with dual-energy X-ray absorptiometry and anthropometric methods in older Englishmen. Am J Clin Nutr 2005;82:980–987.
33 Kensara OA, Wooton SA, Phillips DI, et al: Substrate-energy metabolism and metabolic risk factors for cardiovascular disease in relation to fetal growth and adult body composition. Am J Physiol Endocrinol Metab 2006;291:E365–E371.
34 Sachdev HS, Fall CH, Osmond C, et al: Anthropometric indicators of body composition in young adults: relation to size at birth and serial measurements of body mass index in childhood in the New Delhi birth cohort. Am J Clin Nutr 2005;82:456–466.

35 Bateson P, Barker D, Clutton-Brock T, et al: Developmental plasticity and human health. Nature 2004;430:419–421.
36 Lillycrop KA, Phillips ES, Jackson AA, Hanson MA, Burdge GC: Dietary protein restriction of pregnant rats induces and folic acid supplementation prevents epigenetic modification of hepatic gene expression in the offspring. J Nutr 2005;135:1382–1386.
37 Bird A: DNA methylation patterns and epigenetic memory. Genes Dev 2002;16:6–21.
38 Gidekel S, Bergman Y: A unique developmental pattern of Oct-3/4 DNA methylation is controlled by a cis-demodification element. J Biol Chem 2002;277:34521–34530.
39 Hershko AY, Kafri T, Fainsod A, Razin A: Methylation of HoxA5 and HoxB5 and its relevance to expression during mouse development. Gene 2003;302;65–72.
40 Fuks F, Hurd PJ, Wolf D, et al: The methyl-CpG-binding protein MeCP2 links DNA methylation to histone methylation. J Biol Chem 2003;278:4035–4040.
41 Turner BM: Histone acetylation and an epigenetic code. Bioessays 2000;22:836–845.
42 Weaver IC, Cervoni N, Champagne FA, et al: Epigenetic programming by maternal behavior. Nat Neurosci 2004;7:847–854.
43 Szyf M, Weaver I, Meaney M: Maternal care, the epigenome and phenotypic differences in behavior. Reprod Toxicol 2007;24:9–19.
44 Pham TD, MacLennan NK, Chiu CT, et al: Uteroplacental insufficiency increases apoptosis and alters p53 gene methylation in the full-term IUGR rat kidney. Am J Physiol Regul Integr Comp Physiol 2003;285:R962–R970.
45 Waterland RA, Jirtle RL: Early nutrition, epigenetic changes at transposons and imprinted genes, and enhanced susceptibility to adult chronic diseases. Nutrition 2004;20:63–68.
46 Langley SC, Jackson AA: Increased systolic blood pressure in adult rats induced by fetal exposure to maternal low protein diets. Clin Sci (Lond) 1994;86:217–222.
47 Lillycrop KA, Slater-Jefferies JL, Hanson MA, et al: Induction of altered epigenetic regulation of the hepatic glucocorticoid receptor in the offspring of rats fed a protein-restricted diet during pregnancy suggests that reduced DNA methyltransferase-1 expression is involved in impaired DNA methylation and changes in histone modifications. Br J Nutr 2007;97:1064–1073.
48 Lillycrop KA, Phillips ES, Torrens C, et al: Feeding pregnant rats a protein-restricted diet persistently alters the methylation of specific cytosines in the hepatic PPAR alpha promoter of the offspring. Br J Nutr 2008;100:278–282.
49 Jackson AA, Dunn RL, Marchand MC, Langley-Evans SC: Increased systolic blood pressure in rats induced by a maternal low-protein diet is reversed by dietary supplementation with glycine. Clin Sci (Lond) 2002;103:633–639.
50 Brawley L, Torrens C, Anthony FW, et al: Glycine rectifies vascular dysfunction induced by dietary protein imbalance during pregnancy. J Physiol 2004;554:497–504.
51 Torrens C, Brawley L, Anthony FW, et al: Folate supplementation during pregnancy improves offspring cardiovascular dysfunction induced by protein restriction. Hypertension 2006;47:982–987.
52 Martin JF, Johnston CS, Han CT, Benyshek DC: Nutritional origins of insulin resistance: a rat model for diabetes-prone human populations. J Nutr 2000;130:741–744.
53 Zambrano E, Martínez-Samayoa PM, Bautista CJ, et al: Sex differences in transgenerational alterations of growth and metabolism in progeny (F2) of female offspring (F1) of rats fed a low protein diet during pregnancy and lactation. J Physiol 2005;566:225–236.
54 Benyshek DC, Johnston CS, Martin JF: Glucose metabolism is altered in the adequately-nourished grand-offspring (F3 generation) of rats malnourished during gestation and perinatal life. Diabetologia 2006;49:1117–1119.
55 Torrens C, Poston L, Hanson MA: Transmission of raised blood pressure and endothelial dysfunction to the F2 generation induced by maternal protein restriction in the F0, in the absence of dietary challenge in the F1 generation. Br J Nutr 2008;100:760–766.
56 Jackson AA: The glycine story. Eur J Clin Nutr 1991;45:59–65.
57 Meakins TS, Persaud C, Jackson AA: Dietary supplementation with L-methionine impairs the utilization of urea-nitrogen and increases 5-L-oxoprolinuria in normal women consuming a low protein diet. J Nutr 1998:128;720–772.
58 Langley-Evans SC, Gardner DS, Jackson AA: Maternal protein restriction influences the programming of the rat hypothalamic-pituitary-adrenal axis. J Nutr 1996;126:1578–1585.
59 Terzolo M, Allasino B, Bosio S, et al: Hyperhomocysteinemia in patients with Cushing's syndrome. J Clin Endocrinol Metab 2004;89:3745–3751.

60 Langley-Evans SC: Hypertension induced by foetal exposure to a maternal low-protein diet, in the rat, is prevented by pharmacological blockade of maternal glucocorticoid synthesis. J Hypertens 1997;15: 537–544.
61 Burdge GC, Slater-Jefferies J, Torrens C, et al: Dietary protein restriction of pregnant rats in the F0 generation induces altered methylation of hepatic gene promoters in the adult male offspring in the F1 and F2 generations. Br J Nutr 2007;97:435–439.
62 Liu L, Wylie RC, Andrews LG, Tollefsbol TO: Aging, cancer and nutrition: the DNA methylation connection. Mech Ageing Dev 2003;124:989–998.
63 Zhu J: DNA methylation and hepatocellular carcinoma. J Hepatobiliary Pancreat Surg 2006;13:265–273.
64 Galm O, Herman JG, Baylin SB: The fundamental role of epigenetics in hematopoietic malignancies. Blood Rev 2006;20:1–13.
65 Lopatina N, Haskell JF, Andrews LG, et al: Differential maintenance and de novo methylating activity by three DNA methyltransferases in aging and immortalized fibroblasts. J Cell Biochem 2002; 84:324–334.
66 Lengauer C: Cancer: an unstable liaison. Science 2003;300:442–443.
67 Strathdee G, Appleton K, Illand M, et al: Primary ovarian carcinomas display multiple methylator phenotypes involving known tumor suppressor genes. Am J Pathol 2001;158:1121–1127.
68 Tollefsbol TO, Andrews LG: Mechanisms for telomerase gene control in aging cells and tumorigenesis. Med Hypotheses 2001;56:630–637.
69 Young JI, Sedivy JM, Smith JR: Telomerase expression in normal human fibroblasts stabilizes DNA 5-methylcytosine transferase I. J Biol Chem 2003; 278:19904–19908.
70 Burdge GC, Lillycrop KA, Jackson AA, Gluckman PD, Hanson MA: The nature of the growth pattern and of the metabolic response to fasting in the rat are dependent upon the dietary protein and folic acid intakes of their pregnant dams and post-weaning fat consumption. Br J Nutr 2008;99:540–549.
71 Burdge GC, Lillycrop KA, Phillips ES, et al: Folic acid supplementation during the juvenile-pubertal period in rats modifies the phenotype and epigenotype induced by prenatal nutrition. J Nutr 2009; 139:1054–1060.
72 Gluckman PD, Lillycrop KA, Vickers MH, et al: Metabolic plasticity during mammalian development is directionally dependent on early nutritional status. Proc Natl Acad Sci USA 2007;104:12796–12800.

Prof. Alan A. Jackson
Institute of Human Nutrition, Southampton General Hospital (MP 113)
Tremona Road
Southampton SO16 6YD (UK)
Tel. +44 23 8079 6317, Fax +44 23 8079 4945, E-Mail aaj@soton.ac.uk

Choline: Clinical Nutrigenetic/Nutrigenomic Approaches for Identification of Functions and Dietary Requirements

Steven H. Zeisel

Nutrition Research Institute, Department of Nutrition, School of Public Health and School of Medicine, University of North Carolina at Chapel Hill, Chapel Hill, N.C., USA

Nutrigenetics/nutrigenomics (the study of the bidirectional interactions between genes and diet) is a rapidly developing field that is changing research and practice in human nutrition. Though eventually nutrition clinicians may be able to provide personalized nutrition recommendations, in the immediate future they are most likely to use this knowledge to improve dietary recommendations for populations. Currently, estimated average requirements are used to set dietary reference intakes because scientists cannot adequately identify subsets of the population that differ in requirement for a nutrient. Recommended intake levels must exceed the actual required intake for most of the population in order to assure that individuals with the highest requirement ingest adequate amounts of the nutrient. As a result, dietary reference intake levels often are set so high that diet guidelines suggest almost unattainable intakes of some foods. Once it is possible to identify common subgroups that differ in nutrient requirements using nutrigenetic/nutrigenomic profiling, targeted interventions and recommendations can be refined. In addition, when a large variance exists in response to a nutrient, statistical analyses often argue for a null effect. If responders could be differentiated from nonresponders based on nutrigenetic/nutrigenomic profiling, this statistical noise could be eliminated and the sensitivity of nutrition research greatly increased.

Challenges for Clinical Nutrigenetics/Nutrigenomics

The first challenge for developing clinical nutrigenetics/nutrigenomics is the growing misconception that only very large studies can develop evidence for associations between single nucleotide polymorphisms (SNPs) and phenotypes. The use of genome-wide profiling of common single nucleotide polymorphisms (SNPs) to identify such associations has become common. These genome-wide association studies (GWAS) often screen thousands to millions of genes and their variants in thousands of subjects. In order to avoid the issue of multiplicity, and because of expected modest effect sizes, the scientific community has adopted strict definitions of statistical significance (e.g. $p < 5 \times 10^{-7}$ [1]), which dictate the need for large sample sizes typically involving thousands of subjects. It is important to note that these definitions were adopted assuming an individual SNP has a small effect size and that large numbers of randomly selected SNPs are being screened for an association with a phenotype. Because of the enormous number of genotype-phenotype associations tested in a genome-wide study, spurious associations will substantially outnumber true ones unless rigorous statistical thresholds are applied; smaller p values generally provide greater support for a true association. However, standard Bonferroni correction is overly conservative because it assumes the independence of all tests performed, but in many association studies markers are not independent because they are in linkage disequilibrium.

Sadly, this growing consensus for requiring p values $< 5 \times 10^{-7}$ makes clinical nutrigenetics/nutrigenomics virtually impossible. Inherently, such studies involve tens to hundreds but not thousands of subjects and often measure phenotype parameters that are not practically measured in large populations. If the phenotype to be explained is not easily detected in thousands of people, a population GWAS approach is not possible. For example, we later discuss studies on fatty liver that require controlled diet conditions and mass resonance imaging. It might be possible to perform such studies on hundreds of people, but certainly not on tens of thousands. For clinical nutrigenetics/nutrigenomics approaches to be viable we need to use study designs that allow less stringent p values than are used for GWAS studies. The appropriate design elements have already been considered by the scientific panel that suggested the rigorous p values for GWAS studies [1].

Reasons that are appropriate for lowering the threshold for calling a finding of a particular SNP-phenotype association are the selection of targeted SNPs based on knowledge of the underlying processes causing the phenotype (e.g. selecting the gene for endogenous biosynthesis of a nutrient when studying the phenotype associated with deficiency of the nutrient), or selecting SNPs that are likely to result in defective protein products (such as non-synonymous coding SNPs) [1]. Selection of SNPs for which there is credible laboratory evidence or a validated in silico prediction a priori permits accepting a less rigorous p value; however, creating a credible biological hypothesis post hoc is not acceptable [1]. The lowering of the threshold for positively identifying a particular SNP-phenotype association must be declared before initiation of the analysis and not once the analysis has begun [1]. Additional information gathered from laboratory techniques, bioinformatic tools and a priori biological insight should be used to provide plausibility for interpreting genetic association findings [1]. It is important to limit the number of candidate SNPs considered as the number of multiple comparisons made in the analysis drives the possibility of false discovery. Inherently, small sample sizes can provide imprecise or incorrect estimates of the magnitude of the observed effects; thus, the effect size must be large enough to stand out from such noise. An estimated effect size that is large (that is, with an odds ratio greater than 2) in a small but well-powered study can lend credence to an association, because unknown confounding factors are less likely to produce large effects [1]. Finally, replication of the association between SNP and phenotype in an independent study is important.

Thus, though some geneticists initially expressed doubts about results generated in clinical nutrigenetics/nutrigenomics because they reflexively expect large population studies with very small p values, there are reasonable study designs under which clinical nutrigenetics/nutrigenomics is not only possible but practical (targeted and small number of SNPs studied based on biological insights with SNPs that have a large effect size and results that can be replicated).

Other Considerations before Undertaking Clinical Nutrigenetics/Nutrigenomics

In GWAS or clinical nutrigenetics/nutrigenomic studies, a haplotype associated with the phenotype of interest can be identified. The identified polymorphism is rarely the actual phenotype-causing variant, but is more likely to be correlated, or in linkage disequilibrium with the functional SNP. Because SNP arrays do not assay every polymorphism in a genomic region, it is not possible to identify all the surrounding genetic variants that are correlated with the identified marker. However, we can define the boundaries within the gene where sequencing or subsequent fine-mapping experiments are appropriate [2].

Prototype Experiment in Nutrigenetics/Nutrigenomics: Studies on Choline Deficiency

The case study of the effects of genetic variation on dietary requirements for choline provides an excellent example of how clinical nutrigenetics/nutrigenomics can be used. In these studies, SNPs in the gene responsible for de novo biosynthesis of choline were associated with the risk for developing choline deficiency (phenotype). When young women were found to be resistant to developing choline deficiency, the role of estrogen in induction of choline biosynthesis was identified. In addition, the effects of choline on epigenetic regulation of gene expression were studied.

Choline Metabolism

Choline is involved in 3 major pathways: acetylcholine synthesis, methyl donation via betaine, and phosphatidylcholine synthesis [3]. Choline, via its irreversible oxidation to betaine [4], methylates homocysteine to form methionine. This is the precursor for synthesis of *S*-adenosylmethionine, the universal methyl donor needed for methylation of DNA, RNA and proteins. It is important to realize that choline, methionine and folate metabolism are inter-related at the step that homocysteine is methylated to form methionine [5]. Perturbing metabolism of one of the methyl-donors results in compensatory changes in the other methyl-donors due to the intermingling of these metabolic pathways [6–8]. Rats treated with the anti-folate, methotrexate, had diminished pools of choline metabolites in liver [7, 9]. Rats ingesting a choline-deficient diet had diminished tissue concentrations of methionine and *S*-adenosylmethionine [10] and doubled plasma homocysteine concentrations [11]. Humans who were choline deficient, even when fed adequate amounts of folic acid, had diminished capacity to methylate homocysteine [12].

Most of the foods we eat contain various amounts of choline, choline esters and betaine [13], and in 2004 the United States Department of Agriculture released a database on choline content in common foods (www.nal.usda.gov/fnic/foodcomp/Data/Choline/Choline.pdf). The foods with greatest abundance of choline are of animal origin, especially eggs and liver. Human breast milk also is a good source of free choline and choline esters [14], and the manufacturers of infant formulas have recently modified the content of choline compounds to levels similar with the ones in human breast milk [14, 15]. The only source of choline other than diet is de novo biosynthesis of phosphatidylcholine catalyzed by phosphatidylethanolamine-*N*-methyltransferase (PEMT) in liver. This enzyme uses *S*-adenosylmethionine as a methyl donor and forms a new choline moiety [16].

Studies in humans show that dietary choline is required (reviewed in [3] and discussed later). In 1998, the US Institute of Medicine (Food and Nutrition Board) established for the first time adequate intake (AI) and tolerable upper intake limit values for choline, based on limited human studies [17] The AI is 550 mg/70 kg body weight, with upward adjustment in pregnant and lactating women; the upper intake limit ranges from 1,000 mg/day in children to 3,500 mg/day in adults [17]. For some age categories for which adequate data were missing, AI values have been set by extrapolating from adult values (for ages 1–18 years), and from infants (for ages 7–12 months) [17]. The 2005 NHANES survey reported that most people do not achieve the recommended AI for choline [18]. In participants from the Framingham Offspring Study the mean intake for total choline (energy adjusted) was below the AI values, with a mean intake of 313 mg/day; moreover, there was an inverse association between choline intake and plasma total homocysteine concentration in subjects with low folate intakes [19].

Consequences of Dietary Choline Deficiency in Humans

Using a clinical methodology for phenotyping individuals with respect to their susceptibility to developing organ dysfunction when fed a low choline diet [12, 20–22], adult men and women (pre- and postmenopausal) aged 18–70 years were admitted to the General Clinical Research Center, UNC Chapel Hill and fed a standard diet containing a known amount of choline (550 mg/70 kg/day; baseline). On day 11, subjects were placed on a diet containing <50 mg choline/day for up to 42 days. Blood and urine were collected to measure various experimental parameters of dietary choline status, and markers of organ dysfunction and liver fat were assessed. If at some point during the depletion period functional markers indicated organ dysfunction associated with choline deficiency, subjects were switched to a diet containing choline until replete. Most men and postmenopausal women fed low choline diets under controlled conditions developed reversible fatty liver (measure by mass resonance spectroscopy) as well as liver and muscle damage, while 56% of premenopausal women were resistant to developing choline deficiency [22]. This observation immediately suggested that estrogen moderated the dietary requirement for choline, and, indeed, estrogen induces the gene *(PEMT)* that makes endogenous synthesis of choline possible [23]. The classic actions of estrogen occur through its receptors ERα and ERβ which bind as homodimers or heterodimers to estrogen response elements (EREs) in the promoters of many estrogen-responsive genes [24]. The consensus ERE (PuGGTCAnnnTGACCPy) [24] and some imperfect ERE half site motifs (ERE1/2) bind with ERα and ERβ [25–27]. There are multiple EREs in the promoter region(s) of the *PEMT* gene [23] and estrogen caused a marked up-regulation in *PEMT* mRNA expression and enzyme activity in human hepatocytes [23]. Thus, premenopausal women have an enhanced capacity for de novo biosynthesis of choline moiety. During pregnancy, estradiol concentration rises from approximately 1 to 60 nM at term [28, 29], suggesting that capacity for endogenous synthesis of choline is highest during the period when females need to support fetal development.

Pregnancy and lactation are times when demand for choline is especially high. Large amounts of choline are delivered to the fetus across the placenta, where choline transport systems pump it against a concentration gradient [30, 31] and deplete maternal plasma choline in humans [32]. Plasma or serum choline concentrations are 6- to 7-fold higher in the fetus and newborn than they are in the adult [33, 34]. High levels of choline circulating in the neonate presumably ensure enhanced availability of choline to tissues. It is interesting that despite enhanced capacity to synthesize choline, the demand for this nutrient is so high that stores are depleted during pregnancy. Pregnant rats had diminished total liver choline compounds compared to non-mated controls and become as sensitive to choline-deficient diets as were male rats [35]. Because milk contains a great deal of choline, lactation further increases maternal demand for choline, resulting in further depletion of tissue stores [35, 36]. These observations suggest that women depend on high rates of PEMT activity, as well as on dietary intake of choline to sustain normal pregnancy. $Pemt^{-/-}$ mice abort pregnancies at around 9–10 days of gestation unless fed supplemental choline (personal observation; [37]). As discussed later, choline nutriture during pregnancy is especially important because it influences brain development in the fetus [38–50].

Genetic Variation in Dietary Requirements for Choline

Though premenopausal women should be resistant to choline deficiency because of estrogen, a significant portion of them (44%) developed organ dysfunction when deprived of choline [22]. Genetic variation likely underlies these differences in dietary requirements. As noted earlier, *PEMT* encodes for a protein responsible for endogenous formation of choline, and 78% of female carriers of the variant (C) allele in a SNP in the promoter region of the *PEMT* gene (rs12325817) developed organ dysfunction when fed a low choline diet (OR 25, $p < 0.00005$; p value based on 64 women studied) [51]. The frequency of this variant allele was 0.74 in North Carolina. The risk haplotype abrogated the induction of *PEMT* by estrogen, while the wild-type haplotype did not [Resseguie et al., manuscript submitted]. The SNP rs12325817 is not located in an estrogen response element but probably is in linkage disequilibrium with a functional SNP within such a response element.

Other SNPs in choline metabolism genes may have some influence on the dietary requirements for choline, though the p values for these associations are not as robust as for rs12325817. The first of 2 SNPs in the coding region of the choline dehydrogenase gene (*CHDH*; rs9001) had a protective effect on susceptibility to choline deficiency, while a second *CHDH* variant (rs12676) was associated with increased susceptibility [51]. We did not have the power in this study to identify any association of a SNP in the betaine:homocysteine methyltransferase gene (*BHMT*; rs3733890) with susceptibility to choline deficiency [51].

Genetic variants of genes in folate metabolism also modified the susceptibility of these subjects to choline deficiency [52]. Premenopausal women who were carriers of the very common 5,10-methylenetetrahydrofolate dehydrogenase-G1958A (*MTHFD1*; rs2236225) gene allele were more than 15 times as likely as non-carriers to develop signs of choline deficiency ($p < 0.0001$) on the low choline diet. Sixty-three percent of our study population had at least 1 allele for this SNP. The rs2236225 polymorphism alters the delicately balanced flux between 5,10-methylene tetrahydrofolate and 10-formyl tetrahydrofolate and thereby influences the availability of 5-methyl THF for homocysteine remethylation [53]. This increases demand for choline as a methyl-group donor. It is of interest that the risk of having a child with a neural tube defect increases in mothers with the rs2236225 SNP [54]. We did not have sufficient power in the study to detect any effects of other folate metabolism SNPs (C677T and A1298C polymorphisms of the 5,10-methylene tetrahydrofolate reductase gene and the A80C polymorphism of the reduced folate carrier 1 gene) [52].

Choline and Neural Development

Rats and mice fed a low choline diet in late pregnancy (gestational days 12 to 17 in mice, days 12 to 18 or 20 in rats) had reduced neural progenitor cell proliferation and increased apoptosis in fetal hippocampus and cortex [38, 44, 55]. Similar outcomes were reported when pregnant mice are fed a low-folate diet [56], suggesting, again, potential synergistic mechanisms of action between folate and choline.

The mechanisms associating choline deficiency with decreased cell proliferation are, in part, related to the over-expression of cyclin-dependent kinase inhibitors (Cdkn) like p27Kip1 [40], p15Ink4b [40, 45] and Cdkn3 [45, 57], suggesting that choline deficiency inhibits cell proliferation by inducing G_1 arrest due to the inhibition of the interaction between cyclin-dependent kinases and cyclins. Using mouse hippocampal and cortical progenitor cells exposed to choline deficiency for 48 h, oligonucleotide-array analysis of gene expression showed expression changes in more than a thousand genes, of which 331 were related to cell division, apoptosis, neuronal and glial differentiation, methyl metabolism, and calcium-binding protein ontology classes [58], consistent with the phenotype of reduced cell proliferation, increased apoptosis, and increased differentiation.

Choline Deficiency Alters Gene Expression via Epigenetic Mechanisms

Neural development is influenced by DNA methylation. Overall levels of methylation decrease as neuronal differentiation proceeds [59] and the treatment of neural progenitor cells with demethylating agents induces them to differentiate into cholinergic and adrenergic neurons [60]. Although the relationship between nutrition and epigenetics has been firmly established in the last few years [61], less is known about the role nutrition has in the epigenetic regulation of fetal brain development. Because dietary choline is an important player in the maintenance of the *S*-adenosylmethionine pool (the methyl donor for DNA methylation), along with folate and methionine, it is reasonable to expect that choline influences the epigenetic status of the developing brain. Global DNA methylation is decreased in the neuroepithelial layer of the hippocampus in choline deficient mouse fetal brains. Along with decreased global methylation, changes in gene-specific methylation were reported, where a cyclin-dependent kinase *(Cdkn3)* was hypo-methylated in its promoter by choline deficiency [45, 57] in the progenitor layer of the hippocampus. These alterations were associated with increased protein expression of this cyclin-dependent kinase inhibitor [45], and this model is consistent with previous findings showing that there is epigenetic regulation of cyclin-dependent kinase inhibitors that regulate cell proliferation [62].

Long-Lasting Consequences of Prenatal Choline Availability

The changes induced by dietary choline in fetal brain have long-lasting effects that alter brain function throughout life. Maternal dietary choline availability during late pregnancy was associated with long-lasting changes in the hippocampal function of the adult offspring. Choline supplementation during this period enhanced visuo-spatial and auditory memory in the adult rats throughout their life-span [63–67]. It also enhanced a property of the hippocampus, long-term potentiation [46, 68, 69]. The offspring from mothers fed a choline-deficient diet manifested opposite outcomes [64, 68].

Implications for Human Brain Development

It is always difficult to extrapolate findings reported using animal models to humans. However, limited data are available to support the hypothesis that similar mechanisms are involved in humans. Due to ethical constraints, no studies are available in children or pregnant mothers to validate the rodent model. Because the 2005 National Health and Nutrition Examination Survey (NHANES) data suggests that pregnant women do not consume adequate amounts of choline [18], and case-control studies in California suggest that women eating lower choline diets are at increased risk for giving birth to babies with neural tube defects [70] and cleft palate [71], the recommendation that pregnant women should attempt to consume diets adequate in choline seems reasonable. In addition, because half of the population has gene polymorphisms that affect choline and folate metabolism [52, 72], it is likely that different individuals may have different dietary requirements for choline and may need to pay special attention to choline intake during pregnancy.

Acknowledgments

This work was funded by grants from the National Institutes of Health (DK55865, AG09525). Support for this work was also provided by grants from the NIH to the UNC Nutrition & Obesity Research Center (DK56350).

References

1 Chanock SJ, Manolio T, Boehnke M, et al: Replicating genotype-phenotype associations. Nature 2007;447: 655–660.
2 Teo YY: Exploratory data analysis in large-scale genetic studies. Biostatistics 2010;11:70–81.
3 Zeisel SH: Choline: critical role during fetal development and dietary requirements in adults. Annu Rev Nutr 2006;26:229–250.
4 Niculescu MD, Zeisel SH: Diet methyl donors and DNA methylation: interactions between dietary folate methionine and choline. J Nutr 2002;132: 2333S–2335S.
5 Finkelstein JD: Pathways and regulation of homocysteine metabolism in mammals. Semin Thromb Hemost 2000;26:219–225.
6 Kim Y-I, Miller JW, da Costa K-A, Nadeau M, Smith D, Selhub J, Zeisel SH, Mason JB: Folate deficiency causes secondary depletion of choline and phosphocholine in liver. J Nutr 1995;124:2197–2203.
7 Selhub J, Seyoum E, Pomfret EA, Zeisel SH: Effects of choline deficiency and methotrexate treatment upon liver folate content and distribution. Cancer Res 1991;51:16–21.
8 Varela-Moreiras G, Selhub J, da Costa K, Zeisel SH: Effect of chronic choline deficiency in rats on liver folate content and distribution. J Nutr Biochem 1992;3:519–522.
9 Pomfret EA, da Costa K, Zeisel SH: Effects of choline deficiency and methotrexate treatment upon rat liver. J Nutr Biochem 1990;1:533–541.

10 Zeisel SH, Zola T, daCosta K, Pomfret EA: Effect of choline deficiency on S-adenosylmethionine and methionine concentrations in rat liver. Biochem J 1989;259:725–729.

11 Varela-Moreiras G, Ragel C, Perez de Miguelsanz J: Choline deficiency and methotrexate treatment induces marked but reversible changes in hepatic folate concentrations serum homocysteine and DNA methylation rates in rats. J Amer Coll Nutr 1995;14:480–485.

12 da Costa KA, Gaffney CE, Fischer LM, Zeisel SH: Choline deficiency in mice and humans is associated with increased plasma homocysteine concentration after a methionine load. Am J Clin Nutr 2005;81:440–444.

13 Zeisel SH, Mar M-H, Howe JC, Holden JM: Concentrations of choline-containing compounds and betaine in common foods. J Nutr 2003;133:1302–1307.

14 Ilcol YO, Ozbek R, Hamurtekin E, Ulus IH: Choline status in newborns, infants, children, breast-feeding women, breast-fed infants and human breast milk. J Nutr Biochem 2005;16:489–499.

15 Holmes-McNary MQ, Cheng WL, Mar MH, Fussell S, Zeisel SH: Choline and choline esters in human and rat milk and in infant formulas. Am J Clin Nutr 1996;64:572–576.

16 Blusztajn JK, Zeisel SH, Wurtman RJ: Developmental changes in the activity of phosphatidylethanolamine N-methyltransferases in rat brain. Biochem J 1985; 232:505–511.

17 Institute of Medicine and National Academy of Sciences USA: CholineIn Dietary Reference Intakes for Folate Thiamin Riboflavin Niacin Vitamin B_{12} Panthothenic Acid Biotin and Choline. Washington, National Academy Press, 1998, vol 1, pp 390–422

18 Jensen HH, Batres-Marquez SP, Carriquiry A, Schalinske KL: Choline in the diets of the US population: NHANES 2003–2004. FASEB J 2007;21: lb219.

19 Cho E, Zeisel SH, Jacques P, et al: Dietary choline and betaine assessed by food-frequency questionnaire in relation to plasma total homocysteine concentration in the Framingham Offspring Stud. Am J Clin Nutr 2006;83:905–911.

20 Busby MG, Fischer L, Da Costa KA, et al: Choline- and betaine-defined diets for use in clinical research and for the management of trimethylaminuria. J Am Diet Assoc 2004;104:1836–1845.

21 da Costa KA, Badea M, Fischer LM, Zeisel SH: Elevated serum creatine phosphokinase in choline-deficient humans: mechanistic studies in C2C12 mouse myoblasts. Am J Clin Nutr 2004;80:163–170.

22 Fischer LM, da Costa K, Kwock L, et al: Sex and menopausal status influence human dietary requirements for the nutrient choline. Am J Clin Nutr 2007; 85:1275–1285.

23 Resseguie M, Song J, Niculescu M, da Costa K, Randall T, Zeisel S: Phosphatidylethanolamine n-methyltransferase (PEMT) gene expression is induced by estrogen in human and mouse primary hepatocytes. FASEB J 2007;21:2822–2832.

24 Walter P, Green S, Greene G, et al: Cloning of the human estrogen receptor cDNA. Proc Natl Acad Sci USA 1985;82:7889–7893.

25 Lopez D, Sanchez MD, Shea-Eaton W, McLean MP: Estrogen activates the high-density lipoprotein receptor gene via binding to estrogen response elements and interaction with sterol regulatory element binding protein-1A. Endocrinology 2002;143: 2155–2168.

26 Agarwal A, Yeung WS, Lee KF: Cloning and characterization of the human oviduct-specific glycoprotein (HuOGP) gene promoter. Mol Hum Reprod 2002;8:167–175.

27 Xie T, Ho SL, Ramsden D: Characterization and implications of estrogenic down-regulation of human catechol-O-methyltransferase gene transcription. Mol Pharmacol 1999;56:31–38.

28 Sarda IR, Gorwill RH: Hormonal studies in pregnancyI: total unconjugated estrogens in maternal peripheral vein cord vein and cord artery serum at delivery. Am J Obstet Gynecol 1976;124:234–238.

29 Adeyemo O, Jeyakumar H: Plasma progesterone estradiol-17beta and testosterone in maternal and cord blood and maternal human chorionic gonadotropin at parturition. Afr J Med Med Sci 1993;22:55–60.

30 Sweiry JH, Yudilevich DL: Characterization of choline transport at maternal and fetal interfaces of the perfused guinea-pig placenta. J Physiol 1985;366: 251–266.

31 Sweiry JH, Page KR, Dacke CG, Abramovich DR, Yudilevich DL: Evidence of saturable uptake mechanisms at maternal and fetal sides of the perfused human placenta by rapid paired-tracer dilution: studies with calcium and choline. J Devel Physiol 1986;8:435–445.

32 McMahon KE, Farrell PM: Measurement of free choline concentrations in maternal and neonatal blood by micropyrolysis gas chromatography. Clin Chim Acta 1985;149:1–12.

33 Zeisel SH, Wurtman RJ: Developmental changes in rat blood choline concentration. Biochem J 1981; 198:565–570.

34 Ozarda IY, Uncu G, Ulus IH: Free and phospholipid-bound choline concentrations in serum during pregnancy after delivery and in newborns. Arch Physiol Biochem 2002;110:393–399.

35 Zeisel SH, Mar M-H, Zhou Z-W, da Costa K-A: Pregnancy and lactation are associated with diminished concentrations of choline and its metabolites in rat liver. J Nutr 1995;125:3049–3054.

36 Holmes-McNary M, Cheng WL, Mar MH, Fussell S, Zeisel SH: Choline and choline esters in human and rat milk and infant formulas. Am J Clin Nutr 1996; 64:572–576.

37 Zhu X, Mar MH, Song J, Zeisel SH: Deletion of the Pemt gene increases progenitor cell mitosis DNA and protein methylation and decreases calretinin expression in embryonic day 17 mouse hippocampus. Brain Res Dev Brain Res 2004;149:121–129.

38 Albright CD, Friedrich CB, Brown EC, Mar MH, Zeisel SH: Maternal dietary choline availability alters mitosis apoptosis and the localization of TOAD-64 protein in the developing fetal rat septum. Brain Res Dev Brain Res 1999;115:123–129.

39 Albright CD, Mar MH, Craciunescu CN, Song J, Zeisel SH: Maternal dietary choline availability alters the balance of netrin-1 and DCC neuronal migration proteins in fetal mouse brain hippocampus. Brain Res Dev Brain Res 2005;159:149–154.

40 Albright CD, Mar MH, Friedrich CB, Brown EC, Zeisel SH: Maternal choline availability alters the localization of p15Ink4B and p27Kip1 cyclin-dependent kinase inhibitors in the developing fetal rat brain hippocampus. Dev Neurosci 2001;23:100–106.

41 Albright CD, Siwek DF, Craciunescu CN, et al: Choline availability during embryonic development alters the localization of calretinin in developing and aging mouse hippocampus. Nutr Neurosci 2003;6:129–134.

42 Albright CD, Tsai AY, Friedrich CB, Mar MH, Zeisel SH: Choline availability alters embryonic development of the hippocampus and septum in the rat. Brain Res Dev Brain Res 1999;113:13–20.

43 Albright CD, Tsai AY, Mar M-H, Zeisel SH: Choline availability modulates the expression of TGFß1 and cytoskeletal proteins in the hippocampus of developing rat brain. Neurochem Res 1998;23:751–758.

44 Craciunescu CN, Albright CD, Mar MH, Song J, Zeisel SH: Choline availability during embryonic development alters progenitor cell mitosis in developing mouse hippocampus. J Nutr 2003;133:3614–3618.

45 Niculescu MD, Craciunescu CN, Zeisel SH: Dietary choline deficiency alters global and gene-specific DNA methylation in the developing hippocampus of mouse fetal brains. FASEB J 2006;20:43–49.

46 Pyapali G, Turner D, Williams C, Meck W, Swartzwelder HS: Prenatal choline supplementation decreases the threshold for induction of long-term potentiation in young adult rats. J Neurophysiol 1998;79:1790–1796.

47 Meck W, Williams C: Perinatal choline supplementation increases the threshold for chunking in spatial memory. Neuroreport 1997;8:3053–3059.

48 Meck WH, Smith RA, Williams CL: Pre- and postnatal choline supplementation produces long-term facilitation of spatial memory. Dev Psychobiol 1988; 21:339–353.

49 Meck WH, Williams CL: Metabolic imprinting of choline by its availability during gestation: implications for memory and attentional processing across the lifespan. Neurosci Biobehav Rev 2003;27:385–399.

50 Mellott TJ, Williams CL, Meck WH, Blusztajn JK: Prenatal choline supplementation advances hippocampal development and enhances MAPK and CREB activation. FASEB J 2004;18:545–547.

51 da Costa KA, Kozyreva OG, Song J, et al: Common genetic polymorphisms affect the human requirement for the nutrient choline. FASEB J 2006;20:1336–1344.

52 Kohlmeier M, da Costa KA, Fischer LM, Zeisel SH: Genetic variation of folate-mediated one-carbon transfer pathway predicts susceptibility to choline deficiency in humans. Proc Natl Acad Sci USA 2005;102:16025–16030.

53 Horne DW: Neither methionine nor nitrous oxide inactivation of methionine synthase affect the concentration of 510-methylenetetrahydrofolate in rat liver. J Nutr 2003;133:476–478.

54 Brody LC, Conley M, Cox C, et al: A polymorphism R653Q in the trifunctional enzyme methylenetetrahydrofolate dehydrogenase/methenyltetrahydrofolate cyclohydrolase/formyltetrahydrofolate synthetase is a maternal genetic risk factor for neural tube defects: report of the Birth Defects Research Group. Am J Human Genet 2002;71:1207–1215.

55 Holmes-McNary MQ, Loy R, Mar MH, Albright CD, Zeisel SH: Apoptosis is induced by choline deficiency in fetal brain and in PC12 cells. Brain Res Dev Brain Res 1997;101:9–16.

56 Craciunescu CN, Brown EC, Mar MH, et al: Folic acid deficiency during late gestation decreases progenitor cell proliferation and increases apoptosis in fetal mouse brain. J Nutr 2004;134:162–166.

57 Niculescu MD, Yamamuro Y, Zeisel SH: Choline availability modulates human neuroblastoma cell proliferation and alters the methylation of the promoter region of the cyclin-dependent kinase inhibitor 3 gene. J Neurochem 2004;89:1252–1259.

58 Niculescu MD, Craciunescu CN, Zeisel SH: Gene expression profiling of choline-deprived neural precursor cells isolated from mouse brain. Brain Res Mol Brain Res 2005;134:309–322.

59 Costello JF: DNA methylation in brain development and gliomagenesis. Front Biosci 2003;8:s175–s184.

60 Mattson MP: Methylation and acetylation in nervous system development and neurodegenerative disorders. Ageing Res Rev 2003;2:329–342.
61 Feil R: Environmental and nutritional effects on the epigenetic regulation of genes. Mutation Research/Fundamental and Molecular Mechanisms of Mutagenesis 2006;600;46–57.
62 Fukai K, Yokosuka O, Imazeki F, et al: Methylation status of p14ARF p15INK4b and p16INK4a genes in human hepatocellular carcinoma. Liver International 2005;25:1209–1216.
63 Meck WH, Williams CL: Perinatal choline supplementation increases the threshold for chunking in spatial memory. Neuroreport 1997;8:3053–3059.
64 Meck WH, Williams CL: Simultaneous temporal processing is sensitive to prenatal choline availability in mature and aged rats. Neuroreport 1997;8:3045–3051.
65 Meck WH, Williams CL: Characterization of the facilitative effects of perinatal choline supplementation on timing and temporal memory. Neuroreport 1997;8:2831–2835.
66 Meck WH, Williams CL: Choline supplementation during prenatal development reduces proactive interference in spatial memory. Brain Res Dev Brain Res 1999;118:51–59.
67 Williams CL, Meck WH, Heyer DD, Loy R: Hypertrophy of basal forebrain neurons and enhanced visuospatial memory in perinatally choline-supplemented rats. Brain Res 1998;794:225–238.
68 Jones JP, Meck W, Williams CL, Wilson WA, Swartzwelder HS: Choline availability to the developing rat fetus alters adult hippocampal long-term potentiation. Brain Res Dev Brain Res 1999;118:159–167.
69 Montoya DA, White AM, Williams CL, et al: Prenatal choline exposure alters hippocampal responsiveness to cholinergic stimulation in adulthood. Brain Res Dev Brain Res 2000;123:25–32.
70 Shaw GM, Carmichael SL, Yang W, Selvin S, Schaffer DM: Periconceptional dietary intake of choline and betaine and neural tube defects in offspring. Am J Epidemiol 2004;160:102–109.
71 Shaw GM, Carmichael SL, Laurent C, Rasmussen SA: Maternal nutrient intakes and risk of orofacial clefts. Epidemiology 2006;17:285–291.
72 da Costa KA, Kozyreva OG, Song J, et al: Common genetic polymorphisms affect the human requirement for the nutrient choline. Faseb J 2006;20:1336–1344.

Steven Zeisel MD, PhD
UNC Nutrition Research Institute, University of North Carolina at Chapel Hill
500 Laureate Way
Kannapolis, NC 28081 (USA)
Tel. +1 704 250 5003, E-Mail steven_zeisel@unc.edu

Dietary Polyphenols, Deacetylases and Chromatin Remodeling in Inflammation

Irfan Rahman · Sangwoon Chung

Department of Environmental Medicine, Lung Biology and Disease Program, University of Rochester Medical Center, Rochester, N.Y., USA

The therapeutic benefits of fruits, vegetables, tea and wine are mostly attributed to the presence of phenolic compounds. Naturally occurring dietary polyphenols, such as curcumin (diferuloylmethane, an active component of spice turmeric) and resveratrol (phytoalexin, a flavanoid found in red wine) can modulate signaling pathways mediated via NF-κB and MAP kinase, and up-regulate glutathione biosynthesis genes through activation of Nrf2. Polyphenols also down-regulate the expression of pro-inflammatory mediators, matrix metalloproteinases and adhesion molecules by inhibiting histone acetyltransferase (HAT) activity and activating histone deacetylases (HDACs)/sirtuins. It has been reported that in severe asthma and in chronic obstructive pulmonary disease (COPD) patients, oxidative stress not only activates the NF-κB pathway but also alters the histone acetylation and deacetylation balance via post-translational modifications of HDACs. Corticosteroids have been one the major modes of therapy against various respiratory diseases, such as asthma and COPD. Failure of corticosteroids to ameliorate such disease conditions is due to the reduction of HDAC2 and SIRT1 levels/activities in lungs of asthmatics and COPD patients. Dietary polyphenols, such as curcumin, resveratrol, and catechins have been reported to modulate epigenetic alterations in various experimental models. The anti-inflammatory property of curcumin, resveratrol, and catechins is associated with their ability to induce HDAC activity and thereby restore the efficacy of glucocorticoids or overcome its resistance. Thus, these polyphenolic compounds have therapeutic value as antioxidants, anti-inflammatory therapy and adjuvant therapy with steroids against chronic inflammatory and epigenetically-regulated diseases. In this chapter we present the current knowledge on the mode of action of these polyphenols in the light of HDACs.

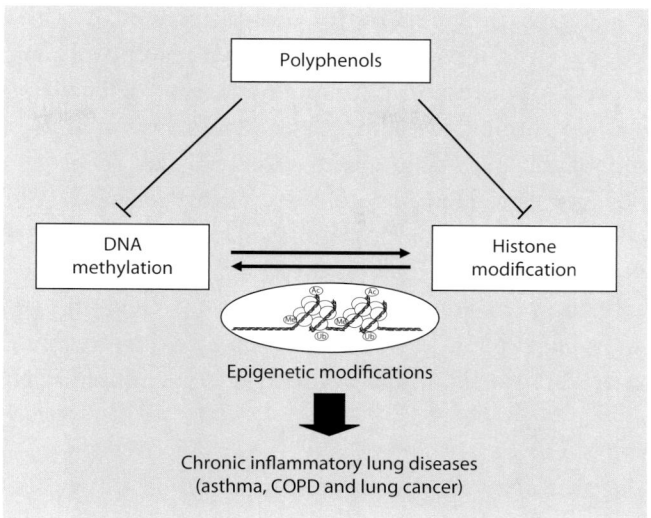

Fig. 1. Regulation of epigenetic events by polyphenols. Dietary polyphenols inhibit epigenetic modifications, such as DNA methylation and histone modification through regulation of DNA methyltransferase, CBP/HAT activity, and deacetylases leading to resolution of inflammation. Thus, this is a possible way forward to design therapeutic strategies for human lung diseases by epigenetic modifications.

Polyphenols: An Overview

A variety of dietary plants contain polyphenols which impart disease prevention abilities to fruits and vegetables. Polyphenols are secondary metabolites of plants and represent a vast group of compounds having aromatic ring(s), characterized by presence of one or more hydroxyl groups with varying structural complexities. The most widely distributed group of plant phenolics are flavonoids. The flavonoids subclasses comprise of flavonols, flavones, flavanols, isoflavones, antocyanidins, and others. In this chapter, we will consider the biological properties, with special reference to epigenetics (histone acetylation/deacetylation) and inflammation, of some well-known and well-studied polyphenols, such as resveratrol, curcumin, and catechins.

Modulation of Inflammation by Polyphenols

Investigations into the mechanism of action of polyphenols have revealed that polyphenols may modulate cellular signaling during inflammation [1–3]. In the following sections, some individual polyphenolic compounds will be discussed, especially their anti-inflammatory properties which impart their effects via chromatin/epigenetics-deacetylase modifications (fig. 1).

Resveratrol
Resveratrol (3,5,4′-trihydroxystilbene) is a phytoalexin and was first discovered in grapes in 1976. It contains 2 phenolic rings connected by a double bond and has

2 isoforms: *trans*-resveratrol and *cis*-resveratrol, with the former being more stable [4]. Recently, it has been reported that resveratrol can inhibit inflammatory cytokine expression in response to lipopolysaccharide challenge in rat lungs [5]. Resveratrol can also inhibit the activation of transcription factors, such as NF-κB and AP-1 in monocytic U937 cells and alveolar epithelial A549 cells [6, 7]. Resveratrol can inhibit phorbol ester (PMA)-induced cyclooxygenase-2 (COX-2) activation, matrix metalloproteinases, adhesion molecules, and inducible nitric oxide synthase gene via down-modulation of NF-κB activation [8, 9]. Furthermore, resveratrol inhibits the activation of c-Jun N-terminal kinases (JNK) [10] and its upstream kinase, mitogen-activated protein kinase [11]. Therefore, it appears that resveratrol can modulate a variety of pro-inflammatory pathways via inhibiting NF-κB and MAPK activation.

Curcumin

Curcumin, a yellow-colored compound, is a member of the curcuminoid family of compounds obtained from the rhizome of *Curcuma longa* L. (family Zingiberaceae). Curcumin is one of the most extensively studied polyphenols and is reported to have a wide variety of effects, such as anti-inflammatory, antibacterial, antiviral, antifungal, antitumor, antispasmodic and hepatoprotective [12].

Curcumin inhibits NF-κB activation, along with suppressing IL-8 release, COX-2 expression, and neutrophil recruitment in the lung [2]. Curcumin inhibits cigarette smoke-induced NF-κB activation by inhibiting IκBα kinase in human lung epithelial cells [13]. Similar to resveratrol, curcumin also down-regulates various NF-κB-regulated genes that are involved in inflammation, such as leukotrienes, phospholipase A2, 5-lipoxygenase, adhesion molecules, inducible nitric oxide synthase and COX-2. In different cell types, various kinase signaling pathways, such as JNK, p38, AKT, JAK, ERK and PKC, are also modulated by curcumin [14]. Therefore, to identify the actual mechanism by which curcumin exerts its anti-inflammatory effects is complicated by its pleiotropic nature due to its ability to target so many different cellular signaling pathways. However, it may be possible that the ability of curcumin to prevent cross-talk between myriad signaling pathways might be a pre-requisite for its anti-inflammatory properties.

Catechins

These are monomeric flavanols comprising of chemically similar compounds, such as catechin, epicatechin, epigallocatechin, epicatechin gallate, and epigallocatechin gallate (EGCG) [15]. EGCG predominates among the various tea polyphenols and is considered to be the major therapeutic agent. EGCG has been shown to inhibit cigarette smoke extract-induced pro-inflammatory cytokine release in lung epithelial cells [16]. EGCG decreased NF-κB activity through hypoacetylation of RelA/p65 by directly inhibiting the activity of HAT [17]. EGCG has also been shown to modulate NF-κB/AP-1 activity in PMA-stimulated mouse epidermal JB6 cells via inactivation of AP-1 [18] and/or NF-κB [19]. Similar to curcumin, green tea polyphenols also modulate myriad inflammatory signaling pathways [9] and therefore a single pathway cannot be assigned to the anti-inflammatory properties of these compounds.

Deacetylases and Inflammation

HDACs remove acetyl moieties from the ε-acetamido group on lysine residues of histones. The resulting deacetylation leads to chromatin condensation and therefore gene silencing. In addition to deacetylation of histones, HDACs can also deacetylate non-histone proteins, such as NF-κB, thus regulating NF-κB-dependent pro-inflammatory gene transcription [20]. Earlier investigations from our laboratory have shown that cigarette smoke-induced reduction in HDAC2 was concomitant to increased levels of total and acetylated RelA/p65 [20, 21]. Furthermore, the study revealed that RelA/p65 interacts with HDAC2 and RelA/p65 is retained in the nucleus, leading to activation of pro-inflammatory gene transcription when HDAC2 is deficient [20, 21]. It is important to note that there is a significant decrement in the expression/activity of HDAC2 in lung parenchyma, bronchial biopsies and alveolar macrophages of COPD patients [22]. Decrease in the expression/activity of HDAC2 negatively correlated with the disease severity and the intensity of lung inflammation [22, 23]. In contrast to increased HAT activity in bronchial biopsies and alveolar macrophages of asthmatics [24], there was no observed alteration in HAT activity in the lungs of COPD subjects [23].

Sirtuins (SIRT) belong to class III HDACs. They were the first to be reported to determine life span in yeast and the nematode. Unlike class I and II deacetylases, sirtuins are NAD^+-dependent and are not inhibited by trichostatin A [25]. Since sirtuins require NAD^+ coming from metabolic reactions, it is hypothesized that sirtuins might act as a molecular link between cellular metabolic status (expressed by the NAD^+/NADH levels) and cellular transcription [26]. The best characterized and studied among the sirtuins is SIRT1, which is activated by polyphenolic compounds such as resveratrol. It is a nuclear deacetylase which primarily but not exclusively deacetylates proteins involved in transcriptional regulation. SIRT1 can therefore influence a wide range of physiological aspects, such as apoptosis/cell survival, autophagy, chromatin remodeling, gene transcription, senescence, endocrine signaling, and differentiation.

HDAC2 and Steroid Resistance
Chronic resistance to glucocorticoids is observed in patients with moderate to severe COPD and in asthmatics who smoke. HDAC2 is an important mediator of glucocorticoid activity and is found to be reduced in lungs of COPD patients and those of rodents exposed to oxidative stress or cigarette smoke. Molecular mechanisms, such as activation of NF-κB and mitogen-activated protein kinase pathways, over-activation AP-1, reduced HDAC2 expression, and increased macrophage migration inhibitory factor have been implicated in onset of glucocorticoid resistance [27].

HDAC2 is required for the anti-inflammatory effects of glucocorticoids in COPD patients. Thus, reduction in the levels/activity of HDAC2 leads to corticosteroid resistance in such patients [22, 28]. Polyphenolic compounds, such as theophylline have been shown to significantly increase HDAC2 activity thereby enhancing dexamethasone-induced suppression of IL-8 release in alveolar macrophage of COPD subjects [29] and exacerbations of COPD patients [30]. Furthermore, the ability of the HDAC2 to deacetylate glucocorticoid receptor (GR) enables GR to associate with RelA/p65, which leads to the attenuation of pro-inflammatory gene transcription [28]. Therefore, therapeutic restoration of HDAC2-dependent deacetylation of RelA/p65 and GR appears to be a good strategy for enhancing glucocorticoid sensitivity.

Sirtuins and Epigenetic Changes
The epigenetic effects of SIRT1 can be appreciated in view of the ability of SIRT1 to deacetylate various transcription factors such as p53, forkhead transcription factor (FOXO), NF-κB, and histone proteins. Some of the physiological phenomena regulated by these transcription factors in response to environmental and toxic challenges include stress resistance, apoptosis, and inflammation [31]. While acetylation of FOXO3 leads to its inactivation, deacetylation by SIRT1 leads to its activation. Therefore, it can be surmised that SIRT1-mediated deacetylation of FOXO3 can induce cell cycle arrest, a phenomena altered in cancer cells. Furthermore, increased transcription of GADD45 (DNA repair system) and MnSOD (reactive oxygen detoxification) is a direct physiological consequence of deacetylation of FOXO3 by SIRT1 [32].

A series of reports have now emphasized the role of SIRT1 in epigenetic regulation of gene expression in cancer cells. Hyperacetylation of H4-K16 and decreased trimethylation of H3-K9 and H4-K20 have been observed after down-regulation of SIRT1 by siRNA in mammalian cells [33]. SIRT1 preferentially deacetylates H4-K16 in vitro [33]. In addition, loss of H4-K16 acetylation and H4-K20 trimethylation has been a hallmark in various tumors and tumor-derived cell lines, suggesting that these modifications may be characteristic epigenetic markers of cancer [34]. Promoter regions of tumor-suppressor genes whose DNA are hypermethylated and are silenced in many types of cancers are characteristic sites of localization of SIRT1 [35]. Such silenced genes were up-regulated in breast and colon cancer sells by down-regulation of SIRT1 levels/activity via increased H4-K16 as well as H3-K9 acetylation in such promoters [35]. Thus SIRT1-mediated epigenetic changes may play an important role in the modulation of various types of cancers and modulation of SIRT1 by polyphenols may serve as a chemopreventive agent.

Modulation of Deacetylases by Dietary Polyphenols

Dietary polyphenols, such as resveratrol, curcumin and catechins are shown to modulate NF-κB activation and chromatin remodeling through modulation of SIRT1 and

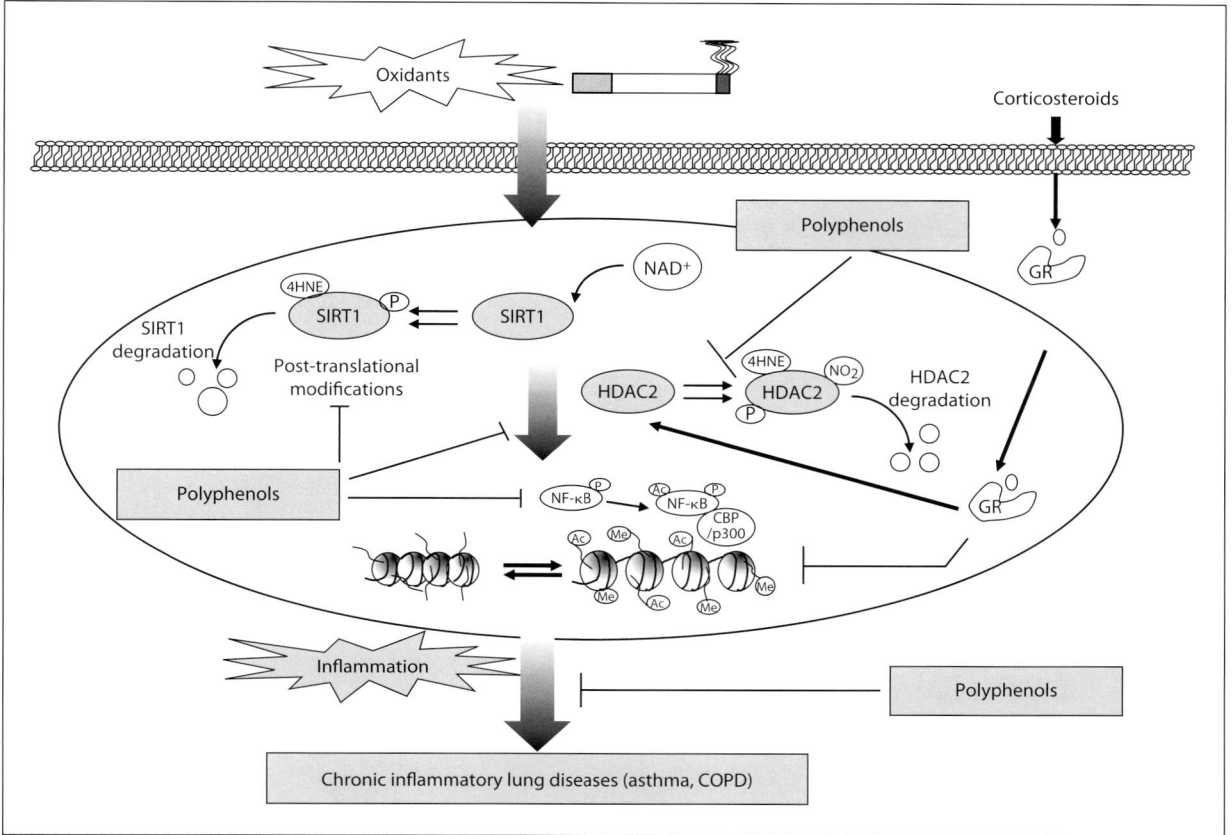

Fig. 2. Regulation of lung inflammation and chromatin remodeling by polyphenols. Dietary polyphenols modulate cigarette smoke and oxidants-mediated human lung inflammation by regulation of histone modifications. Cigarette smoke/oxidants inhibit histone deacetylases, such as SIRT1 and HDAC2 (by post-translational modifications), and/or trigger cellular signaling process leading to histone modifications. These epigenetic changes can cause abnormal activation or silencing of genes subsequent transcriptional repression or activation. Dietary polyphenols inhibit degradation of SIRT1 and HDAC2, and restore glucocorticoid efficacy, culminating in inhibition of chronic inflammatory response in the lung. Ac = acetylated, p = phosphorylated, NO_2 = nitric oxide, GR = glucocorticoid receptor.

HDAC2 activity attenuating inflammatory gene expression in lung epithelium and macrophages (fig. 2). NF-κB (due to intrinsic HAT activity) can lead to acetylation of histones thus causing epigenetic effects.

Modulation of SIRT1
A wide variety of compounds have now been identified, which can inhibit and/or activate sirtuins. Resveratrol, which activates SIRT1, deactivates p53 by significantly inhibiting p53 acetylation or by increased deacetylation of p53 [36] and protects from p53-mediated cellular apoptosis. In addition, resveratrol can also impart protection

against Bax-induced apoptosis by favoring SIRT1-induced formation of Ku70-Bax complex [37]. Resveratrol has also been reported to increase DNA repair capacity and stress resistance by FOXO1/3-dependent expression of GADD43 and p27^{kip1} [38]. Such an effect has also been reported for other sirtuin-activating natural products, such as quercetin. Thus, resveratrol can impart cellular protection via modulating multiple targets.

Alternatively, cancer cells might be targeted using sirtuin inhibitors. These inhibitors induce cell damage by sensitizing the cells to p53-dependent apoptosis [36]. Pharmacological inhibition of SIRT1 decreases cellular resistance to stress and hence promotes cellular apoptosis due to reduced constraint on FOXO3/4 otherwise inhibited by SIRT1 [39]. SIRT1 is known to sensitize tumor cells to TNF-α-induced cell death via inhibiting transactivation of NF-κB [40]. Thus it appears that SIRT1 inhibitors might yield cytoprotective effects by desensitizing the cells to TNF-α and therefore prevent cell death. Recently, it has been shown that SIRT1 activators also inhibit NF-κB-mediated inflammatory mediators release and possibly overcome steroid-resistance in response to oxidative stress [41–43]. Therefore, it can be surmised that modulators of sirtuins might act as novel anti-inflammatory drugs via modulation of NF-κB. Furthermore, reports emerge it is becoming increasingly attractive to consider whether a combination of sirtuin inhibitors and DNA damaging anti-tumor drugs might offer a novel strategy for effective chemotherapeutic cancer therapy.

Modulation of HDACs
Inhibition of HDACs is a new concept in cancer chemoprevention. Of the many HDAC inhibitors known, butyrate, diallyl disulfide, and sulforaphane (SFN) are reported to exhibit anticancer properties [44]. However, in contrast to the traditional HDAC inhibitors, such as trichostatin A or SAHA, which are effective at lower concentrations (nanomolar range), the new range of dietary HDAC inhibitors are required in greater concentrations (micromolar range) [45]. Therefore, it is important to determine whether or not the concentrations of the new class of inhibitors are achieved under normal physiological conditions.

Of all the types of HDAC inhibitors known, butyrate is the smallest in size and can fully fit into the HDAC active site. The inhibitory effect of butyrate is exhibited in vitro between the high micromolar to low millimolar range, which might be achievable in the intestinal tract. The possibility of achievement of such a high concentration within the intestinal tract arises from the fact that colonocytes use butyrate as an oxidative fuel. Diallyl disulfide, found in garlic, is another HDAC inhibitor [46]. In vivo, it is metabolically converted to *S*-allylmercaptocysteine and its structure is similar to butyrate except that it has a 'spacer' ending with a carboxylate group [47]. SFN-cysteine contains a similar spacer and is a metabolite of SFN found in broccoli and broccoli sprouts. In the concentration range 3–15 mM, SFN-cysteine significantly inhibits HDAC activity [48]. In contrast, the parent compound SFN alone had no effect on HDAC activity. However, little is known about the distribution and concentrations of SFN and its active form(s) in different tissues. Although there are many dietary compounds that have HDAC inhibitory properties, more investigations are required in order to understand their bioavailability and the achievable concentrations of these compounds within the body.

Restoration of glucocorticoid function by curcumin is mediated through up-regulation of HDAC2 activity and restoration of HDAC1 and HDAC3 levels [20, 21]. Therefore, polyphenol-dependent redressing of HAT-HDAC imbalance has a significant impact on the epigenome and therefore inflammation, a concept that is corroborated by another report showing the ability of curcumin to inhibit HAT activity at very high concentration (100 mM) and stalling NF-κB-mediated histone acetylation [49]. Alternative mechanisms of polyphenol-mediated inhibition of inflammatory response could be through the reversing post-translational protein modifications of HDAC2 induced by oxidants and reactive aldehydes.

Corticosteroids have been one the major modes of therapy against various respiratory diseases, such as asthma and COPD. Failure of corticosteroids to ameliorate such disease conditions has been attributed to their failure to either recruit HDAC2 and SIRT1 or to the presence of an oxidatively modified HDAC2/SIRT1 in asthmatics and COPD patients. As discussed above, modulation of HDAC2/SIRT1 by dietary polyphenolic compounds may be useful in overcoming the steroid resistance in patients with asthma and COPD.

Conclusions

Epigenetics changes are increasingly believed to modulate the development and progression of many diseases including cancer and chronic respiratory disorders. It is important to understand whether or not a common target is shared by the class I & II HDACs and sirtuins, so that a common therapeutic agent may be designed. Recent reports highlight the pharmacological significance of sirtuin-modulating drugs, and also suggest that identification of substrates specifically targeted by a single class of deacetylases, e.g. SIRT1 would have considerable therapeutic implications in chronic inflammatory diseases.

There are emerging reports that epigenetic alterations might be associated with chronic lung diseases. Recent advances in asthma and COPD research have suggested that epigenetic mechanisms, such as genomic imprinting, histone modification, DNA methylation of regulatory sequences other genes, and regulation by microRNA may also contribute to the susceptibility and complexity of the disease (including in utero) and hence dietary polyphenols may play a pivotal role in regulating these epigenetic modifications. The anti-inflammatory property of curcumin, resveratrol, and catechins may be due to their ability to induce HDAC2 activity and thereby restore the efficacy of glucocorticoids or overcome its resistance. Thus, regulation of inflammation by dietary polyphenols is potential therapeutic value against chronic inflammatory epigenetically-regulated diseases.

Acknowledgments

Supported by the NIH-NHLBI grants RO1-HL-085613, RO1-HL-097751-01, and NIEHS Environmental Health Sciences Center Grant ES-01247.

References

1 Aggarwal BB, Shishodia S: Suppression of the nuclear factor-kappaB activation pathway by spice-derived phytochemicals: reasoning for seasoning. Ann NY Acad Sci 2004;1030:434–441.
2 Biswas SK, McClure D, Jimenez LA, Megson IL, Rahman I: Curcumin induces glutathione biosynthesis and inhibits NF-kappaB activation and interleukin-8 release in alveolar epithelial cells: mechanism of free radical scavenging activity. Antioxid Redox Signal 2005;7:32–41.
3 Rahman I, Biswas SK, Kirkham PA: Regulation of inflammation and redox signaling by dietary polyphenols. Biochem Pharmacol 2006;72:1439–1452.
4 Sovak M: Grape extract, resveratrol, and its analogs: a review. J Med Food 2001;4:93–105.
5 Birrell MA, McCluskie K, Wong S, et al: Resveratrol, an extract of red wine, inhibits lipopolysaccharide induced airway neutrophilia and inflammatory mediators through an NF-kappaB-independent mechanism. FASEB J 2005;19:840–841.
6 Donnelly LE, Newton R, Kennedy GE, et al: Anti-inflammatory effects of resveratrol in lung epithelial cells: molecular mechanisms. Am J Physiol Lung Cell Mol Physiol 2004;287:L774–L783.
7 Manna SK, Mukhopadhyay A, Aggarwal BB: Resveratrol suppresses TNF-induced activation of nuclear transcription factors NF-kappa B activator protein-1, and apoptosis: potential role of reactive oxygen intermediates and lipid peroxidation. J Immunol 2000;164:6509–6519.
8 Leiro J, Arranz JA, Fraiz N, et al: Effect of cis-resveratrol on genes involved in nuclear factor kappa B signaling. Int Immunopharmacol 2005;5:393–406.
9 Biesalski HK: Polyphenols and inflammation: basic interactions. Curr Opin Clin Nutr Metab Care 2007;10:724–728.
10 Yang YT, Weng CT, Ho CT, Yen GC: Resveratrol analog-3,5,4'-trimethoxy-trans-stilbene inhibits invasion of human lung adenocarcinoma cells by suppressing the MAPK pathway and decreasing matrix metalloproteinase-2 expression. Mol Nutr Food Res 2009;53:407–416.
11 Venkatesan B, Ghosh-Choudhury N, Das F, et al: Resveratrol inhibits PDGF receptor mitogenic signaling in mesangial cells: role of PTP1B. FASEB J 2008;22:3469–3482.
12 Aggarwal BB, Kumar A, Bharti AC: Anticancer potential of curcumin: preclinical and clinical studies. Anticancer Res 2003;23:363–398.
13 Shishodia S, Potdar P, Gairola CG, Aggarwal BB: Curcumin (diferuloylmethane) down-regulates cigarette smoke-induced NF-kappaB activation through inhibition of IkappaBalpha kinase in human lung epithelial cells: correlation with suppression of COX-2 MMP-9 and cyclin D1. Carcinogenesis 2003;24:1269–1279.
14 Duvoix A, Blasius R, Delhalle S, et al: Chemopreventive and therapeutic effects of curcumin. Cancer Lett 2005;223:181–190.
15 Beecher GR: Overview of dietary flavonoids: nomenclature occurrence and intake. J Nutr 2003;133:3248S–3254S.
16 Syed DN, Afaq F, Kweon MH, et al: Green tea polyphenol EGCG suppresses cigarette smoke condensate-induced NF-kappaB activation in normal human bronchial epithelial cells. Oncogene 2007;26:673–682.
17 Choi KC, Jung MG, Lee YH, et al: Epigallocatechin-3-gallate a histone acetyltransferase inhibitor inhibits EBV-induced B lymphocyte transformation via suppression of RelA acetylation. Cancer Res 2009;69:583–592.
18 Dong Z, Ma W, Huang C, Yang CS: Inhibition of tumor promoter-induced activator protein 1 activation and cell transformation by tea polyphenols, (-)-epigallocatechin gallate, and theaflavins. Cancer Res 1997;57:4414–4419.

19 Nomura M, Ma W, Chen N, Bode AM, Dong Z: Inhibition of 12-O-tetradecanoylphorbol-13-acetate-induced NF-kappaB activation by tea polyphenols (-)-epigallocatechin gallate and theaflavins. Carcinogenesis 2000;21:1885–1890.

20 Yang SR, Chida AS, Bauter MR, et al: Cigarette smoke induces proinflammatory cytokine release by activation of NF-kappaB and posttranslational modifications of histone deacetylase in macrophages. Am J Physiol Lung Cell Mol Physiol 2006; 291:L46–L57.

21 Meja KK, Rajendrasozhan S, Adenuga D, et al: Curcumin restores corticosteroid function in monocytes exposed to oxidants by maintaining HDAC2. Am J Respir Cell Mol Biol 2008;39:312–323.

22 Ito K, Ito M, Elliott WM, et al: Decreased histone deacetylase activity in chronic obstructive pulmonary disease. N Engl J Med 2005;352:1967–1976.

23 Adenuga D, Yao H, March TH, Seagrave J, Rahman I: Histone deacetylase 2 is phosphorylated, ubiquitinated, and degraded by cigarette smoke. Am J Respir Cell Mol Biol 2009;40:464–473.

24 Barnes PJ, Adcock IM, Ito K: Histone acetylation and deacetylation: importance in inflammatory lung diseases. Eur Respir J 2005;25:552–563.

25 Imai S, Armstrong CM, Kaeberlein M, Guarente L: Transcriptional silencing and longevity protein Sir2 is an NAD-dependent histone deacetylase. Nature 2000;403:795–800.

26 Bordone L, Guarente L: Calorie restriction, SIRT1 and metabolism: understanding longevity. Nat Rev Mol Cell Biol 2005;6:298–305.

27 Barnes PJ, Adcock IM: Glucocorticoid resistance in inflammatory diseases. Lancet 2009;373:1905–1917.

28 Ito K, Yamamura S, Essilfie-Quaye S, et al: Histone deacetylase 2-mediated deacetylation of the glucocorticoid receptor enables NF-kappaB suppression J Exp Med 2006;203:7–13.

29 Cosio BG, Tsaprouni L, Ito K, et al: Theophylline restores histone deacetylase activity and steroid responses in COPD macrophages. J Exp Med 2004; 200:689–695.

30 Cosio BG, Iglesias A, Rios A, et al: Low-dose theophylline enhances the anti-inflammatory effects of steroids during exacerbations of COPD. Thorax 2009;64:424–429.

31 Yang T, Sauve AA: NAD metabolism and sirtuins: metabolic regulation of protein deacetylation in stress and toxicity. AAPS J 2006;8:E632–E643.

32 Kobayashi Y, Furukawa-Hibi Y, Chen C, et al: SIRT1 is critical regulator of FOXO-mediated transcription in response to oxidative stress. Int J Mol Med 2005;16:237–243.

33 Vaquero A, Scher M, Lee D, et al: Human SirT1 interacts with histone H1 and promotes formation of facultative heterochromatin. Mol Cell 2004;16:93–105.

34 Fraga MF, Ballestar E, Villar-Garea A, et al: Loss of acetylation at Lys16 and trimethylation at Lys20 of histone H4 is a common hallmark of human cancer. Nat Genet 2005;37:391–400.

35 Pruitt K, Zinn RL, Ohm JE, et al: Inhibition of SIRT1 reactivates silenced cancer genes without loss of promoter DNA hypermethylation. PLoS Genet 2006;2:e40

36 Howitz KT, Bitterman KJ, Cohen HY, et al: Small molecule activators of sirtuins extend *Saccharomyces cerevisiae* lifespan. Nature 2003;425:191–196.

37 Cohen HY, Miller C, Bitterman KJ, et al: Calorie restriction promotes mammalian cell survival by inducing the SIRT1 deacetylase. Science 2004;305:390–392.

38 Daitoku H, Hatta M, Matsuzaki H, et al: Silent information regulator 2 potentiates Foxo1-mediated transcription through its deacetylase activity. Proc Natl Acad Sci USA 2004;101:10042–10047.

39 Brunet A, Sweeney LB, Sturgill JF, et al: Stress-dependent regulation of FOXO transcription factors by the SIRT1 deacetylase. Science 2004;303:2011–2015.

40 Yeung F, Hoberg JE, Ramsey CS, et al: Modulation of NF-kappaB-dependent transcription and cell survival by the SIRT1 deacetylase. Embo J 2004;23:2369–2380.

41 Nakamaru Y, Vuppusetty C, Wada H, et al: A protein deacetylase SIRT1 is a negative regulator of metalloproteinase-9. FASEB J 2009;23:2810–2819.

42 Rajendrasozhan S, Yang SR, Kinnula VL, Rahman I: SIRT1 an antiinflammatory and antiaging protein is decreased in lungs of patients with chronic obstructive pulmonary disease. Am J Respir Crit Care Med 2008;177:861–870.

43 Yang SR, Wright J, Bauter M, et al: Sirtuin regulates cigarette smoke-induced proinflammatory mediator release via RelA/p65 NF-kappaB in macrophages in vitro and in rat lungs in vivo: implications for chronic inflammation and aging. Am J Physiol Lung Cell Mol Physiol 2007;292:L567–L576.

44 Myzak MC, Dashwood RH: Histone deacetylases as targets for dietary cancer preventive agents: lessons learned with butyrate diallyl disulfide and sulforaphane. Curr Drug Targets 2006;7:443–452.

45 Dashwood RH, Myzak MC, Ho E: Dietary HDAC inhibitors: time to rethink weak ligands in cancer chemoprevention? Carcinogenesis 2006;27:344–349.

46 Druesne N, Pagniez A, Mayeur C, et al: Diallyl disulfide (DADS) increases histone acetylation and p21(waf1/cip1) expression in human colon tumor cell lines Carcinogenesis 2004;25:1227–1236.

47 Guyonnet D, Bergès R, Siess MH, et al: Post-initiation modulating effects of allyl sulfides in rat hepatocarcinogenesis. Food Chem Toxicol 2004;42:1479–1485.

48 Myzak MC, Karplus PA, Chung FL, Dashwood RH: A novel mechanism of chemoprotection by sulforaphane: inhibition of histone deacetylase. Cancer Res 2004;64:5767–5774.

49 Kang J, Chen J, Shi Y, Jia J, Zhang Y: Curcumin-induced histone hypoacetylation: the role of reactive oxygen species. Biochem Pharmacol 2005;69:1205–1213.

Irfan Rahman, PhD
Department of Environmental Medicine, Lung Biology and Disease Program
University of Rochester Medical Center
Box 850, 601 Elmwood Ave
Rochester, NY 14642 (USA)
Tel. +1 585 275 6911, Fax +1 585 276 0239, E-Mail irfan_rahman@urmc.rochester.edu

Dietary Manipulation of Histone Structure and Function

Emily Ho[a,b] · Roderick H. Dashwood[b,c]

[a]Department of Nutrition and Exercise Sciences, [b]Linus Pauling Institute, [c]Department of Environmental and Molecular Toxicology, Oregon State University, Corvallis, Oreg., USA

Epigenetics is the study of the regulation of gene activity that is not dependent on nucleotide sequence; this may include heritable changes in gene activity and expression, but also long-term alterations in the transcriptional potential of a cell that are not heritable. These features are potentially reversible and may affect genomic stability and expression of genes. In recent years, great strides have been made in understanding the many molecular sequences and patterns that determine which genes can be turned on and off. This work has made it increasingly clear that in addition to genetic changes, the epigenome is just as critical as the DNA sequence itself for healthy human development. Importantly, dietary factors and specific nutrients can modulate epigenetic alterations and alter susceptibility to disease. As the field of epigenetics grows, a whole new level of thinking has emerged as to the impact of nutrients on regulation of gene expression and disease susceptibility. For example, the classic view of cancer etiology is that genetic alterations (via genotoxic agents) damage DNA structure and induce mutations resulting in non-functional proteins that lead to disease progression. Aberrant epigenetic events such as DNA hypermethylation and altered histone acetylation have been observed in cancer. To control histone acetylation, a balance exists in normal cells between histone acetyltransferase and histone deacetylase (HDAC) activities, and when this balance is disrupted, cancer development can ensue. HDAC activity increases in metastatic cells compared with normal prostate, and global changes in acetylation pattern predict prostate cancer risk and recurrence [1]. Targeting the epigenome, including the use of HDAC and DNA methyltransferase (DNMT) inhibitors, is an evolving strategy for cancer chemoprevention and both have shown promise in cancer clinical trials [2]. Essential micronutrients such as biotin, B_{12} and folate, and phytochemicals such as sulforaphane and allyl compounds can impact epigenetic events as a novel mechanism of action. This chapter highlights the interactions among nutrients, epigenetics and cancer susceptibility. In particular, we focus on the impact of specific nutrients and food components, such as sulforaphane, on histone modifications that can alter gene expression and influence cancer progression.

Use of Histone Deacetylase Inhibitors in Cancer Prevention

Post-translational modifications to histone proteins have been linked to the transcriptional status of chromatin. Modifications of histones include, but are not limited to, phosphorylation, biotinylation, methylation and acetylation. The reversible acetylation of nuclear histones is one of the better characterized histone modifications and is an important mechanism of gene regulation. In general, addition of acetyl groups to histones by histone acetyltransferase enzymes results in an 'open' chromatin conformation, facilitating gene expression by allowing transcription factors access to DNA. Removal of acetyl groups by HDACs results in a 'closed' conformation, which represses transcription. The HDACs can be divided into 4 classes based on their structure and sequence homology: class I consists of HDACs 1, 2, 3 and 8; class II includes HDACs 4, 5, 6, 7, 9 and 10; class III enzymes comprise the NAD-dependent Sir2-related proteins, and class IV contains HDAC11. Class I and II HDACs belong to the classical HDACs and their activities are inhibited by trichostatin A. Class III HDACs are homologous to the yeast Sir2 deacetylases and are a family of proteins classified as sirtuins that are not affected by trichostatin A. Class I HDACs are homologous to the yeast Rpd3 and are primarily found in nuclear complexes. Class II HDACs are homologous to the yeast protein Hda1, and are capable of translocating in and out of the nucleus. In addition to histone core proteins, several non-histone proteins have been identified that are targeted, especially by class II HDAC enzymes. Targets include cellular proteins such as transcription factors (e.g. p53, androgen receptor, NF-κB), structural (e.g. tubulin) and chaperone proteins (e.g. hsp90), to name a few. Thus, the effects of HDAC inhibitors may be attributed to mechanisms that involve both direct chromatin remodeling and specific modifications to other (non-histone) proteins. When dealing with agents that effect both histone and non-histone acetylation status, the term 'KDAC' has been proposed for 'lysine deacetylase' inhibitors (the letter 'K' being the biochemical abbreviation for lysine).

Increased HDAC activity and expression is common in many cancer malignancies, and can result in repression of transcription that results in a deregulation of differentiation status, cell cycle checkpoint controls and apoptotic mechanisms. Moreover, tumor suppressor genes, such as *p21* appear to be targets of HDACs and are 'turned off' by deacetylation. Prostate cancer cells also exhibit aberrant acetylation patterns. In human patient samples, global decreases in histone acetylation state corresponded with increased grade of cancer and risk of prostate cancer recurrence [1]. Importantly, inhibitors of HDAC, including suberoylanilide hydroxamic acid (SAHA), valproic acid, depsipeptide, and sodium butyrate have been demonstrated to be effective against prostate cancer cell lines and xenograft models [3, 4]. Specific genes associated with prostate cancer, such as tubulin, coxsackie and adenovirus receptor, liver cancer-1 (DLC-1) and KLF-6, have also shown to be hypoacetylated and repressed in prostate cancers [5–7]. The use of class I and II HDAC inhibitors in cancer chemoprevention and therapy has gained significant interest. Several ongoing clinical trials are attempting to establish the chemotherapeutic efficacy of HDAC inhibitors, based on evidence that cancer cells undergo cell cycle arrest, differentiation and apoptosis in vitro, and that tumor volume and/or number may be reduced in animal models. HDAC inhibitors have been shown to increase global acetylation as well as acetylation associated with specific gene promoters. Although the equilibrium is shifted toward greater histone acetylation after treatment with HDAC inhibitors, the expression of only a relatively small number of genes is altered in an upward or downward direction [8]. Importantly, only neoplastically transformed cells appear to respond to increased acetylation by undergoing differentiation, cell cycle arrest or apoptosis; normal cells, despite the increased acetylation, do not respond in this manner to HDAC inhibitors [9]. Thus, effects of HDAC inhibitors on apoptosis and anti-proliferation appear to be selective to cancer, not normal cells, although the mechanism is poorly understood. In general, HDAC inhibitors have been subdivided into several classifications: short chain fatty acids, hydroxamic acids, cyclic tetrapeptides, and benzamides [10, 11]. Most have a conserved structure and act by blocking the HDAC catalytic site. Many of these pharmacological HDAC inhibitors have been used in phase I and I/II clinical trials, with promising results [12]. However, many of these compounds also exhibit several associated side-effects and toxicities. For example, valproic acid and trichostatin A have been associated with developmental abnormalities such as neural tube defects [13]. The use of SAHA has also been associated with several hematologic toxicities such as myelosuppression and thrombocytopenia [14]. Many of these drugs must also be administered i.v., a less than ideal route of administration for patients. Although there has been some attempt to develop oral HDAC inhibitor drugs, these also have side-effects such as fatigue, anorexia, dehydration and GI upset [14, 15]. The identification of HDAC inhibitors, with low toxicity but therapeutic efficacy, is an important area of research.

Dietary Inhibitors of Histone Deacetylases

Recent studies also suggest that sulforaphane (SFN), an isothiocyanate derived from cruciferous vegetables, is an inhibitor of HDAC activity and offers protection against tumor development during the 'post-initiation' phase of carcinogenesis. The general structure of HDAC inhibitors is comprised of a functional group at one end that interacts with a zinc atom and neighboring amino acids at the base of the HDAC active site, a spacer that fits into the channel of the active site, and a cap group which is hypothesized to interact with external amino acid residues [16, 17]. Based on the similarity of SFN metabolites to the conserved structure of HDAC inhibitors, we hypothesized that SFN could effectively inhibit HDAC activity. SFN is metabolized via the mercapturic acid pathway, starting with glutathione conjugation by glutathione-S-transferase (GST). Subsequent steps generate SFN-cysteine (SFN-Cys) followed by SFN-N-acetylcysteine. Based on modeling and in vitro work [18–20], it has been hypothesized that SFN-N-acetylcysteine or SFN-cysteine are the active HDAC inhibitors. This was supported by metabolite studies, showing significant levels of SFN-cysteine generated in SFN-treated prostate cancer cells [Clark J, Ho E, unpubl data]. Molecular modeling in the active site of an HDAC enzyme provided evidence that SFN-cysteine docked in the HDAC pocket as a competitive inhibitor [21]. In BPH1, PC3 and LnCap prostate cancer cells, SFN inhibited HDAC activity with a concomitant increase in global histone acetylation, increased acetylated histone H4 interactions with the *P21* and *Bax* promoter, and induced p21 and Bax mRNA and protein levels [22]. SFN also decreased the expression of HDAC6, a class II HDAC and induced concomitant increases in acetyl-tubulin levels [unpubl. data]. HDAC inhibition coincided with the induction of G_2/M phase cell cycle arrest and apoptosis, as indicated by multi-caspase activation [22]. HDAC inhibition by SFN has also been established in several other cancer cell lines, including breast and colon [21, 23], suggesting the effects are not specific to the prostate. In HCT116 human colorectal cancer cells treated with SFN there were decreases in HDAC activity, increased global histone acetylation, and a selective increase in histone acetylation at the *p21* promoter [21]. HT29 colon cancer cells, which lack endogenous Nrf2 protein, as well as $Nrf2^{-/-}$ mouse embryonic fibroblasts, both exhibited an HDAC inhibitory response to SFN treatment. These results indicated the possibility of a separate SFN chemoprevention pathway distinct from the classic Nrf2 pathway [24]. Importantly, the effects of SFN do appear to be tumor cell specific. We have found that 3–15 μM SFN induces potent HDAC inhibition and G_2/M arrest in PC3 cancer cells, but have no effect on normal prostate epithelial cells [unpubl. data]. These data support the hypothesis that HDAC inhibition may be an important mechanism of chemoprevention for SFN and similar pharmacological HDAC inhibitors, the cytotoxic effects are specific to cancer, not normal cells.

In vivo, dietary SFN supplementation resulted in slower tumor growth and significant HDAC inhibition in the PC3 xenografts, as well as HDAC inhibition in the prostate and circulating peripheral blood mononuclear cells [25]. In other dietary studies examining intestinal cancer, Apc^{min} mice were fed ~6 μmol SFN per day for 10 weeks. In these experiments a significant decrease in intestinal polyps and an increase in global acetylated histones H3 and H4 were observed, with specific increases at the *Bax* and *p21* promoters [26]. From these studies it can be concluded that HDAC inhibition represents a novel chemoprevention mechanism by which SFN might promote cell cycle arrest and apoptosis in vivo. To date very few human clinical trials have evaluated the effects of SFN on cancer outcome; however, several pilot and phase I human SFN trials have been conducted utilizing different sources of SFN. In our laboratory, a small intervention study was performed to determine if the HDAC inhibition effects observed in cell culture and mice could be translated into humans. In clinical trials using pharmacological HDAC inhibitors such as SAHA, alterations in acetylated histone status in peripheral blood cell samples are used as a biomarker for HDAC inhibitory efficacy. In normal healthy volunteers, after the ingestion of 68 g of broccoli sprouts, a significant decrease in HDAC activity was evident in peripheral blood mononuclear cells with a concomitant increase in acetylated histones H3 and H4 [25]. Broccoli sprouts are a rich source of glucoraphanin, the precursor of SFN; thus, these data give preliminary evidence for the ability of dietary SFN to inhibit HDAC activity in humans. Follow-up studies will examine the relationship between specific SFN metabolites in the circulation and HDAC inhibition.

In addition to SFN, there are many other known and putative diet-derived HDAC inhibitors. Experiments with structurally related isothiocyanates such as sulforaphene, erucin and phenylbutyl isothiocyanate, had comparable HDAC inhibitory activities [20]. Butyrate is the smallest known HDAC inhibitor [reviewed in 27], and contains a simple 3-carbon 'spacer' attached to a carboxylic acid group. This compound is derived from the fermentation of dietary fiber and represents the primary metabolic fuel for the colonocytes, where it is present at millimolar concentrations. Recent studies have confirmed that butyrate acts as a competitive HDAC inhibitor [28]. A second class of dietary agents reported to inhibit HDAC activity in vitro is the garlic organosulfur compounds, such as DADS and *S*-allylmercaptocysteine [29], which can be metabolized to allyl mercaptan, a competitive HDAC inhibitor [29]. Treatment of human colon cancer cells with allyl mercaptan induced rapid histone acetylation along with HDAC inhibition, resulting in increased association of acetylated histones and Sp3 transcription factor binding to the promoter element of *P21Waf1*, thereby increasing both p21 mRNA and protein expression and triggering cell cycle arrest [30]. More recently, α-keto acid metabolites of organoselenium compounds have also been identified as novel HDAC inhibitors in both colon and prostate cancer cells. In particular, the metabolite methylselenopyruvate caused HDAC inhibition, increases in acetylated histone and p21 promoter activity, and concomitant increases in apoptosis and cell cycle arrest at concentrations as low as 2 μM [31, 32].

Future Directions and Conclusions

In addition to histone modifications, methylation of CpG islands in promoter elements is a major epigenetic controlling event for gene silencing [33–35]. In fact, transcriptional silencing by aberrant hypermethylation of CpG islands has been reported in nearly every tumor type [36, 37]. Many of the commonly silenced genes include tumor-suppressor genes and genes involved in carcinogen detoxification, hormonal responses and cell cycle control [37–40]. Both DNA hypermethylation and histone modifications are closely related aspects of chromatin remodeling. Epigenetic control of gene expression often requires the cooperation and interaction of both mechanisms, and disruption in these processes can lead to genomic instability and gene silencing, resulting in cancer progression. Interestingly, DNMT1 also appears to direct histone modifications by recruiting HDACs [41]. Methylation of CpG sequences by DNMT1 binds specific methylated DNA binding (MBD) proteins such as MeCP2 and MBD2. This MBD binding complex recruits a complex of transcriptional repressors, including HDACs, which results in chromatin-associated gene silencing [42, 43]. This relationship between DNA methylation and chromatin remodeling suggests significant cross-talk among distinct epigenetic pathways that control gene silencing/unsilencing. Indeed, the combination of pharmacological DNMT inhibitors and HDAC inhibitors has been explored as a potential anti-tumor therapy [44, 45]. However, DNMT inhibitor drugs have potential hazards and side effects because they often require incorporation into DNA, thereby targeting cells dividing in S phase, leading to greater toxicity [46, 47]. Recently, dietary agents that have dual action of promoter methylation and HDAC inhibition have been identified. Phenethyl isothiocyanate (PEITC), an isothiocyanate related to SFN and which is found in cruciferous vegetables such as watercress, was shown to reverse hypermethylation of *GSTP1* promoter elements in androgen-dependent and androgen-independent prostate cancer cells. Concurrent with demethylation effects, phenethyl isothiocyanate (2–5 µM) inhibited HDAC activity and increase acetylated histone status. At the doses tested, phenethyl isothiocyanate was more effective towards promoter demethylation and HDAC inhibition than chemical DNMT and HDAC inhibitors, 5-aza and trichostatin A [48]. Different epigenetic modifications clearly appear to work together to coordinate and maintain gene expression patterns in the cell. Further work examining the possible cross-talk between various epigenetic modifications after exposure to dietary epigenetic modulators appears to be warranted.

Overall, the identification of dietary agents that target HDAC and/or DNA methylation with few side effects is an important area of research [reviewed in 20, 49, 50], and aligns with the National Institutes of Health's Roadmap priority area on 'epigenetics'. Many of these dietary agents have multiple actions on various pathways during carcinogenesis, and their ability to target several mechanisms, including epigenetic targets, may increase their efficacy as chemoprevention agents. Further, the use of dietary strategies to inhibit HDACs or other epigenetic modifiers as chemoprevention agents is significant because of the ease of implementation into clinical trials, due to their relatively non-toxic nature. Ultimately, these types of study have the potential to decrease prevalence of various cancers and/or increase survival through simple dietary choices, such as incorporating easily accessible foods into a patient's diet.

Acknowledgments

This work was supported in part by the Oregon Agricultural Experiment Station, supported in part by funds provided through the Hatch Act. Additional support was provided by NIH grants CA090890, CA065525, CA122906, CA122959 and the Environmental Health Sciences Center (National Institute of Environmental Health Sciences) P30 ES00210.

References

1 Seligson DB, Horvath S, Shi T, et al: Global histone modification patterns predict risk of prostate cancer recurrence. Nature 2005;435:1262–1266.
2 Sigalotti L, Fratta E, Coral S, et al: Epigenetic drugs as pleiotropic agents in cancer treatment: biomolecular aspects and clinical applications. J Cell Physiol 2007;212:330–344.
3 Fronsdal K, Saatcioglu F: Histone deacetylase inhibitors differentially mediate apoptosis in prostate cancer cells. Prostate 2005;62:299–306.
4 Butler LM, Agus DB, Scher HI, et al: Suberoylanilide hydroxamic acid, an inhibitor of histone deacetylase, suppresses the growth of prostate cancer cells in vitro and in vivo. Cancer Res 2000;60:5165–5170.
5 Li D, Yea S, Dolios G, et al: Regulation of Kruppel-like factor 6 tumor suppressor activity by acetylation. Cancer Res 2005;65:9216–9225.
6 Guan M, Zhou X, Soulitzis N, Spandidos DA, Popescu NC: Aberrant methylation and deacetylation of deleted in liver cancer-1 gene in prostate cancer: potential clinical applications. Clin Cancer Res 2006;12:1412–9.
7 Soucek K, Kamaid A, Phung AD, et al: Normal and prostate cancer cells display distinct molecular profiles of alpha-tubulin posttranslational modifications. Prostate 2006;66:954–965.
8 Mitsiades CS, Mitsiades NS, McMullan CJ, et al: Transcriptional signature of histone deacetylase inhibition in multiple myeloma: biological and clinical implications. Proc Natl Acad Sci USA 2004;101:540–545.
9 Brinkmann H, Dahler AL, Popa C, et al: Histone hyperacetylation induced by histone deacetylase inhibitors is not sufficient to cause growth inhibition in human dermal fibroblasts. J Biol Chem 2001;276:22491–22499.
10 Vannini A, Volpari C, Filocamo G, et al: Crystal structure of a eukaryotic zinc-dependent histone deacetylase, human HDAC8, complexed with a hydroxamic acid inhibitor. Proc Natl Acad Sci USA 2004;101:15064–15069.
11 Balasubramanian S, Verner E, Buggy JJ: Isoform-specific histone deacetylase inhibitors: the next step? Cancer Lett 2009;280:211–221.
12 Garcia-Manero G, Issa JP: Histone deacetylase inhibitors: a review of their clinical status as antineoplastic agents. Cancer Invest 2005;23:635–642.
13 Wiltse J: Mode of action: inhibition of histone deacetylase, altering WNT-dependent gene expression, and regulation of beta-catenin: developmental effects of valproic acid. Crit Rev Toxicol 2005;35:727–738.
14 O'Connor OA, Heaney ML, Schwartz L, et al: Clinical experience with intravenous and oral formulations of the novel histone deacetylase inhibitor suberoylanilide hydroxamic acid in patients with advanced hematologic malignancies. J Clin Oncol 2006;24:166–173.
15 Kelly WK, O'Connor OA, Krug LM, et al: Phase I study of an oral histone deacetylase inhibitor, suberoylanilide hydroxamic acid, in patients with advanced cancer. J Clin Oncol 2005;23:3923–3931.
16 Finnin MS, Donigian JR, Cohen A, et al: Structures of a histone deacetylase homologue bound to the TSA and SAHA inhibitors. Nature 1999;401:188–93.
17 Furumai R, Komatsu Y, Nishino N, et al: Potent histone deacetylase inhibitors built from trichostatin A and cyclic tetrapeptide antibiotics including trapoxin. Proc Natl Acad Sci USA 2001;98:87–92.
18 Dashwood RH, Ho E: Dietary histone deacetylase inhibitors: from cells to mice to man. Semin Cancer Biol 2007;17:363–369.
19 Myzak MC, Karplus PA, Chung F-L, Dashwood RH: A novel mechanism of chemoprotection by sulforaphane: inhibition of histone deacetylase. Cancer Res 2004;64:5767–5774.
20 Myzak MC, Ho E, Dashwood RH: Dietary agents as histone deacetylase inhibitors. Mol Carcinog 2006;45:443–446.
21 Myzak MC, Karplus PA, Chung FL, Dashwood RH: A novel mechanism of chemoprotection by sulforaphane: inhibition of histone deacetylase. Cancer Res 2004;64:5767–5774.
22 Myzak MC, Hardin K, Wang R, Dashwood RH, Ho E: Sulforaphane inhibits histone deacetylase activity in BPH-1, LnCaP and PC-3 prostate epithelial cells. Carcinogenesis 2006;27:811–819.
23 Pledgie-Tracy A, Sobolewski MD, Davidson NE: Sulforaphane induces cell type-specific apoptosis in human breast cancer cell lines. Mol Cancer Ther 2007;6:1013–1021.
24 Dashwood RH, Ho E: Dietary histone deacetylase inhibitors: from cells to mice to man. Semin Cancer Biol 2007;17:363–369.
25 Myzak MC, Tong P, Dashwood WM, Dashwood RH, Ho E: Sulforaphane retards the growth of human PC-3 xenografts and inhibits HDAC activity in human subjects. Exp Biol Med (Maywood) 2007;232:227–234.
26 Myzak MC, Dashwood WM, Orner GA, Ho E, Dashwood RH: Sulforaphane inhibits histone deacetylase in vivo and suppresses tumorigenesis in Apc-minus mice. Faseb J 2006;20:506–508.
27 Davie JR: Inhibition of histone deacetylase activity by butyrate. J Nutr 2003;133:2485S–2493S.

28 Sekhavat A, Sun JM, Davie JR: Competitive inhibition of histone deacetylase activity by trichostatin A and butyrate. Biochem Cell Biol 2007;85:751–758.
29 Druesne N, Pagniez A, Mayeur C, et al.: Diallyl disulfide (DADS) increases histone acetylation and p21(waf1/cip1) expression in human colon tumor cell lines. Carcinogenesis 2004;25:1227–1236.
30 Nian H, Delage B, Pinto JT, Dashwood RH: Allyl mercaptan, a garlic-derived organosulfur compound, inhibits histone deacetylase and enhances Sp3 binding on the P21WAF1 promoter. Carcinogenesis 2008;29:1816–1824.
31 Lee JI, Nian H, Cooper AJ, et al: Alpha-keto acid metabolites of naturally occurring organoselenium compounds as inhibitors of histone deacetylase in human prostate cancer cells. Cancer Prev Res 2009; 2:683–693.
32 Nian H, Bisson WH, Dashwood WM, Pinto JT, Dashwood RH: Alpha-keto acid metabolites of organoselenium compounds inhibit histone deacetylase activity in human colon cancer cells. Carcinogenesis 2009;30:1416–1423.
33 Turker MS, Bestor TH: Formation of methylation patterns in the mammalian genome. Mutat Res 1997;386:119–130.
34 Jones PA, Baylin SB: The fundamental role of epigenetic events in cancer. Nat Rev Genet 2002;3:415–428.
35 Wolffe AP, Matzke MA: Epigenetics: regulation through repression. Science 1999;286:481–486.
36 Baylin SB: DNA methylation and gene silencing in cancer. Nat Clin Pract Oncol 2005;2(suppl 1):S4–S11.
37 Baylin SB, Esteller M, Rountree MR, et al: Aberrant patterns of DNA methylation, chromatin formation and gene expression in cancer. Hum Mol Genet 2001;10:687–692.
38 Herman JG, Baylin SB: Gene silencing in cancer in association with promoter hypermethylation. N Engl J Med 2003;349:2042–2054.
39 Baylin SB, Ohm JE: Epigenetic gene silencing in cancer: a mechanism for early oncogenic pathway addiction? Nat Rev Cancer 2006;6:107–116.
40 Li LC, Carroll PR, Dahiya R: Epigenetic changes in prostate cancer: implication for diagnosis and treatment. J Natl Cancer Inst 2005;97:103–115.
41 Dobosy JR, Selker EU: Emerging connections between DNA methylation and histone acetylation. Cell Mol Life Sci 2001;58:721–727.
42 Ng HH, Zhang Y, Hendrich B, et al: MBD2 is a transcriptional repressor belonging to the MeCP1 histone deacetylase complex. Nat Genet 1999;23:58–61.
43 Fuks F, Burgers WA, Brehm A, Hughes-Davies L, Kouzarides T: DNA methyltransferase Dnmt1 associates with histone deacetylase activity. Nat Genet 2000;24:88–91.
44 Gore SD, Baylin S, Sugar E, et al: Combined DNA methyltransferase and histone deacetylase inhibition in the treatment of myeloid neoplasms. Cancer Res 2006;66:6361–6369.
45 Cameron EE, Bachman KE, Myohanen S, Herman JG, Baylin SB: Synergy of demethylation and histone deacetylase inhibition in the re-expression of genes silenced in cancer. Nat Genet 1999;21:103–107.
46 Ghoshal K, Bai S: DNA methyltransferases as targets for cancer therapy. Drugs Today (Barc) 2007; 43:395–422.
47 Juttermann R, Li E, Jaenisch R: Toxicity of 5-aza-2'-deoxycytidine to mammalian cells is mediated primarily by covalent trapping of DNA methyltransferase rather than DNA demethylation. Proc Natl Acad Sci USA 1994;91:11797–11801.
48 Wang LG, Beklemisheva A, Liu XM, et al: Dual action on promoter demethylation and chromatin by an isothiocyanate restored GSTP1 silenced in prostate cancer. Mol Carcinog 2007;46:24–31.
49 Myzak MC, Dashwood RH: Chemoprotection by sulforaphane: keep one eye beyond Keap1. Cancer Lett 2006;233:208–218.
50 Nian H, Delage B, Ho E, Dashwood RH: Modulation of histone deacetylase activity by dietary isothiocyanates and allyl sulfides: studies with sulforaphane and garlic organosulfur compounds. Environ Mol Mutagen 2009;50:213–221.

Emily Ho, PhD
103 Milam Hall, Dept. of Nutrition & Exercise Sciences, Oregon State University
Corvallis, OR 97331 (USA)
Tel. +1 541 737 9559, Fax +1 541 737 6914, E-Mail Emily.ho@oregonstate.edu

Changes in Human Adipose Tissue Gene Expression during Diet-Induced Weight Loss

Per-Arne Svensson · Anders Gummesson · Lena M.S. Carlsson · Kajsa Sjöholm

Sahlgrenska Center for Cardiovascular and Metabolic Research, Department of Molecular and Clinical Medicine, The Sahlgrenska Academy at University of Gothenburg, Gothenburg, Sweden

Obesity

Obesity can be described as the accumulation of adipose tissue to the extent that health may be impaired. An excess of body fat, and in particular of abdominal fat, is associated with multiple complications, leading to poor health. With increasing degrees of obesity there are increasing risks of a wide range of obesity complications and premature death [1–3]. The definition of obesity is based on BMI, which is calculated as weight in kilograms divided by height in meters squared (kg/m^2). Obesity is defined as a BMI greater than 30 kg/m^2, and overweight is defined as a BMI between 25 and 30 kg/m^2. In Europe, the prevalence of obesity in men ranges from 4 to 28% and in women from 6 to 36%. There is considerable geographic variation, with prevalence rates in Central, Eastern and Southern Europe being higher than those in Western and Northern Europe [4]. In the United States, it is estimated that about one third of the adult population is obese [5].

The metabolic syndrome is a term that refers to a collection of obesity-related metabolic abnormalities/risk factors that often co-occur in the same individuals [6]. The metabolic syndrome is defined in various ways, but the essential components are obesity, glucose intolerance, insulin resistance, lipid disturbances and hypertension, all well documented risk factors for cardiovascular disease [7–10]. The available evidence suggests that even modest weight reductions in obese subjects lead to improvement in health outcomes [11–13]. Perhaps weight reduction has the most pronounced effects on diabetes risk. Studies have shown that intensive lifestyle modification can reduce the risk of developing diabetes in subjects with impaired glucose tolerance [13, 14], and the Swedish Obese Subjects study found drastic reduction in diabetes incidence 10 years after bariatric surgery [15].

Obesity Treatment

Obesity is a chronic condition that is difficult to treat. Unless adipose tissue is surgically removed (e.g. liposuction or omentectomy), the only way to lose fat is through negative energy balance. Theoretically this can be achieved by reduced food intake, reduced energy uptake, increased energy expenditure, or a combination of these.

A very low calorie diet (VLCD) or a very low energy diet is defined as a diet with an energy content of less than 800 kcal/day but which still contains adequate amounts of proteins, essential fatty acids, carbohydrates and the recommended daily allowances of vitamins and minerals. Ordinary food is replaced by 3–5 VLCD meals together with 2–2.5 l of non-energy fluid per day. At the end of the VLCD period, ordinary food is gradually reintroduced over 2–4 weeks. In medical treatment programs, VLCD is often used over 12–16 weeks and results in average weight losses of 1.5–2.5 kg/week [16, 17]. VLCDs are mainly indicated in obese patients with disorders or risk factors that can be immediately improved by weight loss (e.g. type 2 diabetes) and when rapid weight loss is needed before a major surgical procedure. There is usually a rebound in weight after VLCD treatment programs, and it is crucial that the VLCD phase is followed by active weight maintenance programs [17].

Obesity surgery provides the greatest degree of sustained weight loss for severely obese patients [18]. On average, surgical treatment for obesity results in 20–40 kg of weight loss and a 10–15 kg/m^2 reduction in BMI [19, 20]. Surgical obesity treatment is generally considered for adult patients if they have a BMI greater than 40 kg/m^2, or a BMI greater than 35 kg/m^2 with serious comorbid conditions such as sleep apnea, diabetes mellitus or joint disease [21].

Adipose Tissue

Adipose tissue plays a key role in the development of obesity and metabolic complications, functioning both as an energy store and as a major endocrine organ. The adipocyte is the main cell type in adipose tissue, but the tissue is also comprised of adipocyte precursor cells, stromal vascular cells, immune cells and nerve cells [22]. In mammals, there are 2 types of adipose tissue: white adipose tissue, which has mainly energy-storing functions, and brown adipose tissue, which is mainly thermogenic. White adipocytes are characterized by a single large lipid droplet that occupies the major part of the cytoplasmic space, whereas brown adipocytes contain multiple smaller lipid droplets and a large number of mitochondria. Brown adipose tissue is abundant in small mammals and in newborns of larger mammals, including humans [23]. In contrast to what was previously believed, a substantial fraction of adult humans possess some amount of active brown adipose tissue [24]. What may also be of physiological significance, although not yet shown in humans, is that white adipocytes have the ability to acquire brown adipocyte features under various stimuli

[25–27]. So far, gene expression in human brown adipose tissue has only been investigated in one study [28].

Expression Profiling of Human Adipose Tissue during Diet-Induced Weight Loss

Expression profiling using microarrays has been used to explore genes and mechanisms that may be implicated in the development of human disease. Microarray technology makes it possible to measure the expression level of thousands of genes simultaneously. The microarray consists of a coated glass surface on which probes for different gene transcripts have been synthesized or spotted onto the glass surface. Samples of labeled RNA are hybridized to the probes on the glass surface and the amount of each specific transcript can be quantified by measuring the amount of florescence emitted from each probe.

Expression profiling has been extensively used in the investigation of human obesity. Several tissues such as the hypothalamus, gut and the liver play key roles in the development of obesity and obesity-related metabolic disorders. The adipose tissue is, due to its importance and relatively easy accessibility, the main site where gene expression has been studied.

Several expression profiling studies have been published describing expression changes in adipose tissue during diet-induced weight loss (table 1). Direct comparison of these studies to get a general answer to the question of which genes in adipose tissue are regulated by diet-induced weight loss is an interesting concept. However, differences between the studies (e.g. in study populations, dietary intervention, degree of weight loss and the microarray system used) makes such direct comparisons challenging. It has also recently been shown that factors such as biopsy collection procedures have an impact on the expression profile [29].

In table 1 we summarize the current literature regarding human adipose tissue expression profiling studies investigating the impact of diet-induced weight loss. Expression profiling after bariatric surgery has not been included in this table. All studies listed used energy-reduced diets and needle aspiration of subcutaneous adipose tissue but they have reported different major findings. This is probably due to the differences in study design and differences in microarray platforms used, but it may also reflect that the different research groups choose to focus on different aspects of the expression profiling results.

The first human adipose tissue expression profiling study of the effects of diet-induced weight loss was published by Clement et al. in 2004 [30]. They show that weight loss improves the inflammatory profile of obese subjects through a decrease of pro-inflammatory factors and an increase of anti-inflammatory molecules in adipose tissue. In a study published in 2005, Dahlman et al. [31] concluded that the weight loss resulted in a coordinated reduction in the expression of genes regulating the production of polyunsaturated fatty acids. In the study by Mutch et al. [32] both responders

Table 1. Human adipose tissue expression profiling studies investigating the impact of diet-induced weight loss

Ref.	Subjects	n[a]	Sex, M/F	Dietary intervention	Time points investigated	Weight loss, kg
Clement, 2004 [30]	Obese	10	0/10	VLCD: 800 kcal/day	0, 4 wks	6
Sjöholm, 2005 [36]	Obese	24	18/6	VLCD: 450 kcal/d (wks 0–16); food reintroduction (wks 16–18)	0, 8, 16, 18 wks	28
Dahlman, 2005 [31]	Obese	23	0/23	IEER-600 kcal/day	0, 10 wks	8
Mutch, 2007 [32]	Obese	27 R	0/27	LF, IEER-600 kcal/day	0, 10 wks	>8
		27 NR	0/27	LF, IEER-600 kcal/day		<4
Capel, 2008 [33]	Obese	24	0/24	LF, IEER-600 kcal/day	0, 10 wks	6.8
		24	0/24	MF, IEER-600 kcal/day		6.9
Kolehmainen, 2008 [34]	Overweight or obese	9	5/4	Weight reduction program (wks 0–12); weight maintenance diet (wks 12–33)	0, 33 wks	8
Capel, 2009 [35]	Obese	8	0/8	VLCD: 800 kcal/day (months 0–1); LCD, IEER-600 kcal/day (months 1–3); weight maintenance diet (months 3–7)	0, 1, 3, 7 months	10.2[b]

IEER = Individually estimated energy requirement; LF = low-fat, high-carbohydrate diet; MF = moderate-fat, low-carbohydrate diet; NR = non-responders to the diet; R = responders to the diet; wks = weeks.
[a] Number and sex of subjects included in the microarray analysis.
[b] All 22 subjects in the study to end of LCD.

and non-responders to the weight loss treatment were included. They conclude that the adipose gene expression profile prior to the intervention differed between the responders and non-responders and that this may be used to predict weight loss [32]. In the study by Chapel et al. from 2008 [33] two different weight loss diets were used (low fat, high carbohydrate or moderate fat, low carbohydrate diet). They conclude that the energy restriction had a more pronounced impact on gene expression than did the macronutrient composition [33]. Kolehmainen et al. used a long-term weight reduction treatment and showed that genes regulating the extracellular matrix and cell death showed a strong down-regulation after weight loss [34]. In a recent study by Chapel et al. it was concluded that adipose tissue macrophages and adipocytes display distinct patterns of gene regulation during various phases of the dietary weight loss program [35]. Together, these studies highlight the large number of processes in

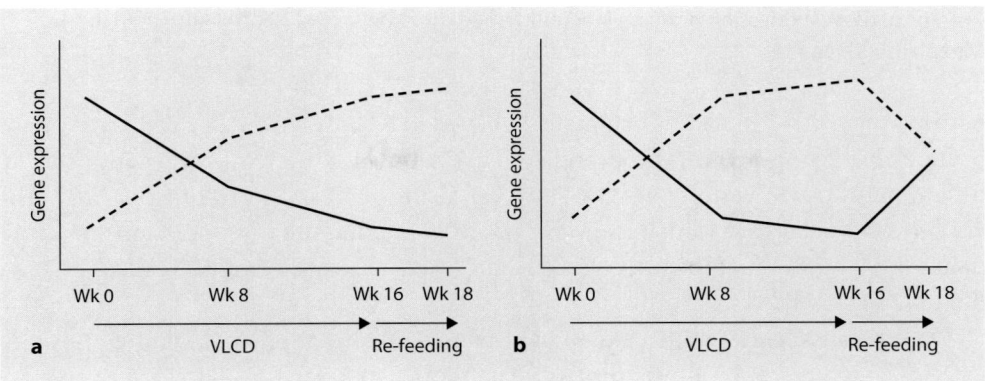

Fig. 1. Schematic illustration of 2 major adipose tissue expression patterns observed in the Gothenburg microarray VLCD study. **a** Gene expression pattern that follows the weight loss of the subjects (solid line) or the inverse pattern of the weight loss of the subjects (dashed line). **b** Gene expression pattern that follows the caloric intake of the subjects (solid line) or the inverse pattern of the caloric intake of the subjects (dashed line). Wk = Week.

the adipose tissue that are affected by dietary-induced weight loss. Furthermore, they illustrate the potential of expression profiling to identify systematic changes in groups of genes that may be of importance for adipose tissue function.

In our study, below denoted the Gothenburg microarray VLCD study, 24 obese subjects were given a VLCD treatment containing 450 kcal/day for 16 weeks, followed by a 2-week period when regular food was gradually reintroduced [36–39]. Study assessments were performed and adipose tissue biopsies were taken at baseline, after 8 weeks of diet, after 16 weeks of diet and at week 18 when regular food had been reintroduced. This dietary intervention resulted in a mean weight loss of 28 kg and a reduction in BMI of 8.7 kg/m^2 after 18 weeks [39]. This weight loss is much larger than in the other adipose tissue expression profiling studies (table 1) and the repeated sampling in this study and the inclusion of the re-feeding time point (week 18) enables the grouping of genes into specific expression patterns. Two commonly observed expression patterns are illustrated in figure 1. These patterns are interesting because they may provide information on the physiological factors controlling the adipose tissue expression of genes included in these groups. The first group (fig. 1a) includes genes that respond to the changes in body weight or improvement in metabolic status during the weight loss treatment. Correlation analysis of the expression level of a gene and the clinical phenotypes of the subjects may provide additional information on parameters relevant for the adipose tissue expression of the gene. The second group (fig. 1b) includes genes that respond to changes in energy intake.

The sections below highlight some of the genes identified as regulated by diet-induced weight loss in the Gothenburg microarray VLCD-study and reviews the current knowledge on these genes in relation to obesity and obesity-related disorders.

Serum Amyloid A Expression in Human Adipose Tissue and Association with Metabolic Disease

Serum amyloid A (SAA) was originally believed to be only a liver-derived acute phase protein displaying up to a thousand-fold concentration increase when induced by inflammation or infection [40, 41]. However, using expression profiling, we and others have revealed that human adipose tissue is a main site of expression for acute phase SAA family members (i.e. SAA1 and SAA2) during conditions of non-acute phase [36, 42, 43].

Obesity is associated with a low-grade chronic inflammation, including slightly elevated circulating levels of inflammatory factors [44, 45]. Several observations suggest that SAA is implicated in both glucose/lipid metabolism and inflammation in adipose tissue [46–49] and it is possible that the increase in circulating levels of SAA contributes to obesity-related complications such as atherosclerosis and thrombosis [50, 51]. Yang et al. [43] have shown that in vitro treatment of isolated human adipocytes with recombinant SAA causes a significant increase in basal lipolysis. Furthermore, they have shown that SAA is a potent pro-inflammatory mediator in adipose tissue stromal-vascular cells, monocytes and endothelial cells [43]. When released into the circulation, SAA rapidly associates with HDL, displacing ApoAI and thereby possibly affecting HDL function. Several lines of evidence point towards a role for SAA-HDL in atherosclerosis [41, 52–54] and serum levels of SAA have been suggested to predict cardiovascular risk [51, 55–57].

It is a well-established fact that weight loss is associated with an improvement of the systemic inflammatory status, and weight loss has been shown to be associated with decreases in C-reactive protein, IL-6 and SAA [36, 58, 59]. In the Gothenburg microarray VLCD study, SAA expression in adipose tissue was down-regulated during the diet-induced weight loss. The expression of SAA remained low also during the re-feeding phase of the study [36]. The adipose tissue SAA expression was also mirrored by decreased SAA levels in serum, and SAA serum levels correlated with total and subcutaneous adipose tissue area, BMI and serum insulin [36]. Yang et al. [43] have shown that SAA mRNA levels and SAA secretion from adipose tissue are correlated with BMI and that serum levels of SAA decrease significantly after weight loss. Furthermore, the improvement in insulin sensitivity correlates with the decrease in circulating SAA levels after weight loss [43]. Changes in SAA concentrations also correlated with the variation in BMI and with changes in inflammatory markers in a study by Poitou et al. [59].

It has been shown that large adipocyte size is associated with insulin resistance and that adipocyte hypertrophy is an independent predictor of type 2 diabetes [60]. We have shown that adipocyte size is important for SAA expression, i.e. large adipocytes express higher levels of SAA than small adipocytes [61]. In addition, we and Poitou et al. have shown that SAA protein expression is also linked to adipocyte size [61, 62]. Hence, it has been speculated that serum levels of SAA could be affected by adipocyte size, but the studies trying to identify such a link have so far produced conflicting results [43, 59, 63]. Based on our results in a recent study, we suggest that it is important to consider measures of glycemic control and gender when analyzing correlations between serum levels of SAA and metabolic and inflammatory parameters [64]. However, we found no evidence that serum levels of SAA are independently associated with adipocyte size. Instead, SAA levels correlated with a general increase in adiposity and inflammation [64].

It is well established that steady-state serum levels of SAA are strongly linked to obesity, insulin resistance, type 2 diabetes and coronary artery disease [51, 65] but further studies are needed to establish whether SAA is just an innocent bystander or an actual cause of obesity-associated diseases such as type 2 diabetes and atherosclerosis.

CIDE Family

The cell death-inducing DNA fragmentation factor-alpha-like effector (CIDE) family consists of 3 highly homologous proteins: CIDEA, CIDEB and CIDEC [66]. The CIDE proteins were originally identified by their sequence homology to the N-terminal region of the DNA fragmentation factor A (DFFA/DFF45) [66], which triggers DNA fragmentation during apoptosis. All 3 CIDE proteins have been found to activate apoptosis in mammalian cells [66, 67]. Gene disruption of these 3 genes in mice has revealed that they also play important roles in various aspects of metabolism. All 3 mice models ($Cidea^{-/-}$, $Cideb^{-/-}$ and $Cidec^{-/-}$) display lean phenotypes and are resistant to diet-induced obesity [68]. In mice, Cidea is specifically expressed in BAT [69], Cideb predominantly expressed in the liver [70] and Cidec is mainly expressed in WAT [69]. It is noteworthy that despite the differences in tissue distribution of Cidea, Cideb and Cidec gene expression, disruption of each of these genes in mice generates a metabolic phenotype with striking similarities, such as reduced plasma triacylglycerol and non-esterified fatty acid levels, decreased leptin levels, decreased lipid content in white adipocytes and increased glucose disposal rates [68]. Proteins of the CIDE family members have been localized to the mitochondria, endoplasmatic reticulum and lipid droplets. The mitochondrial function of CIDE-family members is most likely related to the apoptotic function of these genes. From a metabolic perspective, the view of CIDE family members as lipid droplet-binding proteins is very interesting [68].

There are also data supporting the idea that members of the CIDE family play important roles also in human metabolism [71–73]. However, one striking difference between humans and mice is the tissue distribution of CIDEA expression. In humans, CIDEA and CIDEC are co-expressed in WAT [74, 75]. In cultured adipocytes, siRNA-mediated knockdown of either CIDEA or CIDEC result in increased lipolysis [71, 75], indicating that the 2 proteins have overlapping functions in the adipocyte. In the Gothenburg microarray VLCD study the expression of CIDEA is up-regulated during the caloric restriction phase and returns towards baseline levels during the re-feeding phase [74]. However, in the same study the expression of CIDEC is down-regulated during the caloric restriction phase [75], indicating that there may be functional differences between CIDEA and CIDEC. The expression pattern of both CIDEA and CIDEC in the Gothenburg microarray VLCD study indicate that it is mainly the caloric restriction per se and not the weight reduction that affects the expression of these genes in WAT. Further studies in human WAT and adipocytes are needed to determine the direct mechanisms controlling the expression of these 2 genes and the functional relevance of the observed differential responses to caloric intake.

A Local Activin B Signaling System in Adipose Tissue?

During a microarray-based search for genes specifically expressed in human adipocytes, we identified the inhibin beta B (INHBB) gene as being very highly expressed in adipocytes. The INHBB gene encodes the activin βB subunit which homodimerizes to form activin B [76]. We have shown that INHBB expression in WAT is higher in obese than lean subjects [77]. This is in line with data from the Gothenburg microarray VLCD study showing that INHBB expression in WAT is reduced both during the caloric restriction phase and the re-feeding phase of the study. This indicates that the caloric intake itself is not a major regulator of INHBB expression [38]. However, Hoggard et al. [78] have recently shown that Inhbb expression in mouse epididymal WAT is down-regulated during a 24-hour fasting period and returns to baseline levels during re-feeding. In the same study they also showed that insulin treatment of primary cultures of differentiated adipocytes results in increased Inhbb expression. This suggests that the decreased insulin levels during the Gothenburg microarray VLCD study may explain why INHBB expression levels are also reduced during the re-feeding phase.

For activin B to have local effects in the adipose tissue it requires the co-expression of activin receptors. Activins interact with receptor complexes consisting of 2 receptors, types I and II, both of which are serine/threonine kinases [79]. There are 7 type I receptors, referred to as activin receptor-like kinases (ALK) 1–7. ALK4 and ALK7 appear to function as type 1 receptors for activin B [79, 80]. We have shown that ALK7 is adipose tissue specific in its expression pattern [77]. The expression of ALK7 in WAT is, in contrast to INHBB, at lower levels in obese subjects than in lean subjects [77]. The adipose tissue ALK7 expression correlated with several measurements of body fat, carbohydrate metabolism and lipid metabolism. The regulation of ALK7 during diet-induced weight loss is still unclear. Available data indicate that human adipose tissue expresses components necessary for a local activin signaling system and that some of these components (INHBB and ALK7) are specific for adipose tissue. The difference in expression between INHBB and ALK7 in obese subjects compared to lean subjects makes it hard to predict if increased or decreased signaling is related to human obesity. The importance of a local activin signaling system is illustrated by studies showing that ALK7 deficient mice have reduced fat accumulation and partial resistance to diet-induced obesity [81], indicating that increased signaling could also be associated with obesity in humans. Further mechanistic studies are needed to reveal how adipocyte function is affected by this local activin signaling system.

Conclusions

Expression profiling of human adipose tissue during diet-induced weight loss has identified several genes that affect human obesity and obesity-related metabolic disease. These studies also highlight the drastic changes that occur in the adipose tissue during the weight loss. The investigation of multiple time points during diet-induced weight loss and the combination of expression profiling data from several sources enable researchers to gain more detailed information on the regulation of gene expression in adipose tissue. In the future, more sophisticated experimental designs and better analytical tools will most likely increase our knowledge of mechanisms of importance for the development of human obesity and obesity-related metabolic disease.

Acknowledgments

This work was supported by grants from the Sahlgrenska Academy, the Swedish Research Council (K2007-55X-11285-13-3, K2008-65X-20753-01-4, K2005-71X-15424-01A), the Swedish Foundation for Strategic Research to the Sahlgrenska Center for Cardiovascular and Metabolic Research, the Swedish Diabetes Foundation, the VINNOVA-VINNMER program, the Jeansson Foundations, the Åke Wiberg Foundation, Dr. P. Håkanssons Foundation, and the Swedish federal government under the LUA/ALF agreement.

References

1. Bray GA: Medical consequences of obesity. J Clin Endocrinol Metab 2004;89:2583–2589.
2. Fontaine KR, Redden DT, Wang C, Westfall AO, Allison DB: Years of life lost due to obesity. JAMA 2003;289:187–193.
3. McTigue K, Larson JC, Valoski A, et al: Mortality and cardiac and vascular outcomes in extremely obese women. JAMA 2006;296:79–86.
4. Berghöfer A, Pischon T, Reinhold T, et al: Obesity prevalence from a European perspective: a systematic review. BMC Public Health 2008;8:200.
5. Ogden CL, Carroll MD, Curtin LR, et al: Prevalence of overweight and obesity in the United States, 1999–2004. JAMA 2006;295:1549–1555.
6. Reaven GM: Banting lecture 1988: role of insulin resistance in human disease. Diabetes 1988;37:1595–1607.
7. Alberti KG, Zimmet PZ: Definition, diagnosis and classification of diabetes mellitus and its complications. Part 1. Diagnosis and classification of diabetes mellitus provisional report of a WHO consultation. Diabet Med 1998;15:539–553.
8. Balkau B, Charles MA: Comment on the provisional report from the WHO consultation. European Group for the Study of Insulin Resistance (EGIR). Diabet Med 1999;16:442–443.

9 Executive Summary of The Third Report of The National Cholesterol Education Program (NCEP) Expert Panel on Detection, Evaluation, and Treatment of High Blood Cholesterol In Adults (Adult Treatment Panel III). JAMA 2001;285:2486–24897.

10 Alberti KG, Zimmet P, Shaw J: The metabolic syndrome: a new worldwide definition. Lancet 2005;366:1059–1062.

11 Douketis JD, Macie C, Thabane L, Williamson DF: Systematic review of long-term weight loss studies in obese adults: clinical significance and applicability to clinical practice. Int J Obes 2005;29:1153–1167.

12 Moore LL, Visioni AJ, Qureshi MM, et al: Weight loss in overweight adults and the long-term risk of hypertension: the Framingham study. Arch Intern Med 2005;165:1298–1303.

13 Knowler WC, Barrett-Connor E, Fowler SE, et al: Reduction in the incidence of type 2 diabetes with lifestyle intervention or metformin. N Engl J Med 2002;346:393–403.

14 Tuomilehto J, Lindstrom J, Eriksson JG, et al: Prevention of type 2 diabetes mellitus by changes in lifestyle among subjects with impaired glucose tolerance. N Engl J Med 2001;344:1343–1350.

15 Sjöström L, Lindroos AK, Peltonen M, et al: Lifestyle, diabetes, and cardiovascular risk factors 10 years after bariatric surgery. N Engl J Med 2004;351:2683–2693.

16 Very low-calorie diets. National Task Force on the Prevention and Treatment of Obesity, National Institutes of Health. JAMA 1993;270:967–974.

17 Saris WH: Very-low-calorie diets and sustained weight loss. Obes Res 2001;9 Suppl 4:295S–301S.

18 Sjöström L: Surgical intervention as a strategy for treatment of obesity. Endocrine 2000;13:213–230.

19 Maggard MA, Shugarman LR, Suttorp M, et al: Meta-analysis: surgical treatment of obesity. Ann Intern Med 2005;142:547–559.

20 Buchwald H, Avidor Y, Braunwald E, et al: Bariatric surgery: a systematic review and meta-analysis. JAMA 2004;292:1724–1737.

21 NIH conference. Gastrointestinal surgery for severe obesity. Consensus Development Conference Panel. Ann Intern Med 1991;115:956–961.

22 Wang P, Mariman E, Renes J, Keijer J: The secretory function of adipocytes in the physiology of white adipose tissue. J Cell Physiol 2008;216:3–13.

23 Sell H, Deshaies Y, Richard D: The brown adipocyte: update on its metabolic role. Int J Biochem Cell Biol 2004;36:2098–2104.

24 Nedergaard J, Bengtsson T, Cannon B: Unexpected evidence for active brown adipose tissue in adult humans. Am J Physiol Endocrinol Metab 2007;293:E444–E452.

25 Yoshida T, Umekawa T, Kumamoto K, et al: Beta 3-Adrenergic agonist induces a functionally active uncoupling protein in fat and slow-twitch muscle fibers. Am J Physiol 1998;274:E469–E475.

26 Mercader J, Ribot J, Murano I, et al: Remodeling of white adipose tissue after retinoic acid administration in mice. Endocrinology 2006;147:5325–5332.

27 Tiraby C, Tavernier G, Lefort C, et al: Acquirement of brown fat cell features by human white adipocytes. J Biol Chem 2003;278:33370–33376.

28 Virtanen KA, Lidell ME, Orava J, et al: Functional brown adipose tissue in healthy adults. N Engl J Med 2009;360:1518–1525.

29 Mutch DM, Tordjman J, Pelloux V, et al: Needle and surgical biopsy techniques differentially affect adipose tissue gene expression profiles. Am J Clin Nutr 2009;89:51–57.

30 Clement K, Viguerie N, Poitou C, et al: Weight loss regulates inflammation-related genes in white adipose tissue of obese subjects. FASEB J 2004;18:1657–1669.

31 Dahlman I, Linder K, Arvidsson Nordström E, et al: Changes in adipose tissue gene expression with energy-restricted diets in obese women. Am J Clin Nutr 2005;81:1275–1285.

32 Mutch DM, Temanni MR, Henegar C, et al: Adipose gene expression prior to weight loss can differentiate and weakly predict dietary responders. PLoS One 2007;2:e1344.

33 Capel F, Viguerie N, Vega N, et al: Contribution of energy restriction and macronutrient composition to changes in adipose tissue gene expression during dietary weight-loss programs in obese women. J Clin Endocrinol Metab 2008;93:4315–4322.

34 Kolehmainen M, Salopuro T, Schwab US, et al: Weight reduction modulates expression of genes involved in extracellular matrix and cell death: the GENOBIN study. Int J Obes 2008;32:292–303.

35 Capel F, Klimcakova E, Viguerie N, et al: Macrophages and adipocytes in human obesity: adipose tissue gene expression and insulin sensitivity during calorie restriction and weight stabilization. Diabetes 2009;58:1558–1567.

36 Sjöholm K, Palming J, Olofsson LE, et al: A microarray search for genes predominantly expressed in human omental adipocytes: adipose tissue as a major production site of serum amyloid A. J Clin Endocrinol Metab 2005;90:2233–2239.

37 Svensson PA, Gabrielsson BG, Jernås M, Gummesson A, Sjöholm K: Regulation of human aldoketoreductase 1C3 (AKR1C3) gene expression in the adipose tissue. Cell Mol Biol Lett 2008;13:599–613.

38 Sjöholm K, Palming J, Lystig TC, et al: The expression of inhibin beta B is high in human adipocytes, reduced by weight loss, and correlates to factors implicated in metabolic disease. Biochem Biophys Res Commun 2006;344:1308–1314.

39 Palming J, Sjöholm K, Jernås M, et al: The expression of NAD(P)H:quinone oxidoreductase 1 is high in human adipose tissue, reduced by weight loss, and correlates with adiposity, insulin sensitivity, and markers of liver dysfunction. J Clin Endocrinol Metab 2007;92:2346–2352.

40 Gabay C, Kushner I: Acute-phase proteins and other systemic responses to inflammation. N Engl J Med 1999;340:448–454.

41 O'Brien KD, Chait A: Serum amyloid A: the 'other' inflammatory protein. Curr Atheroscler Rep 2006;8:62–68.

42 Poitou C, Viguerie N, Cancello R, et al: Serum amyloid A: production by human white adipocyte and regulation by obesity and nutrition. Diabetologia 2005;48:519–528.

43 Yang RZ, Lee MJ, Hu H, et al: Acute-phase serum amyloid A: an inflammatory adipokine and potential link between obesity and its metabolic complications. PLoS Med 2006;3:e287.

44 Clement K, Langin D: Regulation of inflammation-related genes in human adipose tissue. J Intern Med 2007;262:422–430.

45 Bastard JP, Maachi M, Lagathu C, et al: Recent advances in the relationship between obesity, inflammation, and insulin resistance. Eur Cytokine Netw 2006;17:4–12.

46 Karlsson HK, Tsuchida H, Lake S, Koistinen HA, Krook A: Relationship between serum amyloid A level and Tanis/SelS mRNA expression in skeletal muscle and adipose tissue from healthy and type 2 diabetic subjects. Diabetes 2004;53:1424–1428.

47 Leinonen E, Hurt-Camejo E, Wiklund O, et al: Insulin resistance and adiposity correlate with acute-phase reaction and soluble cell adhesion molecules in type 2 diabetes. Atherosclerosis 2003;166:387–394.

48 Walder K, Kantham L, McMillan JS, et al: Tanis: a link between type 2 diabetes and inflammation? Diabetes 2002;51:1859–1866.

49 Lin Y, Rajala MW, Berger JP, et al: Hyperglycemia-induced production of acute phase reactants in adipose tissue. J Biol Chem 2001;276:42077–42083.

50 Urieli-Shoval S, Linke RP, Matzner Y: Expression and function of serum amyloid A, a major acute-phase protein, in normal and disease states. Curr Opin Hematol 2000;7:64–69.

51 Johnson BD, Kip KE, Marroquin OC, et al: Serum amyloid A as a predictor of coronary artery disease and cardiovascular outcome in women: the National Heart, Lung, and Blood Institute-Sponsored Women's Ischemia Syndrome Evaluation (WISE). Circulation 2004;109:726–732.

52 Maier W, Altwegg LA, Corti R, et al: Inflammatory markers at the site of ruptured plaque in acute myocardial infarction: locally increased interleukin-6 and serum amyloid A but decreased C-reactive protein. Circulation 2005;111:1355–1361.

53 Meek RL, Urieli-Shoval S, Benditt EP: Expression of apolipoprotein serum amyloid A mRNA in human atherosclerotic lesions and cultured vascular cells: implications for serum amyloid A function. Proc Natl Acad Sci USA 1994;91:3186–3190.

54 Lewis KE, Kirk EA, McDonald TO, et al: Increase in serum amyloid a evoked by dietary cholesterol is associated with increased atherosclerosis in mice. Circulation 2004;110:540–545.

55 Katayama T, Nakashima H, Takagi C, et al: Serum amyloid a protein as a predictor of cardiac rupture in acute myocardial infarction patients following primary coronary angioplasty. Circ J 2006;70:530–535.

56 Kosuge M, Ebina T, Ishikawa T, et al: Serum amyloid A is a better predictor of clinical outcomes than C-reactive protein in non-ST-segment elevation acute coronary syndromes. Circ J 2007;71:186–190.

57 Liuzzo G, Biasucci LM, Gallimore JR, et al: The prognostic value of C-reactive protein and serum amyloid A protein in severe unstable angina. N Engl J Med 1994;331:417–424.

58 Salas-Salvado J, Bullo M, Garcia-Lorda P, et al: Subcutaneous adipose tissue cytokine production is not responsible for the restoration of systemic inflammation markers during weight loss. Int J Obes (Lond) 2006;30:1714–1720.

59 Poitou C, Coussieu C, Rouault C, et al: Serum amyloid A: a marker of adiposity-induced low-grade inflammation but not of metabolic status. Obesity (Silver Spring) 2006;14:309–318.

60 Weyer C, Foley JE, Bogardus C, Tataranni PA, Pratley RE: Enlarged subcutaneous abdominal adipocyte size, but not obesity itself, predicts type II diabetes independent of insulin resistance. Diabetologia 2000;43:1498–1506.

61 Jernås M, Palming J, Sjöholm K, et al: Separation of human adipocytes by size: hypertrophic fat cells display distinct gene expression. FASEB J 2006;20:1540–1542.

62 Poitou C, Divoux A, Faty A, et al: Role of serum amyloid A in adipocyte-macrophage cross talk and adipocyte cholesterol efflux. J Clin Endocrinol Metab 2009;94:1810–1817.

63 Lappalainen T, Kolehmainen M, Schwab U, et al: Serum concentrations and expressions of serum amyloid A and leptin in adipose tissue are interrelated: the Genobin Study. Eur J Endocrinol 2008; 158:333–341.
64 Sjöholm K, Lundgren M, Olsson M, Eriksson JW: Association of serum amyloid A levels with adipocyte size and serum levels of adipokines: differences between men and women. Cytokine 2009;48:260–266.
65 Pickup JC, Mattock MB, Chusney GD, Burt D: NIDDM as a disease of the innate immune system: association of acute-phase reactants and interleukin-6 with metabolic syndrome X. Diabetologia 1997;40:1286–1292.
66 Inohara N, Koseki T, Chen S, Wu X, Nunez G: CIDE, a novel family of cell death activators with homology to the 45 kDa subunit of the DNA fragmentation factor. Embo J 1998;17:2526–2533.
67 Liang L, Zhao M, Xu Z, Yokoyama KK, Li T: Molecular cloning and characterization of CIDE-3, a novel member of the cell-death-inducing DNA-fragmentation-factor (DFF45)-like effector family. Biochem J 2003;370:195–203.
68 Gong J, Sun Z, Li P: CIDE proteins and metabolic disorders. Curr Opin Lipidol 2009;20:121–126.
69 Zhou Z, Yon Toh S, Chen Z, et al: Cidea-deficient mice have lean phenotype and are resistant to obesity. Nat Genet 2003;35:49–56.
70 Li JZ, Ye J, Xue B, et al: Cideb regulates diet-induced obesity, liver steatosis, and insulin sensitivity by controlling lipogenesis and fatty acid oxidation. Diabetes 2007;56:2523–32.
71 Nordström EA, Ryden M, Backlund EC, et al: A human-specific role of cell death-inducing DFFA (DNA fragmentation factor-alpha)-like effector A (CIDEA) in adipocyte lipolysis and obesity. Diabetes 2005;54:1726–1734.
72 Dahlman I, Kaaman M, Jiao H, et al: The CIDEA gene V115F polymorphism is associated with obesity in Swedish subjects. Diabetes 2005;54:3032–3034.
73 Zhang L, Miyaki K, Nakayama T, Muramatsu M: Cell death-inducing DNA fragmentation factor alpha-like effector A (CIDEA) gene V115F (G→T) polymorphism is associated with phenotypes of metabolic syndrome in Japanese men. Metabolism 2008;57:502–505.
74 Gummesson A, Jernås M, Svensson PA, et al: Relations of adipose tissue CIDEA gene expression to basal metabolic rate, energy restriction, and obesity: population-based and dietary intervention studies. J Clin Endocrinol Metab 2007;92:4759–4765.
75 Magnusson B, Gummesson A, Glad CA, et al: Cell death-inducing DFF45-like effector C is reduced by caloric restriction and regulates adipocyte lipid metabolism. Metabolism 2008;57:1307–1313.
76 Woodruff TK: Regulation of cellular and system function by activin. Biochem Pharmacol 1998;55:953–963.
77 Carlsson LM, Jacobson P, Walley A, et al: ALK7 expression is specific for adipose tissue, reduced in obesity and correlates to factors implicated in metabolic disease. Biochem Biophys Res Commun 2009; 382:309–314.
78 Hoggard N, Cruickshank M, Moar KM, et al: Inhibin betaB expression in murine adipose tissue and its regulation by leptin, insulin and dexamethasone. J Mol Endocrinol 2009;43:171–177.
79 Tsuchida K, Nakatani M, Uezumi A, Murakami T, Cui X: Signal transduction pathway through activin receptors as a therapeutic target of musculoskeletal diseases and cancer. Endocr J 2008;55:11–21.
80 Rodgarkia-Dara C, Vejda S, Erlach N, et al: The activin axis in liver biology and disease. Mutat Res 2006;613:123–137.
81 Andersson O, Korach-Andre M, Reissmann E, Ibanez CF, Bertolino P: Growth/differentiation factor 3 signals through ALK7 and regulates accumulation of adipose tissue and diet-induced obesity. Proc Natl Acad Sci USA 2008;105:7252–7256.

Per-Arne Svensson, PhD
Department of Molecular and Clinical Medicine, The Sahlgrenska Academy at University of Gothenburg
SOS-sekr, Vita Stråket 15
SE–413 45 Gothenburg (Sweden)
Tel. +46 31 342 6736, Fax +46 31 418 527, E-Mail per-arne.svensson@medic.gu.se

Toxicogenomics and Studies of Genomic Effects of Dietary Components

Karol Thompson

Center for Drug Evaluation and Research, US Food and Drug Administration, Silver Spring, Md., USA

During the past 10 years, the use of transcriptomics, or genome-wide measurements of gene expression, has become more routine in toxicology studies. In the area of drug discovery and development, expression profiling is recognized to add value to preclinical studies for certain types of toxicities [1]. Preclinical, multiple dose studies on drug candidates are performed to identify toxicities that are dose limiting in order to estimate a therapeutic margin of safety for clinical studies. Genomics data can provide mechanistic information for assessing the relevance of nonclinical findings to humans. In many cases, toxicogenomic changes occur prior to the appearance of microscopic lesions observed by histopathologic examination and provide earlier detection of the adverse drug effects that can be seen using traditional endpoints only after longer exposure times. One area of toxicology where genomics technology could potentially have a great impact is carcinogenicity testing. Genomic approaches could be used to modernize the current paradigm of lifetime dosing studies in rodents through the application of more mechanistic approaches [2].

An increased use of pharmacogenomics in drug development was spurred on by guidelines issued by the US Food and Drug Administration (FDA), which defined the process for the submission and review of genomics data on new drug candidates [3]. Significant advancements in toxicogenomics have been made by research consortia that joined the collective experience of industry, government and academic scientists in investigating some of the fundamental issues that influence the technical and biological variation in expression data. These consortia include the ILSI Health and Environmental Sciences Institute (HESI) Technical Committee on the Application of Genomics in Mechanism-Based Risk Assessment [4], the NIEHS Toxicogenomics Research Consortium [5], the MicroArray Quality Control (MAQC) project [6], and an FDA collaborative project on universal reference materials [7]. Key findings from these collaborative programs that are important for reproducibility and interpretability of gene expression profiling between centers and which can be extrapolated to other biomedical investigations are summarized below.

Reference Materials and Methods to Improve and Monitor Laboratory Proficiency in Microarray Assays

Technical variation in microarray assays can be significant if not controlled by the use of unified metrics and standards to index performance levels and monitor for drift in performance over time. A system for evaluating laboratory performance and process improvement for microarray assays has been developed that uses 2 reference samples that are composed of mixes of different tissue or cell line RNAs that are easily prepared by laboratories that conduct rodent studies or from commercial sources [7]. The 2 reference samples are composed of total RNA from 4 rat tissues with dissimilar expression and contain tissue-selective analytes at defined target ratios for measuring performance on rat whole-genome arrays [7]. Certain tissues that contain higher numbers of specifically expressed genes compared to other tissues in global gene expression analyses (e.g. liver, brain, skeletal muscle and heart [8]) can be used as components of a mixed tissue RNA control for the organism under study. When these tissue RNAs are mixed in different proportions, the ratio in signal level of the identified tissue-selective genes can be predicted from the ratios of the tissue RNA in the mixes. Mixing several different tissue RNAs within one sample allows measurement of several target ratios between just 2 samples. The rat mixed-tissue RNA reference material (MTRRM) contains 1 sample (Mix1) of 10% testis, 40% brain, 30% liver and 20% kidney RNA and the second sample (Mix2) that is composed of 40% testis, 20% brain, 20% liver and 20% kidney RNA. This design allows 4 defined target ratios (4, 2, 1.5, and 1) to be measured using a subset of probes for transcripts predominantly expressed in 1 of the 4 tissues. A proof of concept study demonstrated that the MTRRM could be applied in performance assessments on multiple rat expression array formats (Affymetrix, Agilent, and CodeLink) using a defined set of tissue-selective probes [7]. A similar approach is currently being developed for human gene expression microarrays. Larger universal sets of external RNA controls that are currently under development will also be of utility for comprehensive indexing of performance on platforms where the corresponding probes have been included in the design [9].

Microarray assay performance can be assessed with the MTRRM using a relevant metric for diagnostic tests: the accuracy of detecting changes in expression, measured as the area under the curve (AUC) from receiver-operating characteristic plots. This method has been used to compare overall performance in a proficiency testing program using rat mixed tissue samples [10] and with the data generated on 5 commercial human whole-genome microarray platforms for the MicroArray Quality Control (MAQC) project [11]. Of the AUCs that are derived to measure the diagnostic accuracy of detection of each set of true positive changes (4-, 2- and 1.5-fold,

Table 1. Number of baseline expression datasets for 4 variables in the Baseline Expression Data Set [13]

Variable	Type	Datasets, n
Array	RGU34A	192
	RAE230A	213
	RAE230 20	131
Tissue	liver	396
	kidney	140
Strain	Sprague-Dawley	302
	Wistar	210
	F344/N	24
Gender	male	436
	female	100

using a 1:1 set as the true negative fraction), the AUC for 1.5-fold change detection was the more sensitive measure for evaluating overall performance, because it approaches the technical limit for reliable discrimination of differences between 2 microarray samples.

Identification of Factors that Increase Biological Noise in Gene Expression Studies

Toxicogenomics studies can be quite variable in design, even when they are a part of routine non-GLP safety studies where expression profiling was included as an additional endpoint. Common variables include the specific dosing regimen (vehicle, route, duration) and factors known to have confounding effects in toxicity studies (strain, supplier, gender, diet and age) [12]. In addition, although fasting has a known strong impact on liver gene expression, it is common practice to fast animals overnight prior to the end of a toxicology study to enhance the evaluation of liver histopathology. To examine the impact of variations in toxicogenomics study design on gene expression, a working group of the HESI Technical Committee on the Application of Genomics in Mechanism-Based Risk Assessment developed a public dataset of microarray expression data from rats that served as controls in toxicity studies [13]. The dataset contains Affymetrix microarray data for over 500 samples of control rat liver and kidney from 16 different institutions and 48 in-life studies, along with 35 biological and technical factors that describe a wide range of study characteristics. The types of data that were collected are listed in table 1. From an analysis of this dataset, it was found that the key sources of variability in expression across control animals were differences in gender, strain, organ section in kidney and fasting state

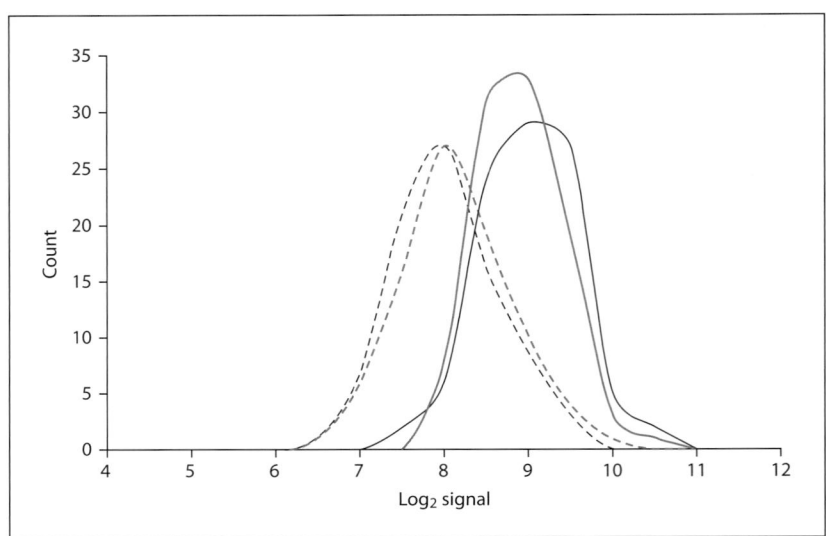

Fig. 1. Baseline levels of expression in rat liver of 2 high variance genes in the cholesterol biosynthesis pathway. Histograms of liver gene expression levels for *Hmgcr* (black lines) and *Sqle* (grey lines) are shown for samples from fasted (dotted line; n = 84) and non-fasted (solid line; n = 96) rats. The data is from 179 control animal samples that were collected on Affymetrix RAE230A arrays and normalized using robust multi-array average.

in liver. These findings can be incorporated into designs of public repositories of microarray data to include factors that should be among the minimal information reported as descriptors of gene profiling studies for data exchange. Additionally, this dataset serves as a resource to generate robust lists of genes with differential expression in liver between certain study factors (e.g. gender or fasting) that are commutable for other applications.

Large sets of control microarray data can also be used to identify gene transcripts and associated pathways that have a high degree of baseline variability (i.e. not attributable to any known study factor). In the human liver transcriptome, the most variable genes are primarily involved in drug and intermediary metabolism, inflammation, and cell cycle control [14]. The genes with the highest variance in control rat liver included 3 gene transcripts that encode proteins involved in bile acid and cholesterol synthesis *(Hmgcr, Sqle* and *Idi)* [13]. These 3 genes have significantly reduced expression in the liver of fasted animals in this dataset. However, as shown in an analysis of 179 control rat samples assayed on Affymetrix RAE230A arrays (fig. 1), significant variation in baseline expression of *Hmgcr* and *Sqle* occurs within groups of fasted and non-fasted liver RNA samples, as well as between fasting and non-fasting groups. Part of this variance could be due to differences in the timing of sample collection. *Hmgcr, Sqle* and *Idi* have been shown to exhibit a circadian oscillation of expression in liver that peaks 4 h into the dark phase [15]. Reference lists of genes regulated by fasting and by the light/dark cycle can be important tools for interpreting observed differences within control groups, as well as between treatment and control groups.

In addition to the use of pathway mapping tools, reference sets of gene expression data ('knowledge sets') help differentiate adverse from adaptive effects in treatment-related gene profiles observed in toxicogenomics studies. For example, in an investigation of the mechanism of skeletal muscle injury induced by treatment with the antimalarial drug chloroquine, a phospholipidotic compound, we observed a dose-related reduction in weight gain due to drug palatability over the 4-week course of the study [16]. To investigate the impact of decreased body weight on the dose-related increase in muscle autophagy observed with chloroquine treatment, gene expression profiling was conducted on soleus, the most affected muscle type, and compared to an internal reference set of genes changed by 24 h fasting in soleus. A subset of genes significantly changed by chloroquine treatment are also regulated by 24 h fasting, but changed in an opposite direction which is characteristic of prolonged reduction in caloric intake. The reference set of fasting-induced changes in type I skeletal muscle was an important tool in identifying adaptive responses within a treatment-induced expression profile.

Phenotypic Anchoring to Supply a Biological Context for Interpreting Gene Expression Data

Phenotypic anchoring in toxicogenomics refers to relating expression values to either traditional measures of toxicity, like histopathology or clinical chemistry values, or to molecular toxicology endpoints, such as the type and incidence of DNA adducts. Biological variability in response to chemicals makes phenotypic anchoring of toxicogenomic data necessary for biologically meaningful meta-analysis of gene expression data [17]. Correlation of gene changes to adverse effects may require the use of endpoints that are more sensitive than routine toxicity measures, as shown by Powell et al. [18] using acetaminophen-induced liver injury as a model. A dose of acetaminophen that significantly increased a set of oxidative stress-associated genes but was sub-toxic on the basis of histopathological change, was found to cause an increased incidence of more sensitive biochemical markers of oxidative stress in liver (i.e. nitrotyrosine adducts and 8-hydroxy-deoxyguanosine lesions).

For toxicogenomic studies, there are certain control groups that can be incorporated into the study design that can aid in linking expression data to biological endpoints of interest. A toxicogenomics study of unusual depth that was designed by a working group in the HESI technical committee on genomics will inform the field on the added value of multiple comparator groups to the mechanistic understanding of toxicity, using doxorubicin cardiotoxicity as the example [19]. Control and treatment groups that were included to provide additional comparisons for linking gene expression changes to toxicity include: (1) a noncardiotoxic drug (etoposide) that has the same therapeutic target activity (inhibition of topoisomerase II) at an equal pharmacologic dose; (2) a cardioprotectant (dexrazoxane) that reduced doxorubicin cardiotoxicity; (3) expression profiling on a non-target tissue (skeletal muscle); (4) a dose range that includes a sub-toxic dose, and (5) a time course that includes time points prior to the detection of histopathological lesions.

Reference Sets that Aid in the Interpretation of Adverse versus Adaptive Effects

Large reference sets of expression changes that contain data for a wide variety of conditions relevant to the biological process under study and that are coupled to traditional measurements of physiological, metabolic or pathologic state can be useful for determining the specificity of transcriptional changes within the context of a study [1]. Reference sets for toxicogenomics contain expression data for a diverse set of drugs and model toxicants, along with histopathology scores and clinical chemistry values. This content can be used to develop gene signature classifiers for pathologic or pharmacologic endpoints, such as was derived with a large commercial set of liver microarray data that is now in the public domain [20]. One example of pharmacologic classifiers is the increase in both *Hmgcr* and *Sqle* expression in liver that is characteristic of the cholesterol-lowering statin drugs, as an adaptive response to their pharmacologic activity as inhibitors of 3-hydroxy 3-methylglutaryl coenzyme A reductase. Pharmacologic signatures can be useful in determinations of whether toxic effects in non-target tissues occur through off-target or on-target mechanisms (e.g. in statin-related rhabdomyolysis) [21].

The Chemical Effects in Biological Systems (CEBS) knowledgebase is a large public database designed for housing and for structured querying of biomedical data from several data streams, including genomics and other -omics data with its associated metadata [22]. In developing CEBS and other toxicogenomics databases, much attention was paid to standardizing the experimental descriptors to facilitate secondary analysis of the database content [23]. For toxicogenomics, these descriptors expand upon the Minimal Information About a Microarray Experiment (MIAME) standard to include, for example, a study timeline of treatments, observations, and sample collecting, and study exit details on the checklist.

Comprehensive datasets developed for pharmacologic research that may also have utility in nutrigenomics research include those that compare basal and induced expression levels of drug metabolism genes in humans and preclinical model species [24–26]. The published catalog of genes in rat liver that exhibit circadian variation in expression is a resource for investigating confounding effects in toxicogenomics or nutrigenomics research [15]. For example, this set would enable testing the hypothesis that dysregulation of circadian oscillations by treatment effects like weight loss is a contributing source of gene expression changes within a study.

Conclusions

Based on the collective experience gained in consortia that were formed to address important issues in toxicogenomics, several key concepts have been formulated that are equally applicable to genomic investigations of other biological endpoints. Following these recommendations will allow investigators to advance the science in other biomedical fields using genomic technology. These observations are that: (1) sources of technical noise should be controlled through the use of reference materials and methods to improve and monitor laboratory proficiency in performing microarray assays; (2) it is important to identify factors that affect biological noise in gene expression studies; (3) with external sources of genomic data, it is important to preserve the biological context of the study, and (4) different areas of biomedical investigation should establish appropriate reference sets that relate expression data to relevant biological endpoints.

Disclaimer

The views presented in this chapter do not necessarily represent those of the US Food and Drug Administration.

References

1 Foster WR, Chen SJ, He A, et al: A retrospective analysis of toxicogenomics in the safety assessment of drug candidates. Toxicol Pathol 2007;35:621–635.
2 Ellinger-Ziegelbauer H, Aubrecht J, Kleinjans JC, Ahr HJ: Application of toxicogenomics to study mechanisms of genotoxicity and carcinogenicity. Toxicol Lett 2009;186:36–44.
3 US Food and Drug Administration: Guidance to industry: pharmacogenomic data submissions. 2005. www.fda.gov/downloads/Drugs/Guidance ComplianceRegulatoryInformation/Guidances/ ucm079849.pdf (accessed January 26, 2010).
4 Pennie W, Pettit SD, Lord PG: Toxicogenomics in risk assessment: an overview of an HESI collaborative research program. Environ Health Perspect 2004;112:417–419.
5 Bammler T, Beyer RP, Bhattacharya S, et al: Standardizing global gene expression analysis between laboratories and across platforms. Nat Methods 2005;2:351–356.
6 Guo L, Lobenhofer EK, Wang C, et al: Rat toxicogenomic study reveals analytical consistency across microarray platforms. Nat Biotechnol 2006;24:1162–1169.
7 Thompson KL, Rosenzweig BA, Pine PS, et al: Use of a mixed tissue RNA design for performance assessments on multiple microarray formats. Nucleic Acids Res 2005;33:e187.
8 Son CG, Bilke S, Davis S, et al: Database of mRNA gene expression profiles of multiple human organs Genome Res 2005;15:443–450.
9 External RNA Controls Consortium: The external RNA controls consortium: a progress report. Nat Methods 2005;2:731–734.
10 Pine PS, Boedigheimer M, Rosenzweig BA, et al: Use of diagnostic accuracy as a metric for evaluating laboratory proficiency with microarray assays using mixed tissue RNA reference samples. Pharmacogenomics 2008;9:1753–1763.
11 Thompson KL, Pine PS: Comparison of the diagnostic performance of human whole genome microarrays using mixed-tissue RNA reference samples. Toxicol Lett 2009;186:58–61.
12 Kacew S: Confounding factors in toxicity testing. Toxicology 2001;160:87–96.

13 Boedigheimer MJ, Wolfinger RD, Bass MB, et al: Sources of variation in baseline gene expression levels from toxicogenomics study control animals across multiple laboratories. BMC Genomics 2008; 9:285.

14 Slatter JG, Templeton IE, Castle JC, et al: Compendium of gene expression profiles comprising a baseline model of the human liver drug metabolism transcriptome. Xenobiotica 2006;36: 938–962.

15 Almon RR, Yang E, Lai W, et al: Circadian variations in rat liver gene expression: relationships to drug actions. J Pharmacol Exp Ther 2008;326:700–716.

16 Thompson K, Miller T, Honchel R, et al: Genomic analysis of skeletal muscle injury induced in the rat by chronic exposure to chloroquine. The Toxicologist, supplement to Toxicol Sci 2009;108: 11.

17 Beyer RP, Fry RC, Lasarev MR, et al: Multicenter study of acetaminophen hepatotoxicity reveals the importance of biological endpoints in genomic analyses. Toxicol Sci 2007;99:326–337.

18 Powell CL, Kosyk O, Ross PK, et al: Phenotypic anchoring of acetaminophen-induced oxidative stress with gene expression profiles in rat liver. Toxicol Sci 2006;93:213–222.

19 Hamadeh H: Exploration of mechanisms of doxorubicin toxicity: a multi-endpoint rodent study. Intl J Toxicol 2008;27:413.

20 Natsoulis G, Pearson CI, Gollub J, et al: The liver pharmacological and xenobiotic gene response repertoire. Mol Syst Biol 2008;4:175.

21 Morikawa S, Murakami T, Yamazaki H, et al: Analysis of the global RNA expression profiles of skeletal muscle cells treated with statins. J Atheroscler Thromb 2005;12:121–131.

22 Waters MD, Fostel JM: Toxicogenomics and systems toxicology: aims and prospects. Nat Rev Genetics 2004;5:936–948.

23 Fostel JM, Burgoon L, Zwickl C, et al: Toward a checklist for exchange and interpretation of data from a toxicology study. Toxicol Sci 2007;99:26–34.

24 Slatter JG, Cheng O, Cornwell PD, et al: Microarray-based compendium of hepatic gene expression profiles for prototypical ADME gene-inducing compounds in rats and mice in vivo. Xenobiotica 2006;36:902–937.

25 Bleasby K, Castle JC, Roberts CJ, et al: Expression profiles of 50 xenobiotic transporter genes in humans and pre-clinical species: a resource for investigations into drug disposition. Xenobiotica 2006;36:963–988.

26 Mattes WB, Daniels KK, Summan M, Xu ZA, Mendrick DL: Tissue and species distribution of the glutathione pathway transcriptome. Xenobiotica 2006;36:1081–1121.

Karol Thompson
10903 New Hampshire Ave.
WO64–2036
Silver Spring, MD 20993 (USA)
Tel. +1 301 796 0126, Fax +1 301 796 9818, E-Mail karol.thompson@fda.hhs.gov

Dietary Methyl Deficiency, microRNA Expression and Susceptibility to Liver Carcinogenesis

Athena Starlard-Davenport[a] · Volodymyr Tryndyak[a] ·
Oksana Kosyk[b] · Sharon R. Ross[c] · Ivan Rusyn[b] ·
Frederick A. Beland[a] · Igor P. Pogribny[a]

[a]Division of Biochemical Toxicology, National Center for Toxicological Research, Jefferson, Ariz., [b]Department of Environmental Sciences and Engineering, University of North Carolina, Chapel Hill, N.C., and [c]Division of Cancer Prevention, National Cancer Institute, Bethesda, Md., USA

MicroRNAs (miRNAs) are small 21–25 nucleotide-long non-coding RNAs that have emerged as key negative post-transcriptional regulators of gene expression [1, 2]. Currently there are more than 700 mammalian miRNAs that can potentially target up to one-third of protein-coding human genes [1] involved in diverse physiological and pathological processes, including cancer [3, 4]. Indeed, aberrant levels of miRNAs have been reported in all major human malignancies [5, 6]. In tumors, altered expression of miRNAs has been demonstrated to inhibit tumor suppressor genes or inappropriately activate oncogenes and has been associated with every aspect of tumor biology, including tumor progression, invasiveness, metastasis, and acquisition of resistance by malignant cells to chemotherapeutic agents [3, 4, 7, 8]. These observations lead to the suggestion that aberrant expression of miRNAs may contribute to tumorigenesis [9]. However, most of the tumor-miRNA-related studies are based on expression analysis of miRNAs in tumors in comparison with corresponding adjacent normal tissues [4–6]. The altered expression of any given miRNA in neoplastic cells is not sufficient to address conclusively the role of these changes in tumorigenesis [10]. Additionally, despite the established biological significance of miRNA dysregulation in neoplastic cells, there is a lack of knowledge on the role of miRNAs during early stages of tumor development, especially if variations in the expression of specific miRNAs are associated with differences in the susceptibility to tumorigenesis.

A.S.-D. and V.T contributed equally to this work.

In light of these considerations, the goals of this study were to: (1) define the role of miRNA dysregulation in early stages of liver carcinogenesis, and (2) determine how these alterations in miRNA expression may be mechanistically linked to the pathogenesis of liver cancer induced by dietary methyl deficiency.

Materials and Methods

Animals, Diets and Experimental Design
Male C57BL/6J and DBA/2J mice (Jackson Laboratory, Bar Harbor, Me., USA) were housed in sterilized cages in a temperature-controlled room (24°C) with a 12-hour light/dark cycle, and given ad libitum access to purified water and NIH-31 pelleted diet (Purina Mills, Richmond, Ind., USA). At 8 weeks of age, the mice from each strain were allocated randomly into 2 groups, 1 control and 1 experimental. The mice in the experimental group were maintained on a low methionine (0.18%) diet, lacking in choline and folic acid (Dyets Inc, Bethlehem, Pa., USA) for 12 weeks. The mice in the control group received a diet supplemented with 0.4% methionine, 0.3% choline bitartrate and 2 mg/kg folic acid. Diets were stored at 4°C and given ad libitum, with twice a week replacement. Five experimental and 5 control mice were sacrificed at 12 weeks after diet initiation. The livers were excised, frozen immediately in liquid nitrogen, and stored at –80°C for subsequent analyses. All animal experimental procedures were carried out in accordance with the animal study protocol approved by the National Center for Toxicological Research Animal Care and Use Committee.

RNA Extraction and miRNA Microarray Expression Analysis
Total RNA was extracted from the liver tissue using miRNAeasy Mini Kit (Qiagen, Valencia, Calif, USA) according to the manufacturer's instructions. The miRNA microarray analysis was performed by LC Sciences (Houston, Tex., USA), as reported previously in detail [11].

miRNA Expression Analysis by Quantitative Reverse Transcription Real-Time PCR
Total RNA (200 ng) was used for qRT-PCRs of the miR-29c, miR-34a, miR-122, miR-155, miR-192, miR-200b, miR-203 and miR-221, utilizing TaqMan miRNA assays (Applied Biosystems, Foster City, Calif., USA), according to the manufacturer's instructions. snoRNA202 was used as an endogenous control. The relative amount of each miRNA was measured using the $2^{-\Delta\Delta Ct}$ method [12]. All qRT-PCR reactions were conducted in triplicate and repeated twice.

Gene Expression Analysis by qRT-PCR
Total RNA (10 μg) was reverse transcribed using random primers and a high-capacity cDNA archive kit (Applied Biosystems), according to the manufacturer's protocol. The expression of the α-smooth muscle actin *(α-Sma)* gene was measured by qRT-PCR, using Taqman® gene expression assay (Mm00725412_s1; Applied Biosystems).

Western Blot Analysis of Protein Expression
The levels of cyclin G1 (Ccng1), cyclogenase 2 (Cox2), E2F transcription factor 3 (E2f3), and CCAAT enhancer binding protein beta (C/ebp-β) proteins were determined by Western immunoblot analysis [13].

Statistical Analysis
Results are presented as mean ± SD. Statistical analyses were conducted by 1-way ANOVA, using treatment and weeks as fixed factors. Pair-wise comparisons were conducted by the Student-Newman-Keuls test. p values <0.05 were considered significant.

Results and Discussion

Dysregulation of miRNAs in the Livers of C57BL/6J Mice Fed a Methyl-Deficient Diet
miRNA microarrays were used to analyze the miRNA expression profiles in the livers of control C57BL/6J mice and C57BL/6J mice fed a methyl-deficient diet that causes a liver pathological state similar to human nonalcoholic fatty liver disease [14]. We identified 74 miRNAs (40 up-regulated and 34 down-regulated) that were differentially expressed ($p < 0.05$), including miR-15a, miR-29c, miR-30a, miR-34a, miR-101a, miR-107, miR-122, miR-155, miR-200b, miR-200c, miR-221, miR-222 and miR-224 in the livers of the C57BL/6J methyl-deficient mice (fig. 1a). The results obtained by miRNA microarray analysis were confirmed by qRT-PCR (fig. 2a).

Functions of Dysregulated miRNAs
Dysregulated miRNAs are known to affect cell proliferation, apoptosis, lipid metabolism, oxidative stress, DNA methylation and inflammation. These processes are substantially compromised in pathological states associated with hepatocarcinogenesis. Specifically, it is well-established that altered lipid metabolism, oxidative stress, apoptosis and epigenetic alterations may directly trigger hepatic steatosis, a condition that has been shown to progress to hepatocellular carcinoma [15–17].

Among the down-regulated miRNAs, miR-15a, miR-30a, miR-101a and miR-122 are of particular interest. Previously, we and other investigators have demonstrated a substantial down-regulation of liver-specific miR-122 during liver carcinogenesis and in primary hepatocellular carcinomas [18–21]. Recently, a significant decrease in miR-122 expression has been observed in individuals with non-alcoholic steatohepatitis [22]. The down-regulation of miR-122 in the livers of C57BL/6J mice fed a methyl-deficient diet was accompanied by increased level of Ccng1 protein (fig. 1b). The altered expression of CCNG1 [19] and other confirmed targets of miR-122, such as fatty acid synthase [22, 23], sterol regulatory element-binding protein-1c [22, 23], cationic amino acid transporter (CAT1; SLC7A1) [24], and BCL-W, an anti-apoptotic member of BCL2 family member [25], has frequently been observed during hepatocarcinogenesis and has been attributed to the pathogenesis of liver cancer.

Feeding C57BL/6J mice a methyl-deficient diet for 12 weeks resulted in decreased expression of miR-101a and miR-101b (fig. 1a). One of the confirmed targets for miR-101a is Cox-2 [26], which is substantially up-regulated in the livers of mice exposed to the methyl-deficient diet (fig. 1b). The increased expression of COX-2 has been detected during human and rodent liver tumor development [27, 28] and is currently considered as an attractive target for chemoprevention during early stages of hepatocarcinogenesis. Additionally, recent evidence has demonstrated that miR-101 targets FBJ murine osteosarcoma viral oncogene homolog (FOS) oncogene [29], a key component of the liver oncogenic network [30].

Another down-regulated miRNA in the livers of mice fed the methyl-deficient diet is miR-15a, one of the first miRNA's discovered to be dysregulated in cancer [31].

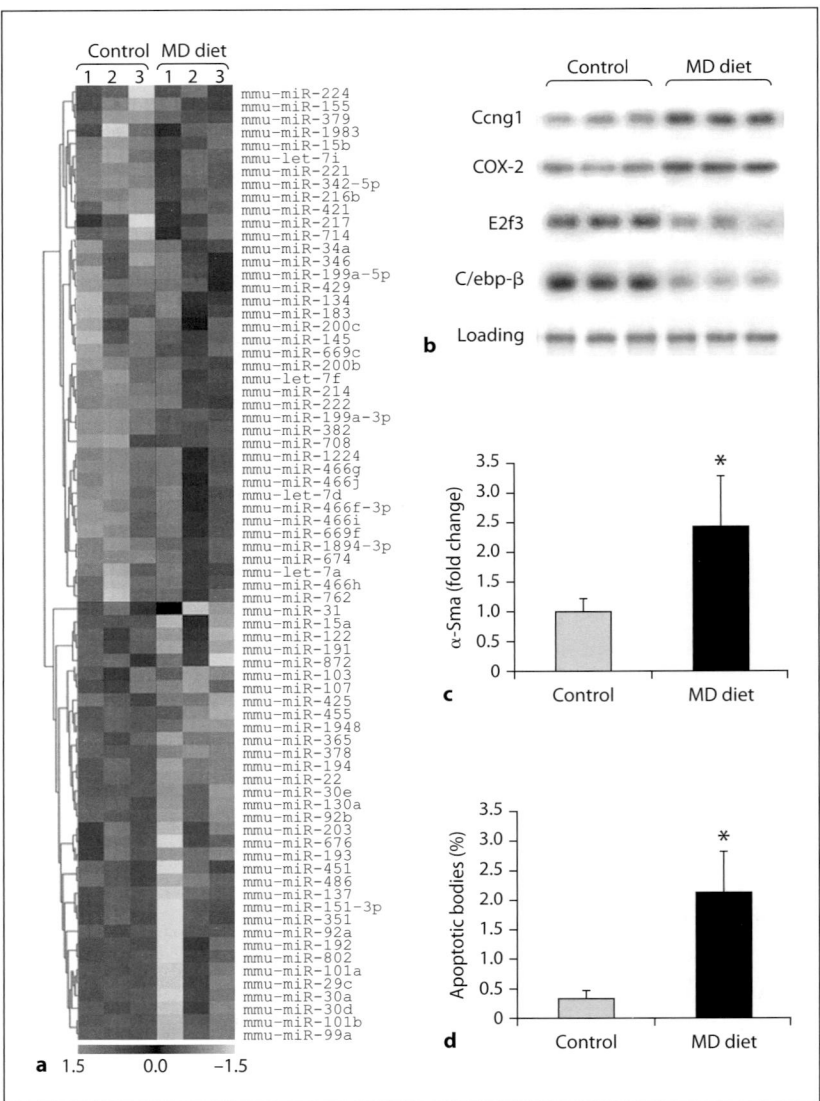

Fig. 1. Dysregulation of miRNA expression in the livers of C57BL/6J mice fed a methyl-deficient diet for 12 weeks. **a** Hierarchical clustering of the differentially expressed miRNA genes (as determined by ANOVA) in the livers of control and methyl-deficient (MD) mice. Rows show miRNA, while columns show independent biological replicates. For each miRNA red indicates high expression levels and green indicates low expression levels. Each miRNA listed is significantly differentially expressed ($p < 0.05$; $n = 3$). **b** Western blot analysis of Ccng1 (miR-122), COX-2 (miR-101a), E2f3 (miR-34a and miR-200b) and Cebp/β (miR-155) proteins in the livers of control and methyl-deficient mice. **c** qRT-PCR analysis of *a-Sma* gene in the livers of control and methyl-deficient mice (mean ± SD; $n = 5$). **d** Apoptotic cell death in the livers of control and methyl-deficient mice as detected by TUNEL assay (mean ± SD; $n = 5$).

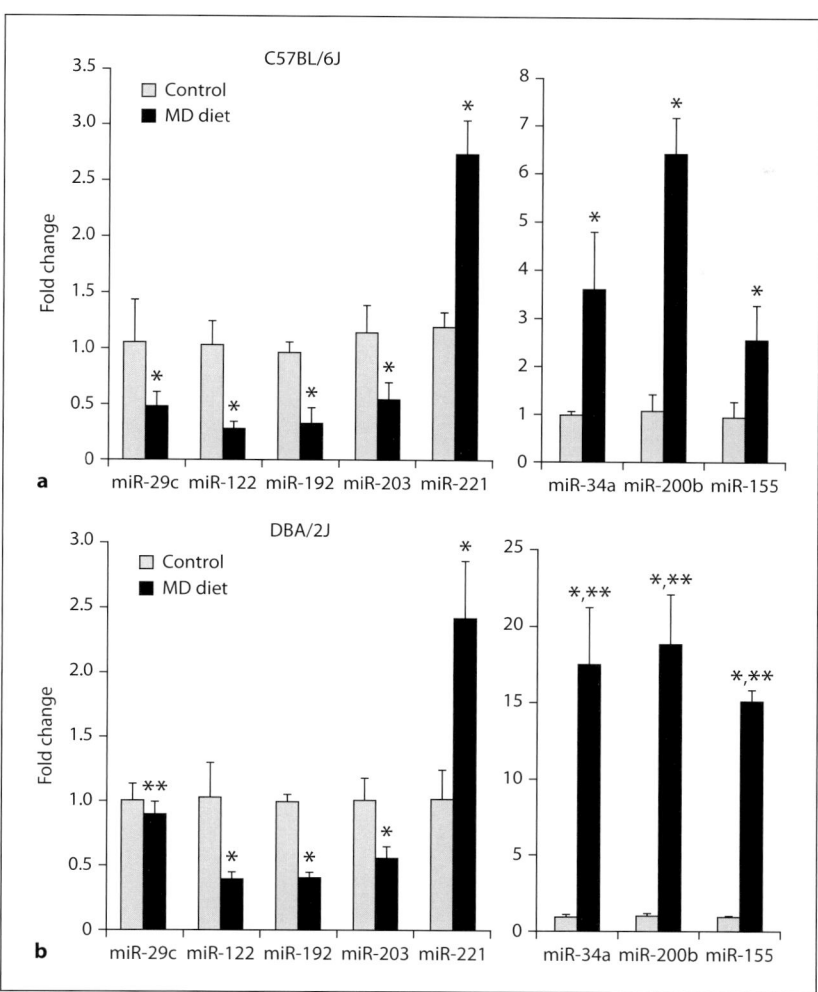

Fig. 2. qRT-PCR analysis of differentially expressed miRNAs in the livers of control C57BL/6J (**a**) and DBA/2J mice (**b**) and mice fed a methyl-deficient diet (MD) for 12 weeks. * Significantly different from control mice. ** Significantly different from C57BL/6J methyl-deficient mice (mean ± SD; n = 5).

miR-15a targets multiple oncogenic pathways, including BCL2, cyclin D1 (CCND1) and WNT3A signaling [31], a pathway that triggers the activation of hepatic stellate cells and progression of hepatic fibrosis [32]. miR-107 [20] and let-7a and let-7d [33], which are down-regulated (miR-107) and up-regulated (let-7a and let-7d) in the livers of methyl-deficient mice (fig. 1a), have also been associated with the pathogenesis of hepatic steatosis, fibrosis and hepatocarcinogenesis. Indeed, figure 1c shows an increase in expression of the *α-Sma* gene, a marker of hepatic stellate cell activation and fibrosis development [34] in the livers of mice fed the methyl-deficient diet.

miR-34a, miR-155, miR-200b and miR-221 were the most up-regulated miRNAs among the differentially expressed miRNAs in the livers of methyl-deficient C57BL/6J mice (figs. 1a and 2). The transcription factor E2f3, a critical regulator of the p53 network, is one of the targets for these miRNAs as reported in Targetscan 5.1 (www.targetscan.org) and in other reports [35, 36]. Furthermore, there is a solid connection between miR-34 and the p53 apoptotic pathway [37–39], which plays a pivotal role in the pathogenesis of liver injury regardless of its etiology, and especially in non-alcoholic hepatosteatitis [40, 41]. Figure 1d shows the increased apoptosis in the livers of C57BL/6J mice fed a methyl-deficient diet. Additionally, recent evidence has demonstrated the importance of miR-34a, not only in apoptosis, but also in non-apoptotic cell death in vivo [42].

The over-expression of miR-155 and miR-221 has been frequently detected during tumor development [43, 44]. The up-regulation of these miRNAs has been associated with activation of the extracellular signal-regulated (ERK) and phosphatidylinositol 3-kinase (PI3)-AKT pathways, 2 pathways frequently disturbed during liver tumorigenesis. Furthermore, the results of a recent study have demonstrated that miR-221 targets and down-regulates pro-apoptotic BCL2-modifying factor during human hepatocarcinogenesis [45]. It is well-established that one of the hallmarks of the carcinogenic process is a dysregulation of cell proliferation and apoptosis [46]. In this context, the altered expression of miR-34a, miR-155, miR-200b and miR-221 in the livers of methyl-deficient mice illustrates the critical role of miRNA in the disruption of the delicate balance between cell division and apoptosis during carcinogenesis.

In a previous study [17], we demonstrated that feeding DBA/2J mice a lipogenic methyl-deficient diet resulted in more prominent pathomorphological and molecular changes in the livers, including DNA hypomethylation, a greater severity of steatosis and necrosis, and oval cell proliferation, as compared to C57BL/6J mice. Interestingly, we detected strain-specific significant differences in the expression of miR-29c, miR-34a, miR-155 and miR-200b in the livers of C57BL/6J (fig. 2a) and DBA/2J methyl-deficient mice (fig. 2b). Specifically, the expression of miR-34a, miR-155 and miR-200b in the livers of DBA/2J mice fed the methyl-deficient diet was, respectively, 4.9, 5.9 and 3.0 times greater than in methyl-deficient C57BL/6J mice. Likewise, the livers of C57BL/6J mice were characterized by a more pronounced down-regulation of miR-29c. The aberrant expression of these miRNAs is associated with an altered DNA methylation status (miR-29c), increased cell death (miR-34a and miR-200b), and liver steatosis and fibrosis (miR-155). miR-155, which was the most differentially expressed miRNA in the livers of DBA/2J and C57BL/6J mice fed the methyl-deficient diet, activates the AKT signaling pathway [47], triggering oval cell proliferation [48], a fundamental event in hepatocarcinogenesis.

In conclusion, these findings demonstrate that alterations in expression of miRNAs are a prominent event during early stages of liver carcinogenesis induced by methyl deficiency and strongly suggest that differences in the susceptibility to liver carcinogenesis may be determined by the variations in miRNA expression response. More importantly, our data provide a mechanistic link between alterations in microRNA expression and the pathogenesis of liver cancer.

Disclaimer

The views presented in this chapter do not necessarily represent those of the US Food and Drug Administration.

References

1 Bartell DP: MicroRNAs: genomics, biogenesis, and function. Cell 2004;116:281–297.
2 Guarnieri DJ, DiLeone RJ: MicroRNAs: a new class of gene regulators. Ann Med 2008;40:197–208.
3 Ventura A, Jacks T: MicroRNAs and cancer: short RNAs go a long way. Cell 2009;136:586–591.
4 Garzon R, Calin GA, Croce CM: MicroRNAs in cancer. Annu Rev Med 2009;60:167–179.
5 Lu J, Getz G, Miska EA, et al: MicroRNA expression profiles classify human cancers. Nature 2005;435:834–838.
6 Calin GA, Croce CM: MicroRNA signatures in human cancers. Nat Rev Cancer 2006;6:857–866.
7 Ma L, Teruya-Feldstein J, Weinberg RA: Tumor invasion and metastasis initiated by microRNA-10b in breast cancer. Nature 2007;449:682–688.
8 Zheng T, Wang J, Chen X, Liu LX: Role of microRNA in anticancer drug resistance. Int J Cancer 2010;126:2–10.
9 Osada H, Takahashi T: MicroRNAs in biological processes and carcinogenesis. Carcinogenesis 2007;28:2–12.
10 Kent OA, Mendell JT: A small piece in the cancer puzzle: microRNAs as tumor suppressors and oncogenes. Oncogene 2006;25:6188–6196.
11 Pogribny IP, Tryndyak VP, Boyko A, et al: Induction of microRNAome deregulation in rat liver by long-term tamoxifen exposure. Mutat Res 2007;619:30–37.
12 Livak KJ, Schmittgen TD: Analysis of relative gene expression data using real-time quantitative PCR and the $2^{-\Delta\Delta Ct}$ method. Methods 2001;25:402–408.
13 Pogribny IP, Muskhelishvili L, Tryndyak VP, Beland FA: The tumor-promoting activity of 2-acetylaminofluorene is associated with disruption of the p53 signaling pathway and the balance between apoptosis and cell proliferation. Toxicol Appl Pharmacol 2009;235:305–311.
14 Anstee QM, Goldin RD: Mouse models in nonalcoholic fatty liver and steatohepatitis research. Int J Exp Pathol 2006;87:1–16.
15 Farrell GC, Larter CZ: Nonalcoholic fatty liver disease: from steatosis to cirrhosis. Hepatology 2006;43:S99–S112.
16 Erickson SK: Nonalcoholic fatty liver disease. J Lipid Res 2009;50:S412–S416.
17 Pogribny IP, Tryndyak VP, Bagnyukova TV, et al: Hepatic epigenetic phenotype predermines individual susceptibility to hepatic steatosis in mice fed a lipogenic methyl-deficient diet. J Hepatol 2009;51:176–186.
18 Kutay H, Bai S, Datta J, et al: Down-regulation of miR-122 in the rodent and human hepatocellular carcinomas. J Cell Biochem 2006;99:671–678.
19 Gramantieri L, Ferrracin M, Fornari F, et al: Cyclin G1 is a target of miR-122a, a microRNA frequently down-regulated in human hepatocellular carcinoma. Cancer Res 2007;67:6092–6099.
20 Ladeiro Y, Couchy G, Balabaud C, et al: MicroRNA profiling in hepatocellular tumors is associated with clinical fetures and oncogene/tumor suppressor gene mutations. Hepatology 2008;47:1955–1963.
21 Coulouarn C, Factor VM, Andersen JB, Durkin ME, Thorgeirsson SS: Loss of miR-122 expression in liver cancer correlates with suppression of the hepatic phenotype and gain of metastatic properties. Oncogene 2009;28:3526–3536.
22 Cheung O, Puri P, Eicken C, et al: Nonalcoholic steatohepatitis is associated with altered hepatic microRNA expression. Hepatology 2008;48:1810–1820.
23 Mitsuyoshi H, Yasui K, Harano Y, et al: Analysis of hepatic genes involved in the metabolism of fatty acids and iron in non-alcoholic fatty liver disease. Hepatol Res 2009;39:366–373.
24 Chang J, Nicolas E, Marks D, et al: miR-122, a mammalian liver-specific microRNA, is processed from hcr mRNA and may downregulate the high affinity cationic amino acid transporter CAT-1. RNA Biol 2004;1:106–113.

25 Lin CJ, Gong HY, Tseng HC, Wang WL, Wu JL: miR-122 targets an anti-apoptotic gene, Bcl-w, in human hepatocellular carcinoma cell lines. Biochem Biophys Res Commun 2008;375:315–320.

26 Tanaka T, Haneda S, Imakawa K, Sakai S, Nagaoka K: A microRNA, miR-101a, controls mammary gland development by regulating cyclooxygenase-2 expression. Differentiation 2009;77:181–187.

27 Denda A, Kitayama W, Murata A, et al: Increased expression of cyloogenase-2 protein during rat hepatocarcinogenesis caused by a choline-deficient, L-amino acid defined diet and chemopreventive efficacy of a specific inhibitor, nimesulide. Carcinogenesis 2002;23:245–256.

28 Sung YK, Hwang SY, Kim JO, et al: The correlation between cyclooxygenase-2 expression and hepatocellular carcinogenesis. Mol Cells 2004;17:35–38.

29 Li S, Fu H, Wang Y, et al: MicroRNA-101 regulates expression of the v-fos FBJ murine osteosarcoma viral oncogene homolog (FOS) oncogene in human hepatocellular carcinoma. Hepatology 2009;49: 1194–1202.

30 Caselmann WH: Transactivation of cellular gene expression by hepatitis B viral proteins: a possible molecular mechanism of hepatocarcinogenesis. J Hepatol 1995;22:34–37.

31 Aqeilan RI, Calin GA, Croce CM: miR-15a and miR-16-1 in cancer: discovery, function and future perspectives. Cell Death Differ 2009;17:215–220.

32 Myung Sj, Yoon JH, Gwak GY, et al: Wnt signaling enhances the activation and survival human hepatic stellate cells. FEBS Lett 2007;581:2954–2958.

33 Mott JL: MicroRNAs involved in tumor suppressor and oncogene pathways: implications for hepatobiliary neoplasia. Hepatology 2009;50:630–637.

34 Lefkowitch JH: Hepatobiliary pathology. Curr Opin Gastroenterol 2006;22:198–208.

35 Welch C, Chen Y, Stallings RL: MicroRNA-34a functions as a potential tumor suppressor by inducing apoptosis in neuroblastoma cells. Oncogene 2007;26:5017–5022.

36 Tazawa H, Tsuchiya N, Izumiya M, Nakagawa H: Tumor-suppressive miR34a induces senescence-like growth arrest through modulation of the E2F pathway in human colon cancer cells. Proc Natl Acad Sci USA 2007;104:15472–15477.

37 He L, He X, Lim LP, et al: A microRNA component of the p53 tumour suppressor network. Nature 2007;447:1130–1134.

38 Raver-Shapira N, Marciano E, Meiri E, et al: Transcriptional activation of miR-34a contributes to p53-mediated apoptosis. Mol Cell 2007;26:731–743.

39 Yamakuchi M, Ferlito M, Lowenstein CJ: miR-34a repression of SIRT1 regulates apoptosis. Pric Natl Acad Sci USA 2008;105:13421–13426.

40 Wieckowska A, Zein NN, Yerian LM, et al: In vivo assessment of liver cell apoptosis as a novel biomarker of disease severity in nonalcoholic fatty liver disease. Hepatology 2006;44:27–33.

41 Farrell GC, Larter CZ, Hou JY, et al: Apoptosis in experimental NASH is associated with p53 activation and TRAIL receptor expression. J Gastroenterol Hepatol 2009;24;443–452.

42 Kato M, Paranjape T, Ullrich R, et al: The miR-34 microRNA is required for the DNA damage response in vivo in C. elegans and in vitro in human breast cancer cells. Oncogene 2009;28:2419–2424.

43 Gramantieri L, Fornari F, Callegari E, et al: MicroRNA involvement in hepatocellular carcinoma. J Cell Mol Med 2008;12:2189–2204.

44 Faraoni I, Antonetti FR, Cardone J, Bonmassar E: miR-155 gene: a typical multifunctional microRNA. Biochim Biophys Acta 2009;1792:497–505.

45 Gramantieri L, Fornari F, Ferracin M, et al: MicroRNA-221 targets Bmf in hepatocellular carcinoma and correlates with tumor multifocality. Clin Cancer Res 2009;15:5073–5081.

46 Hanahan D, Weinberg RA: The hallmarks of cancer. Cell 2000;100:57–70.

47 Yamanaka Y, Tagawa H, Takahashi N, et al: Aberrant overexpression of microRNAs activate AKT signaling via downregulation of tumor suppressors in NK-cell lymphoma/leukemia. Blood 2009;114:3265–3275.

48 Okano J, Shiota G, Matsumoto K, et al: Hepatocyte growth factor exerts a proliferative effect on oval cells through the PI3/AKT signaling pathway. Biochem Biophys Res Commun 2003;309:298–304.

Igor P. Pogribny
Division of Biochemical Toxicology, National Center for Toxicological Research
Jefferson, AR 72079 (USA)
Tel. +1 870 543 7096, Fax +1 870 543 7520, E-Mail igor.pogribny@fda.hhs.gov

Redox Dysregulation and Oxidative Stress in Schizophrenia: Nutrigenetics as a Challenge in Psychiatric Disease Prevention

Kim Q. Do[a,b] · Philippe Conus[a,c] · Michel Cuenod[a,b]

[a]Department of Psychiatry, [b]Center for Psychiatric Neuroscience, and [c]Service of General Psychiatry, Lausanne University Hospital, Lausanne, Switzerland

Schizophrenia is a major psychiatric brain disease with potentially devastating effects. It strikes in adolescence and young adulthood and can last a lifetime. It affects about 1% of the world's population, is destructive for the individual, family and society, and constitutes a major costly public health problem. It develops progressively, most often undetected during childhood and adolescence in a pre-morbid phase. This usually leads to the onset of psychosis at between 18 and 25 years of age, often evolving toward invalidity. Approximately two-thirds of those who develop schizophrenia require assistance from health care providers (such as government and social security systems) within a few years of onset. The majority of people who develop schizophrenia are unable to return to work or school and may have difficulties in maintaining normal social interactions [1].

The symptoms of schizophrenia are classically divided into categories of positive symptoms (delusions, hallucinations, thought disorder) and negative ones (e.g. deficits in social abilities, poverty of speech, affective flattening). The patients also present other discrete, but more permanent dysfunctions, such as cognitive deficits (problems with attention, specific forms of memory, executive functions) and perceptual instability (basic symptoms) that are now thought to be central to patients' behavioral disturbances and functional disability. Moreover, patients with schizophrenia also present non-specific symptoms such as anxiety, depression, obsessive behavior, drug and alcohol abuse and suicidal tendency (10% incidence). While present antipsychotic treatments are relatively effective against positive symptoms, they are almost ineffectual for negative and cognitive ones. Indeed, even in patients stabilized with present antipsychotics, these negative and cognitive symptoms are impediments to the social and professional integration of young individuals from the time of disease onset [1–3].

Despite a growing understanding of its neurochemical anomalies, schizophrenia remains an elusive and multifaceted disorder and available evidence regarding its onset and etiology point to a complex interplay of genetic, environmental and developmental factors. Various pathophysiological hypotheses have been put forward, which account for available evidence to varying degrees. Globally, they involve dysfunctions in neurotransmission and impairments of functional connectivity.

Genetic Factors

It is well established from twin and adoption studies that schizophrenia is highly heritable, but in a complex manner, with a concordance rate of ~50% for monozygotic twins and a heritability of 80% [4]. Numerous studies have focused on identifying genetic vulnerability factors. Results from several genome-wide scans [5–8] have identified chromosomal regions of interest, and cumulative evidence from replication efforts suggest that schizophrenia susceptibility genes may be found on chromosomes 1, 6, 8, 10, 13 and 22 [see reviews in 9–11]. Very recent studies from large genome-wide scans in multiple, large cohorts that have identified both rare high-risk mutations (RR: 2–14) [12–15] and common low-risk variations on chromosome 2 (ZnF804A) and 11 (RR: 1.09–1.19) [16] and in the HLA and histone regions on chromosome 6 [17]. Similarly, studies that have adopted a family-based approach have identified a balanced translocation that disrupts the DISC1 gene [18], as well as the neuregulin gene [19], while hypothesis-driven approaches based on biological findings of deficits in the ability to cope with oxidative stress in patients with schizophrenia have implicated gene variants in the biosynthesis of glutathione as susceptibility factors of the illness [20, 21]. Moreover, understanding how genetic variation at each locus confers susceptibility and/or protection, or what is the contribution of each gene, their relationship with the phenotype and their interaction with environmental risk factors [22, 23] remains a great challenge.

Environmental Factors

These include exposure to viral infections [24], autoimmune, toxic or traumatic insults and stress during gestation, birth or childhood [25–27] that have been implicated in the pathogenesis of schizophrenia. Recently, models based on epigenetic factors and an interaction between a susceptible genotype and environmental factors have been proposed for this puzzlingly complex disease [28].

Developmental Factors

In attempting to produce a unifying concept of the etiology of schizophrenia, researchers have posited that these biological mechanisms have their origins in developmental processes that emerge prior to the onset of clinical symptoms. Indeed, evidence for pre- and perinatal epidemiological risk factors of schizophrenia, and for premorbid dysfunction during infancy and childhood have led to the formulation of the so-called neurodevelopmental hypothesis: schizophrenia is viewed as resulting from etiological events acting between conception and birth, and interfering with normal maturational processes of the central nervous system [29–31]. Moreover, it is also hypothesized that the interaction between a hereditary predisposition and early neurodevelopmental insults results in defective connectivity between a number of brain regions, including the midbrain, nucleus accumbens, thalamus, temporo-limbic (including hippocampus) and prefrontal cortices [2, 32–34]. This defective neural circuitry is then vulnerable to dysfunction when unmasked by developmental processes and events of adolescence (myelination, synaptic pruning and hormonal effects of puberty on the central nervous system) and exposure to stressors as the individual enters high-risk ages [3, 31, 35].

Neurotransmission Dysfunction

A number of theories implicate aberrant neurotransmission systems in schizophrenia, in particular, aberrant dopaminergic [36–38], glutamatergic [39–41] and γ-aminobutyric acid (GABA)-ergic systems [42–46] involving dysfunctions in presynaptic storage, vesicular transport, release, re-uptake and metabolic mechanisms [3, 47]. It is unclear, however, to what extent such neurochemical findings reflect primary causes rather than secondary effects of the pathology, including compensatory mechanisms or environmental interactions.

Impaired Structural Connectivity

Multiple lines of evidence suggest that schizophrenia is associated with abnormalities in neural circuitry and impaired structural connectivity. Post-mortem histological studies have shown anomalies at the level of dendritic spines [48–51] and decreases in numbers of inhibitory GABA-parvalbumin interneurons in the prefrontal cortex [46, 52]. Moreover, recent advances in diffusion tensor imaging have allowed in vivo explorations of anatomical connectivity in the human brain. These have pointed to connectivity abnormalities in fronto-parietal and fronto-temporal circuitry in schizophrenia [for reviews see 53, 54]. Further evidence for anomalies in information integration across brain networks is accumulating.

Impaired Functional Connectivity

This is based on the study of dynamic, context-dependent processes, which require the preferential recruitment of context-relevant networks over others [55–57]. Evidence is emerging in schizophrenia for an impairment in both local and long-range synchronization in a range of cognitive and perceptual tasks [58–61]. Such perturbation of brain connectivity might be associated with functional anomalies of dopaminergic, glutamatergic and GABA-ergic systems [62–64]. The connectivity argument is reinforced by the fact that the age of onset of full-blown psychosis corresponds to the maturation of myelinated pathways, in particular those involving the prefrontal cortex.

In summary, existing neuroanatomical, neurochemical, neurophysiological and psychopathological arguments converge to suggest that schizophrenia may be considered as a developmental syndrome involving faulty connectivity and neurotransmission and it is likely to have complex origins deriving from multiple genetic and environmental factors.

Redox/Glutathione Dysregulation Is a Vulnerability Factor in Schizophrenia

In the present review, we will emphasize the need to identify a 'hub' or 'final common pathway' leading to schizophrenia, a hub on which various known causal factors converge and from which established patho-physiological impairments originate. Through a reverse translational approach [65], we have identified a candidate hub related to redox dysregulation. The hub of redox dysregulation/oxidative stress resulting from a genetic impairment of glutathione (GSH) synthesis fulfills such requirements: it represents a complex interplay between genetic and environmental factors during brain development, which leads to impaired neuronal integrity and connectivity and sets off a cascade of events that extend into adult life (fig. 1).

The tripeptide GSH (γ-glutamyl-cysteine-glycine), known as the major intracellular non-protein antioxidant, is required (1) for protection against cellular damage due to reactive oxygen and nitrogen species (ROS and RNS) and detoxification of environmental toxins and reactive metabolites [66], and (2) for the maintenance of the thiol redox status which is critical for redox-sensitive processes [67] such as cell cycle regulation and cell differentiation [68], receptor activation (e.g. N-methyl-D-aspartate, NMDA, receptor [69]), signal transduction (e.g. H-Ras, PTP-1B) and transcription factor binding to DNA (e.g. Nrf-2, NF-κB) [67]. GSH deficiency will induce oxidative stress, leading to deleterious peroxidations of lipids, proteins and DNAs, altering lipid metabolism and affecting mitochondrial function [70].

Substantial evidence of oxidative damage has been observed in peripheral tissues and post-mortem brain of schizophrenia patients [71–78]. However, variability in these results highlights the contribution of the diverse genotypes and tissues studied [for review see 79]. It remains unclear if the responsible oxidative stress was due to environmental factors or was of genetic origin, preventing the affected brain areas from reacting adequately to oxidative stress. We propose that a primary genetic defect of GSH synthesis is at the origin of the failure of antioxidant defenses in schizophrenia. This implies the involvement of a critical neurodevelopmental component

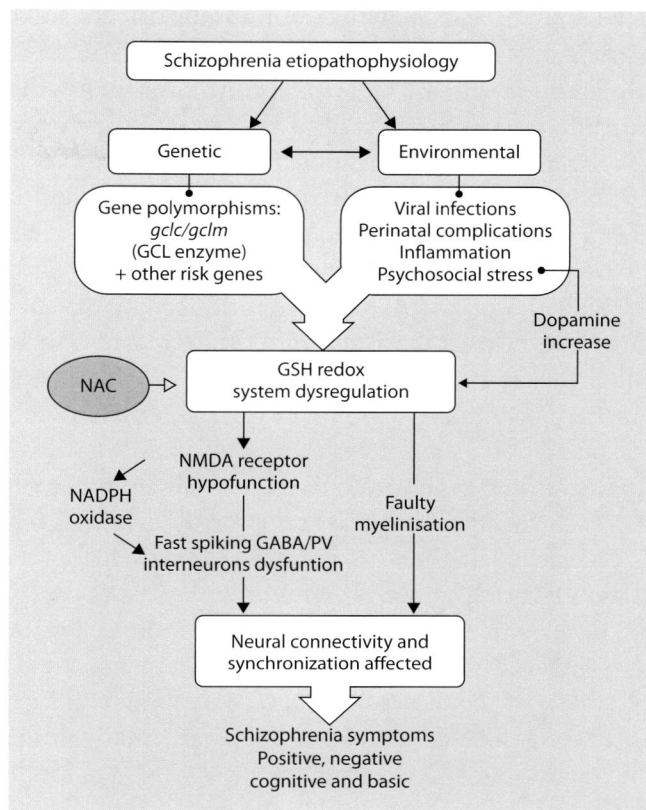

Fig. 1. Role of GSH/redox dysregulation in schizophrenia, focusing on genetic and environmental causal factors and their pathophysiological consequences. GABA =: γ-aminobutyric acid; GCL = glutamate-cysteine ligase; gclc = catalytic unit of GCL gene; gclm = modulatory unit of GCL; NAC = N-acetyl-cysteine; NADPH = nicotinamide adenine dinucleotide phosphate; NMDAR = N-methyl-D-aspartate receptor; PV = parvalbumine.

in schizophrenia when compared with neurodegenerative disorders. Indeed, there is also increasing evidence for the involvement of oxidative stress-induced cellular damage in the pathogenesis of various neurodegenerative diseases such as Parkinson's, Alzheimer's and Huntington's. However, in these cases, ROS/RNS increase and GSH depletion appears to be a downstream consequences of other primary causes (such as mitochondrial complex I dysfunction in Parkinson's disease, amyloid-β peptide toxicity in Alzheimer's disease, and huntingtin-related mitochondrial dysfunction in Huntington's disease) [70].

An association between schizophrenia and a trinucleotide repeat polymorphism in the key gene responsible for GSH synthesis has been recently demonstrated, which suggests a genetic origin for the dysregulation of the redox system seen in the disease [21]. Indeed, patients suffering from schizophrenia present a brain deficit in the GSH system which is of genetic origin: (1) GSH levels in the brain and cerebrospinal fluid are decreased [80–82]; (2) glutamate cysteine ligase (GCL) activity and GSH synthesis are decreased in patients' fibroblasts under oxidative stress conditions [21], and (3) allelic variants of the key GSH-synthesizing enzyme the GCL-modulatory subunit

(GCLM) [20] and catalytic subunit (GCLC) [21] are associated with the disease. In particular, in 2 case-control studies with a total of 570 patients and 797 controls, a GAG trinucleotide with 7, 8 or 9 repeat polymorphisms in the GCLC gene showed a significant intergroup difference regarding the overall genotype distribution [21]: the GCLC genotypes 7/7 and 7/9 are more frequent in controls ('low risk' genotypes), while 8/7, 8/8, 8/9 and 9/9 are more frequent in patients ('high risk' genotypes). This polymorphism has functional consequences: the high-risk genotypes had lower GCL activity, GCLC protein expression and GSH content than subjects with low risk. Interestingly, the high-risk genotype is present in 36–40% of patients and is 3 times more frequent in patients. This is consistent with the decreased GSH levels in the cerebrospinal fluid and medial prefrontal cortex in vivo [80, 82], as well as in post-mortem striatum [81]. Furthermore, high-risk genotype patients have lower fibroblast GSH levels and higher plasmatic free oxidized cysteine levels than low-risk ones (Gysin et al., in preparation), pointing to generalized oxidative systemic conditions [76, 83].

Taken together, these results provide evidence that polymorphisms in the key GSH-synthesizing genes are associated with schizophrenia, leading to a redox dysregulation favoring oxidative and nitrosative stress consequences. These results inspired the development of the 'glutathione hypothesis' [84]: brain deficits in the GSH system would lead to both a functional and a structural disconnectivity, which could be a basis of the disease etiology. Moreover, results gathered in experimental models, revealed that a decrease in GSH, particularly during development, induces morphological [85, 86], electrophysiological [87, 88] and behavioral [89–91] anomalies analogous to those observed in the disease (see 'Developmental animal models with redox dysregulation', below), thus providing additional support to the hypothesis.

Pathophysiological Mechanisms

We thus propose that a redox/antioxidant dysregulation due to GSH deficit could represent a vulnerability factor in the early phase of brain development in schizophrenia. Combined with other genetic and environmental factors, it could favor the development of the disease [84]. Life event stresses, through hypothalamic-pituitary-adrenal axis stimulation, induce substantial dopamine release [92–94]. This could result, when combined with GSH deficit, in an increase in ROS and thus in oxidative damage to lipids, proteins and DNA [95], leading during brain development and maturation to progressive structural and functional disconnectivity.

Low GSH and Structural Problems

As GSH is the main non-protein cellular redox regulator, protecting against cell damage due to ROS, this deficit would be particularly damaging in brain regions rich in dopamine (e.g. prefrontal cortex), whose metabolism generates ROS. This mechanism could be responsible for morphological alterations such as anomalies of dendritic spines and of parvalbumin-positive inhibitory interneurones in prefrontal cortex [46, 49, 96].

Low GSH and Functional Problems

A GSH deficit would also depress NMDA (glutamate) receptor responses [97], a phenomenon known to be involved in perturbations of sensory and cognitive functions in schizophrenia [64], as demonstrated by the psychotomimetic action of the NMDA antagonist phencyclidine [98]. Indeed, GSH potentiates the glutamate response of the NMDA receptor (NMDAR) through interaction at the redox site [97]. This action could be depressed in case of a GSH deficit, leading to effects similar to those induced by phencyclidine. In summary, the framework of the 'glutathione hypothesis' can integrate both dopamine and glutamate theories.

Hub of GSH Deficit

The etiological hub of GSH deficit can have many causes via an interaction between genetic and environmental factors [84] (fig. 1). Besides the GSH regulatory genes described above, some other genetic factors identified as implicated in schizophrenia could also lead to a redox imbalance and an oxidative stress. Indeed, a positive association with schizophrenia has been found for a SNP in *PRODH* which increases the proline oxidase (PRODH) activity, reported to promote ROS generation [99, 100]. On the other hand, various environmental insults known to be schizophrenia risk factors all lead to a GSH deficit: viral infections [24], inflammation, toxic or traumatic insults and stress during gestation or birth or childhood, psycho-social stress and perhaps even diet and post-natal exposure to toxins [25–27]. It is thus likely that such insults, particularly when combined with a genetically deficient redox system, will cause oxidative stress and damaging peroxidations. Impacts during early development may become apparent only in adulthood. Exposure to oxidative stress at various developmental stages affects at least 2 essential cerebral processes that are dysfunctional in schizophrenia (fig. 1): (1) reductions in parvalbumin (PV) fast spiking GABAergic interneurons (FSGI) [46] known to be crucial for brain oscillatory activity [101], and (2) deficient myelination [102].

Reductions in PV FSGI
The NMDAR, which is essential for synaptic plasticity, learning and memory, possesses a redox site which modulates its activity: it is depressed under oxidizing conditions and thus hypoactive when GSH is low [97]. Antagonists of the NMDAR

(phencyclidine, ketamine) are known to induce psychotic states in normal subjects and worsen the symptoms of patients [98]. At the cellular level, the prefrontal cortex FSGI show a decrease of PV and GAD67 in post-mortem brains of patients [46]. The same result is obtained in animal models under low GSH conditions [85] or after treatment with NMDAR antagonists [103, 104, 105]. It thus appears that GSH deficit induces an impaired function in FSGI, particularly during brain development. This NMDAR hypofunction induced FSGI defect is mediated by activation of NAPDH oxidases [106, 107]. The latter also produces ROS, which will not be sufficiently reduced when GSH is low. The FSGI are critically involved in the functional cortical circuitry responsible for synchronization and gamma band EEG oscillations during cognitive tasks [59, 101, 108]. Their impairment could potentially lead to decreased synchronization and γ-oscillation power and to cognitive deficits both in patients and in animal models. This chain of events is likely to be causally involved in the generation of schizophrenia phenotype.

Deficient Myelination
In addition, oxidative stress is likely to affect the development of progenitor cells in the central nervous system, and the precursors of oligodendrocytes are particularly sensitive to redox balance. A tendency toward the oxidative side of the balance favors differentiation over proliferation, leading to a deficit in oligodendrocytes and to anomalies of myelination [109, 110]. The development of appropriate levels of myelin is affected in the schizophrenic brain and the resulting errors in conduction speed of action potentials is likely to contribute to the deficits in connectivity and synchronization in diverse pathways which would underlie the cognitive and negative symptoms.

Developmental Animal Models with Redox Dysregulation

As noted above, schizophrenia is a multifaceted disorder, with evidence concerning its onset and etiology pointing to a complex interplay of genetic, environmental and developmental factors. Several approaches have been taken to develop animal models of schizophrenia [for review see 111, 112]. These include:
– Specific pharmacological or genetic manipulations that aim at modeling a particular aspect of the pathophysiology observed in schizophrenia in order to assess the consequences of these defects. These are applicable to post-pubertal and chronic stages of the disease.
– Disruptions of normal brain development and maturation, focusing on those which lead to behavioral impairments related to schizophrenia that only appear after puberty.
– Animal models with obstetrical complications and prenatal maternal infections, two conditions known to increase the risk of schizophrenia.

However, none of these models by itself addresses in a comprehensive manner the complexity and heterogeneity of schizophrenia and its multiple stages of development. Integration of results obtained from models of these different elements are needed to determine the conditions and defects that can produce the various symptoms of schizophrenia. It is becoming apparent that several different defects independently or in combination can converge to provoke similar behavioral dysfunctions related to schizophrenia. There is thus a strong need to develop new models that combine several manipulations (e.g. combining genetic or pharmacological manipulations with a developmental environmental factor). A unifying pathogenesis concept was proposed [31]: 'genetic susceptibility in concert with particular stressors during development, may lead to a critical threshold that, when crossed, produces the clinical syndrome at a later stage in life.'

We review here results concerning 2 animal models which explore such convergence of both genetic and environmental risk factors during development, based on impairment of GSH synthesis, redox dysregulation and increased oxidative stress.

BSO-Induced Glutathione Deficit

We have established a pharmacological model in rats based on inducing transient redox dysregulation during development involving specific inhibition of GSH synthesis with t-butyl sulfoximide (BSO) leading to a 50–60% decrease of brain GSH levels from postnatal days (PN) 5 to 16. Alone or combined with oxidative stress (induced by a blockade of dopamine uptake with GBR12909 leading to high levels of extracellular dopamine and thus to ROS production), this treatment leads to following morphological, electrophysiological and behavioral anomalies:

- In prefrontal cortex neurons, we observed a decrease in dendritic spine density [86, 113], as well as in parvalbumin immunoreactivity [85]. These observations are similar to those reported in the brain of schizophrenia patients [49, 96].
- Memory and sensory integration are perturbed (later in female rats than in males [89–91]), reproducing some of the cognitive deficits observed in schizophrenia.
- In rat hippocampal slices, GSH depletion impairs NMDA-dependent synaptic plasticity [87]. In neuronal cultures, while dopamine enhanced NMDA responses in control, it depressed them in GSH-depleted neurons. Antagonist of D2-Rs prevented this depression, a mechanism contributing to the efficacy of antipsychotics [88].

All of these anomalies are quite similar to those reported in schizophrenia and show that an insult imposed in the developmental period of PN 5–16 has long-term behavioral consequences. This pharmacological model has, however, some technical limitations, in particular bound to the fact that the period at which BSO can be applied systemically is restricted by its transitory permeability across the blood brain barrier.

GCLM$^{-/-}$ Knockout Mice

This preclinical animal model permits exploration of how interaction between this susceptibility gene and environmental insults during brain development will result in impaired neuronal integrity and connectivity, setting off a cascade of events that extend to adult life. As discussed above, the fact that the GCLM gene has allelic variations associated with schizophrenia in patients [20] indicates that the GCLM$^{-/-}$ mouse is a useful model. Its GSH level is low (20% of wild type) throughout development, rendering it at permanent risk for oxidative stress (note that a knockout of the gene coding the catalytic subunit GCLC is lethal in mice). At the other end, environmental stress, through hypothalamic-pituitary-adrenal axis stimulation, induces substantial dopamine release [92–94]. This would result in an augmentation in ROS and thus further increase oxidative stress. We thus investigated an animal model which involves *GCLM* as a risk gene causing redox dysregulation and employ hyperdopaminergia as an environmental stressor which can be applied at various stages during neural development. GCLM$^{-/-}$ mice showed selective and region-specific anomalies in the GABAergic system. As in the BSO-treated rats, PV immunoreactive interneurons in GCLM$^{-/-}$ mice were particularly affected.

In anterior cingulate of GCLM$^{-/-}$ mice, concomitantly to an increase in oxidative stress as revealed by 8-oxo-dG (marker of DNA oxidation), the developmental expression of PV was impaired at PN 10, but normalized at PN 20. Additional stress (GBR treatment) during postnatal development (from PN 10–20) prevents this normalization at PN 20 [114]. Moreover, myelination is also impaired as revealed by a weaker myelin basic protein immunolabelling intensity and thinner myelin basic protein immunoreactivity profiles [114].

In ventral but not dorsal hippocampus of adult GCLM$^{-/-}$ mice, oxidative stress marker 8-hydroxy-2-deoxyguanosine was increased while PV immunoreactivity of GABA interneurons and kainate-induced γ-oscillations were reduced. These effects were severe in the dentate gyrus and CA3 region but not CA1. Furthermore, GCLM$^{-/-}$ had no impairment in dorsal hippocampus-related spatial learning and memory (rewarded alternation and Morris water maze) while they display novelty-induced hyperactivity, reduced anxiety, alterations in social behavior and deficiency in object memory, all tasks related to ventral hippocampus [114, 115].

Altogether, these observations confirm that PV immunoreactive interneurons are particularly sensitive to a GSH deficit but their vulnerability depends on brain region and correlates with the level of oxidative stress. This also supports the notion that PV immunoreactive fast-spiking interneurons are highly vulnerable to oxidative stress [116]. As noted above, patients with schizophrenia are characterized by decreases in PV containing GABAergic interneurons that are crucially involved in the generation of high-frequency oscillations. Moreover the synchronization of such oscillatory activity which is at the basis of neural activity coordination during perceptual and cognitive processes is also impaired in schizophrenia [108, for review see 117].

The impairment of PV interneurons and neural synchronization in GCLM$^{-/-}$ mice suggests that GSH deficit and redox dysregulation underly cognitive and behavioral anomalies observed in schizophrenia, at least in high-risk GCLC genotype patients.

The myelination anomalies observed in GCLM$^{-/-}$ mice are consistent with the impairment of oligodendroglia-mediated myelination in schizophrenia as evidenced from gene expression profiling, neurocytochemical and neuroimaging studies [54, 118, 119]. A deficit in myelination would influence the axonal conduction velocity and thus prevent precise synchronizations. It also would have an impact on the association pathways essential for intermodal sensory integration and the 'binding' process [117], underlying the cognitive and negative symptoms. As cortical myelination extends until late adolescence for the temporal and prefrontal regions, its deficit could be related to the delayed onset of the disease in early adulthood. As discussed above, intracellular redox state appears to be a necessary and sufficient modulator of the balance between self-renewal and differentiation in dividing oligodendrocyte-type-2 astrocyte progenitor cells [109, 110]. More specifically, cells that are more oxidized tend to differentiate, whereas those that are more reduced undergo self-renewal. Therefore the redox dysregulation observed in schizophrenia may lead to myelination perturbation through oligodendrocytes mitogenic signaling disruption [109].

Therapeutic and Preventive Perspectives

Proof-of-Concept Clinical Trial with N-Acetyl-Cysteine

N-acetyl cysteine (NAC) is a commercial drug approved as an add-on treatment for bronchitis and as an antidote in paracetamol intoxication. Recently, biological effects of NAC have been studied in order to explore potential additional clinical indications, such as graft rejection [120], cystic fibrosis [121], chronic obstructive pulmonary disease [122], arthritis [120], some forms of cancer [120], neurodegenerative disorders [123–125] and cocaine and heroin dependency [126, for review see 127]. Various NAC characteristics suggest it is a very promising candidate in the context of a potential GSH-redox dysregulation linked to schizophrenia, through its influence on the GSH system as well as through a direct antioxidant effect. These characteristics can be defined as follows:
– Induction of in vivo biosynthesis of GSH: cysteine, an NAC metabolite, is essential for GSH synthesis. Availability of cysteine is therefore a crucial factor for constitution of adequate intracerebral reserves of GSH, considering glutathione itself does not cross the blood-brain barrier.
– Gene expression modulation by oxidative stress: NAC plays an important modulating role in expression of genes linked to oxidative stress through its effect on transcription factors such as NF-κB and AP1 [128].

- Antioxidant effect of NACNAC reduces concentration of free radicals and other oxidants through direct inactivation of reactive oxygenated compounds through the molecule's free thiol group and formation of NAC-disulfide as the final product.
- Protection of nerve cells: numerous studies, both in vitro and in vivo, have shown that administration of NAC protects nervous cells against free radicals [120, 128].

In a double-blind, placebo-controlled study, NAC has proven to be efficient at improving schizophrenia symptoms. Indeed, NAC, as an add-on treatment to antipsychotics, decreased negative symptoms and reduced side effects (akathisia) in a cohort of 140 chronic patients [129]. Moreover, this GSH precursor is also effective in improving mismatch negativity [130], an auditory related, NMDA-dependent evoked potential typically impaired in schizophrenia [62, 131]. This is encouraging since present antipsychotic treatments are rather ineffective against cognitive and negative symptoms and have no effect on certain biomarkers like mismatch negativity, a pre-attentional component which is proposed to gate some cognitive and functional modules.

It is of interest to note that the high-risk GAG trinucleotide polymorphism is also associated with bipolar patients [Gysin et al., unpubl. observations], but not with major depression, supporting the view that various genetic anomalies are common to several psychoses. This is consistent with the observation that NAC supplementation improves bipolar patients [132], and is consistent with the concept of a psychosis continuum, as proposed by Crow [133].

Early Intervention and Prevention

Early intervention in psychosis has become an important focus of interest in psychiatry [134, 135]. Prospective studies conducted in first episode psychosis patients [136–139] have identified long delays between onset of psychotic symptoms and initiation of adequate treatment and lack of specificity in treatment of the early phase of psychosis (fig. 2). Two additional concepts emerged from this research: first, that full-blown psychosis is preceded by a 'prodromal phase' [140–143], and second, that the first few years after onset of the major symptoms constitute a 'critical phase' where outcome is more likely to be influenced [144]. However, the diagnosis of the prodromal phase still relies exclusively on clinical assessment [145] with limited specificity and hence a high rate of false positives, which raises important ethical issues when designing therapeutic strategies [146, 147] and underlines the need for valid biomarkers.

Our present knowledge indicates that the maximal efficacy of our treatments would be in the early psychosis and prodromal phase before redox dysregulation/oxidative stress has done major damage. Considering NAC has negligible side effects, its efficacy in early psychosis and prodromal phase will be a first step towards identifying pharmacological agents that are much more acceptable to patients and may

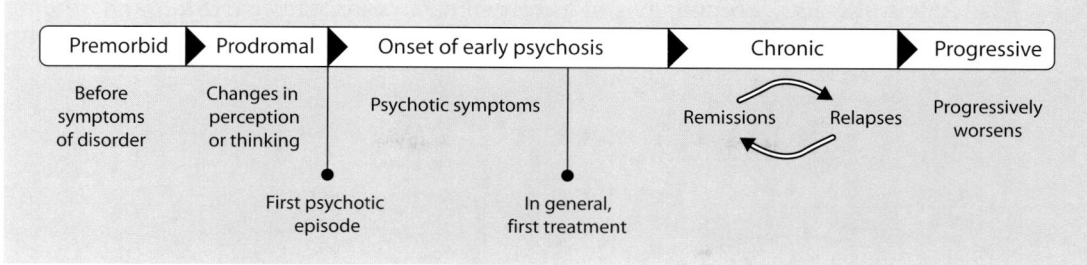

Fig. 2. Phases of schizophrenia.

therefore improve adherence to treatment. Moreover, NAC supplementation has very promising potential in children and adolescents who suffer from neurodevelopmental psychotic disorders, because neuroprotection could be crucial at the critical ages of adolescence when pathological processes are interfering with ongoing brain development. Finally, the presence of a GSH-redox dysregulation or its genetic correlates may prove to be a useful marker in the frame of early detection of schizophrenia.

Nutrients and Antioxidants for Prevention and Treatment

Glutathione and C1 Metabolism
Disturbances in single-carbon metabolism appear to be related to a variety of neuropsychiatric disorders, covering a broad spectrum that includes depression [148], autism [149] and psychosis [150, 151]. Indeed, the enzymes and metabolites of the methionine and folate cyle are associated with schizophrenia [152–155]. However, we do not know yet whether an observed disturbance is a primary event that is fundamentally related to the pathogenesis or a secondary phenomenon reflecting a non-pathogenic mechanism.

Interestingly, methionine given per os has been shown to be the only amino acid that exacerbates the psychotic symptoms in schizophrenic patients [154]. Experimental methionine loading brings about various effects on the single-carbon cycle as it lowers serum folate concentration [156], induces oxidative stress [157], and lowers the amino acid cysteine [158], the rate-limiting precursor in the GSH synthesis. The exacerbation of psychosis could thus be the consequences of an aggravation of the impairment of the GSH deficit and redox dyregulation hub, at least in the high-risk GCLC genotype schizophrenia patients. Moreover, GSH is a cofactor for the function of methionine adenosyltransferase (MAT), which is a sensitive target for oxidation, and MAT activity is therefore strongly dependent on cellular GSH levels [159]. MAT has been reported to be significantly underactive in red blood cells and brains of schizophrenic patients [160]. In addition, GSH deficit, through methionine and

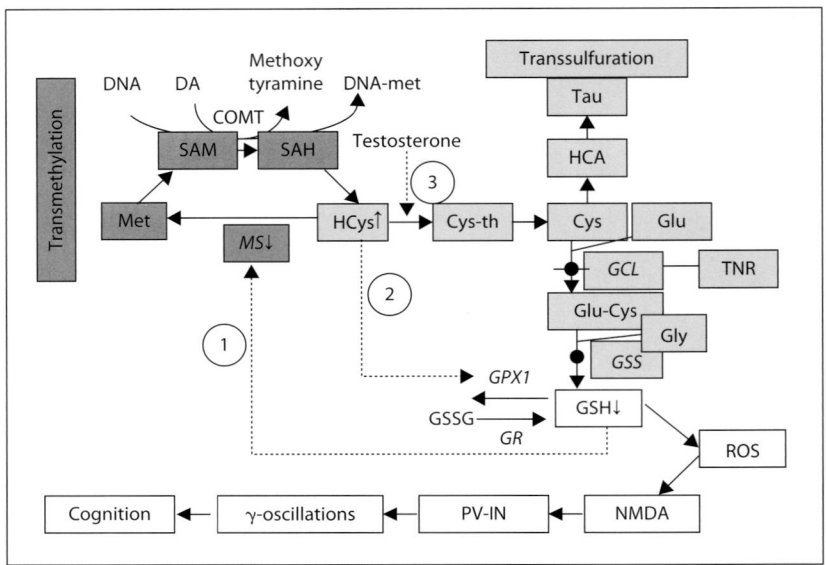

Fig. 3. Single-carbon metabolism and glutathione in schizophrenia. GSH dysregulation might play a role in the framework of the single-carbon hypothesis of schizophrenia originally proposed by Smythies et al. [183]. In the transmethylation pathway, methionine is converted to homocysteine providing methyl groups to DNA, lipids and proteins. Homocysteine can be either remethylated to methionine through activation of methionine synthase, which depends on folate and vitamin B_{12}, or metabolized to cystathionine and cysteine through the transsulfuration pathway. Cysteine can then be used as a precursor of GSH. Thus, homocysteine is in a central position, going either to transmethylation or to transsulfuration and GSH synthesis. Deth et al. [155] proposed that methionine synthase can act as a 'redox sensor'. Under oxidative stress conditions, methionine synthase is inactivated (dotted arrow line 1), allowing homocysteine to be shunted into the transsulfuration pathway to increase GSH synthesis and thus neutralize oxidative stress. This mechanism is of particular interest in the perspective of schizophrenia, as hyperhomocysteinemia has been reported in subgroups of patients. Such a hyperhomocysteinemia could be related to a partial block of both transmethylation and transsulfuration pathways. A GSH deficit due to the impairment of GCL could thus interfere with the transsulfuration pathway, and inhibit the methionine synthase affecting the transmethylation pathway. In addition, hyperhomocysteinemia exercises an inhibition on GPX1 activity (dotted arrow line 2), further depressing the reduction effect of GSH [184], and testosterone has been shown to depress the β-cystationase (dotted arrow line 3), possibly contributing to gender differences in severity [185]. These mechanisms are likely to be exacerbated by an enhancement of oxidative stress during the acute phases of psychosis.

the transmethylation pathway could contribute to the dysregulation of DNA methylation thus affecting epigenetic processes (fig. 3). Indeed, under oxidative stress conditions, methionine synthase is inactivated, allowing homocysteine to be shunted into the transsulfuration pathway in order to favour GSH synthesis [161]. As GSH synthesis is impaired in the high-risk genotype, both transmethylation and transsulfuration pathways will be depressed, leading to perturbations of the DNA methylation process and increase of homocysteine levels often observed in schizophrenia [28, 162, 163].

A most encouraging feature of single-carbon metabolism is its potential modification by natural means, such as B vitamins and antioxidants. In one case report, cobalamine treatment alleviated psychotic symptoms [152]. However, this clinical effect diminished with time, and the metabolic abnormality was thus not wholly cobalamin dependent. In a double-blind, placebo-controlled trial, methylfolate supplementation significantly improved clinical and social recovery among both depressed and schizophrenic patients [164].

Polyunsaturated Fatty Acids
Another potential alternative and adjunctive to current antipsychotic treatments is the use of certain polyunsaturated fatty acids (PUFA), the omega-3 and omega-6, which play key roles in brain structure and function but which must be derived from dietary sources [165]. A high dietary ratio of omega-6, found in soft margarine, most vegetable oils and animal fats, to omega-3, found principally in oily fish and seafood, has been linked with vulnerability to many disorders of physical and mental health [166].

In our context, GSH deficit and redox dysregulaton in schizophrenia could lead to oxidative stress and ROS-mediated injury as supported by increased lipid peroxidation products and reduced membrane PUFAs. Decrease in membrane phospholipids in blood cells of psychotic patients [167, 168] and fibroblasts from drug-naïve patients [169] and in post-mortem brain [170] were indeed reported. It has been also suggested that peripheral membrane anomalies correlate with abnormal central phospholipid metabolism in first-episode and chronic schizophrenia patients [171, 172]. Recently, a microarray and proteomic study on post-mortem brain showed anomalies of mitochondrial function and oxidative stress pathways in schizophrenia [76]. Mitochondrial dysfunction in schizophrenia has also been observed [74, 173]. As main ROS producers, mitochondria are particularly susceptible to oxidative damage. Since the brain is highly vulnerable to oxidative damage because of its high oxygen consumption, its high content of oxidizable PUFAs and the presence of redox-active metals (Cu, Fe), a deficit in GSH could be particularly damaging to the neuronal function.

There is increasing evidence that dietary supplementation with omega-3 fatty acids may be beneficial in psychiatric conditions [174]. This evidence includes randomized controlled trials in conditions such as schizophrenia, depression and borderline personality disorder [175–178]. However, recent meta-analyses of these studies show little evidence of a robust clinically relevant effect of omega-3 PUFA in schizophrenia, while the most convincing evidence for beneficial effects of omega-3 PUFA is to be found in depression [179]. Moreover, supplementation with omega-3 PUFA and vitamins C and E appear to exacerbate the positive symptoms in a subgroup of schizophrenia patients with low plasma PUFA [180]. These puzzling results might be explained by assuming an intrinsic GSH deficit of genetic origin in these patients. Indeed, antioxidants such as vitamins C and E might become pro-oxidants in an oxidizing environment [181, 182] as they require GSH to be reduced and regenerated

[70]. The same argument can be applied for the short-term effect of the above-described cobalamine treatment. Thus, nutritional approachs must take into account the genetic and epigenetic background of individual patients. Nutrigenetics research will offer a strong foundation for future clinical investigations towards alternative treatment and prevention of psychiatric diseases.

Conclusion

Redox dysregulation may constitute a hub where genetic and environmental vulnerability factors converge, and their timing in brain development is likely to play a decisive role in the phenotype of schizophrenia patients. In experimental models, such redox dysregulation induces anomalies strikingly similar to those observed in patients. A treatment restoring redox balance, deprived of side-effects, yields improvements in chronic patients. Its application in early psychosis and prodrome, intended to halt pathological developmental processes, is promising. The proposed mechanisms should provide biomarkers for early detection, paving the way for prevention perspectives in which nutrigenetics would play a primordial role.

Acknowledgments

We thank all patients and controls who participated in the studies and all collaborators involved in the study: R. Gysin, C. Butticaz, A. Cottier, F. Gheorghita, J.P. Hornung, S. Lavoie, H. Moser, A. Polari, M. Preisig, D. Preissmann, T. Teichmann. This work was supported by the Swiss National Foundation (310000-116689 and 320000-122419/1), Loterie Romande, NARSAD, the Stanley Thomas Johnson Foundation and the Alamaya Foundation.

References

1 Insel TR: Disruptive insights in psychiatry: transforming a clinical discipline. J Clin Invest 2009;119:700–705.
2 Andreasen NC: Schizophrenia: the fundamental questions. Brain Res Brain Res Rev 2000;31:106–112.
3 Lewis DA, Lieberman JA: Catching up on schizophrenia: natural history and neurobiology. Neuron 2000;28:325–334.
4 Cardno AG, Gottesman II: Twin studies of schizophrenia: from bow-and-arrow concordances to star wars Mx and functional genomics. Am J Med Genet 2000;97:12–17.
5 Barr CL, Kennedy JL, Pakstis AJ, et al: Progress in a genome scan for linkage in schizophrenia in a large Swedish kindred. Am J Med Genet 1994;54:51–58.
6 Coon H, Jensen S, Holik J, et al: Genomic scan for genes predisposing to schizophrenia. Am J Med Genet 1994;54:59–71.
7 Blouin JL, Dombroski BA, Nath SK, et al: Schizophrenia susceptibility loci on chromosomes 13q32 and 8p21. Nat Genet 1998;20:70–73.
8 Brzustowicz LM, Honer WG, Chow EW, et al: Linkage of familial schizophrenia to chromosome 13q32. Am J Hum Genet 1999;65:1096–1103.
9 Pulver AE : Search for schizophrenia susceptibility genes. Biol Psychiatry 2000;47:221–230.
10 Mcguffin P, Tandon K, Corsico A: Linkage and association studies of schizophrenia. Curr Psychiatry Rep 2003;5:121–127.
11 Carlson CS, Eberle MA, Kruglyak L, Nickerson DA: Mapping complex disease loci in whole-genome association studies. Nature 2004;429:446–452.

12 Stefansson H, Rujescu D, Cichon S, et al: Large recurrent microdeletions associated with schizophrenia. Nature 2008;455:232–236.
13 Rujescu D, Ingason A, Cichon S, et al: Disruption of the neurexin 1 gene is associated with schizophrenia. Hum Mol Genet 2009;18:988–996.
14 International Schizophrenia Consortium: Rare chromosomal deletions and duplications increase risk of schizophrenia. Nature 2008;455:237–241.
15 Hoogendoorn ML, Vorstman JA, Jalali GR, et al: Prevalence of 22q11 2 deletions in 311 Dutch patients with schizophrenia. Schizophr Res 2008;98:84–88.
16 O'Donovan MC, Craddock N, Norton N, et al: Identification of loci associated with schizophrenia by genome-wide association and follow-up. Nat Genet 2008;40:1053–1055.
17 Sklar P: Genomewide association for schizophrenia: the Broad/Stanley study. World Congress of Psychiatric Genetics, 2008.
18 Blackwood DH, Fordyce A, Walker MT, et al: Schizophrenia and affective disorders: cosegregation with a translocation at chromosome 1q42 that directly disrupts brain-expressed genes: clinical and P300 findings in a family. Am J Hum Genet 2001;69:428–433.
19 Tosato S, Dazzan P, Collier D: Association between the neuregulin 1 gene and schizophrenia: a systematic review. Schizophr Bull 2005;31:613–617.
20 Tosic M, Ott J, Barral S, et al: Schizophrenia and oxidative stress: glutamate cysteine ligase modifier as a susceptibility gene. Am J Hum Genet 2006;79:586–592.
21 Gysin R, Kraftsik R, Sandell J, et al: Impaired glutathione synthesis in schizophrenia: convergent genetic and functional evidence. Proc Natl Acad Sci USA 2007;104:16621–16626.
22 Caspi A, Moffitt TE, Cannon M, et al: Moderation of the effect of adolescent-onset cannabis use on adult psychosis by a functional polymorphism in the catechol-O-methyltransferase gene: longitudinal evidence of a gene X environment interaction. Biol Psychiatry 2005;57:1117–1127.
23 Nicodemus KK, Straub RE, Egan MF, Weinberger DR: Evidence for statistical epistasis between (COMT) Val158Met polymorphism and multiple putative schizophreia susceptibility genes. Am J Med Genet B Neuropsychiatr Genet 2005;138B:130–131.
24 Leweke FM, Gerth CW, Koethe D, et al: Antibodies to infectious agents in individuals with recent onset schizophrenia. Eur Arch Psychiatry Clin Neurosci 2004;254:4–8.
25 Cannon TD, Rosso IM, Hollister JM, et al: A prospective cohort study of genetic and perinatal influences in the etiology of schizophrenia. Schizophr Bull 2000;26:351–366.
26 Rosso IM, Cannon TD, Huttunen T, et al: Obstetric risk factors for early-onset schizophrenia in a Finnish birth cohort. Am J Psychiatry 2000;157:801–807.
27 Marcelis M, Van Os J, Sham P, et al: Obstetric complications and familial morbid risk of psychiatric disorders. Am J Med Genet 1998;81:29–36.
28 Petronis A: The origin of schizophrenia: genetic thesis, epigenetic antithesis and resolving synthesis. Biol Psychiatry 2004;55:965–970.
29 Weinberger DR: Implications of normal brain development for the pathogenesis of schizophrenia. Arch Gen Psychiatry 1987;44:660–669.
30 Murray RM, Lewis SW: Is schizophrenia a neurodevelopmental disorder? Br Med J (Clin Res Ed) 1987;295:681–682.
31 Lewis DA, Levitt P: Schizophrenia as a disorder of neurodevelopment. Annu Rev Neurosci 2002;25:409–432.
32 Selemon LD, Goldman-Rakic PS: The reduced neuropil hypothesis: a circuit based model of schizophrenia. Biol Psychiatry 1999;45:17–25.
33 Parnas J, Bovet P, Innocenti GM: Schizophrenic trait features binding and cortico-cortical connectivity: a neurodevelopmental pathogenetic hypothesis. Neurol Psychiatry Brain Res 1996;4:185–196
34 Friston KJ: The disconnection hypothesis. Schizophrenia Res 1998;30:115–125.
35 Raedler TJ, Knable MB, Weinberger DR: Schizophrenia as a developmental disorder of the cerebral cortex. Curr Opin Neurobiol 2000;8:157–161.
36 Matthysse S: Antipsychotic drug actions: a clue to the neuropathology of schizophrenia? Fed Proc 1973;32:200–205.
37 Carlsson A: The current status of the dopamine hypothesis of schizophrenia. Neuropsychopharmacology 1988;1:179–186.
38 Lewis DA, Gonzalez-Burgos G: Pathophysiologically based treatment interventions in schizophrenia. Nat Med 2006;12:1016–1022.
39 Tamminga CA, Lahti AC, Medoff DR, Gao XM, Holcomb HH: Evaluating glutamatergic transmission in schizophrenia. Ann NY Acad Sci 2003;1003:113–118.
40 Moghaddam B: Bringing order to the glutamate chaos in schizophrenia. Neuron 2003;40:881–884.
41 Coyle JT: Glutamate and schizophrenia: beyond the dopamine hypothesis. Cell Mol Neurobiol 2006;26:365–384.

42 Benes FM, Berretta S: GABAergic interneurons: implications for understanding schizophrenia and bipolar disorder. Neuropsychopharmacology 2001;25:1–27.

43 Volk DW, Pierri JN, Fritschy JM, et al: Reciprocal alterations in pre- and postsynaptic inhibitory markers at chandelier cell inputs to pyramidal neurons in schizophrenia. Cereb Cortex 2002;12:1063–1070.

44 Beasley CL, Zhang ZJ, Patten I, Reynolds GP: Selective deficits in prefrontal cortical GABAergic neurons in schizophrenia defined by the presence of calcium-binding proteins. Biol Psychiatry 2002;52:708–715.

45 Hashimoto T, Volk DW, Eggan SM, et al: Gene expression deficits in a subclass of GABA neurons in the prefrontal cortex of subjects with schizophrenia. J Neurosci 2003;23:6315–6326.

46 Lewis DA, Hashimoto T, Volk DW: Cortical inhibitory neurons and schizophrenia. Nat Rev Neurosci 2005;6:312–324.

47 Ross CA, Margolis RL, Reading SA, Pletnikov M, Coyle JT: Neurobiology of schizophrenia. Neuron 2006;52:139–153.

48 Garey LJ, Ong WY, Patel TS, et al: Reduced dendritic spine density on cerebral cortical pyramidal neurons in schizophrenia. J Neurol Neurosurg Psychiatry 1998;65:446–453.

49 Glantz LA, Lewis DA: Decreased dendritic spine density on prefrontal cortical pyramidal neurons in schizophrenia. Arch Gen Psychiatry 2000;57:65–73.

50 Rosoklija G, Toomayan G, Ellis SP, et al: Structural abnormalities of subicular dendrites in subjects with schizophrenia and mood disorders: preliminary findings. Arch Gen Psychiatry 2000;57:349–356.

51 Kolluri N, Sun Z, Sampson AR, Lewis DA: Lamina-specific reductions in dendritic spine density in the prefrontal cortex of subjects with schizophrenia. Am J Psychiatry 2005;162:1200–1202.

52 Volk DW, Austin MC, Pierri JN, Sampson AR, Lewis DA: Decreased glutamic acid decarboxylase67 messenger RNA expression in a subset of prefrontal cortical gamma-aminobutyric acid neurons in subjects with schizophrenia. Arch Gen Psychiatry 2000;57:237–245.

53 Lim KO, Helpern JA: Neuropsychiatric applications of DTI-a review. NMR Biomed 2002;15:587–593.

54 Kanaan RA, Kim JS, Kaufmann WE, et al: Diffusion tensor imaging in schizophrenia. Biol Psychiatry 2005;58:921–929.

55 Engel AK, Konig P, Kreiter AK, Singer W: Interhemispheric synchronization of oscillatory neuronal responses in cat visual cortex. Science 1991;252:1177–1179.

56 Singer W, Gray CM: Visual feature integration and the temporal correlation hypothesis. Annu Rev Neurosci 1995;18:555–586.

57 Tallon-Baudry C, Bertrand O: Oscillatory gamma activity in humans and its role in object representation. Trends Cogn Sci 1999;3:151–162.

58 Spencer KM, Nestor PG, Niznikiewicz MA, et al: Abnormal neural synchrony in schizophrenia. J Neurosci 2003;23:7407–7411.

59 Uhlhaas PJ, Singer W: Neural synchrony in brain disorders: relevance for cognitive dysfunctions and pathophysiology. Neuron 2006;52:155–168.

60 Jalili M, Lavoie S, Deppen P, et al: Dysconnection topography in schizophrenia revealed with state-space analysis of EEG. PLoS ONE 2007;2:e1059.

61 Knyazeva MG, Jalili M, Meuli R, et al: Alpha rhythm and hypofrontality in schizophrenia. Acta Psychiatr Scand 2008;118:188–199.

62 Shelley AM, Ward PB, Catts SV, et al: Mismatch negativity: an index of a preattentive processing deficit in schizophrenia. Biol Psychiatry 1991;30:1059–1062.

63 Umbricht D, Javitt D, Novak G, et al: Effects of clozapine on auditory event-related potentials in schizophrenia. Biol Psychiatry 1998;44:716–725.

64 Umbricht D, Schmid L, Koller R, et al: Ketamine-induced deficits in auditory and visual context-dependent processing in healthy volunteers: implications for models of cognitive deficits in schizophrenia. Arch Gen Psychiatry 2000;57:1139–1147.

65 Insel TR: Translating scientific opportunity into public health impact: a strategic plan for research on mental illness. Arch Gen Psychiatry 2009;66:128–133.

66 Lu SC: Regulation of glutathione synthesis. Mol Aspects Med 2008;30:42–59.

67 Jones DP: Radical-free biology of oxidative stress. Am J Physiol Cell Physiol 2008;295:C849–C868.

68 Shi ZZ, Osei-Frimpong J, Kala G, et al: Glutathione synthesis is essential for mouse development but not for cell growth in culture. Proc Natl Acad Sci USA 2000;97:5101–5106.

69 Lipton SA, Choi YB, Takahashi H, et al: Cysteine regulation of protein function as exemplified by NMDA-receptor modulation. Trends Neurosci 2002;25:474–480.

70 Valko M, Leibfritz D, Moncol J, et al: Free radicals and antioxidants in normal physiological functions and human disease. Int J Biochem Cell Biol 2007;39:44–84.

71 Mahadik SP, Mukherjee S: Free radical pathology and antioxidant defense in schizophrenia: a review. Schizophrenia Res 1996;19:1–17.

72 Yao JK, Reddy RD, van Kammen DP: Oxidative damage and schizophrenia: an overview of the evidence and its therapeutic implications. CNS Drugs 2001;15:287–310.

73 Herken H, Uz E, Ozyurt H, et al: Evidence that the activities of erythrocyte free radical scavenging enzymes and the products of lipid peroxidation are increased in different forms of schizophrenia. Mol Psychiatry 2001;6:66–73.

74 Ben-Shachar D: Mitochondrial dysfunction in schizophrenia: a possible linkage to dopamine. J Neurochem 2002;83:1241–1251.

75 Zhang XY, Tan YL, Cao LY, et al: Antioxidant enzymes and lipid peroxidation in different forms of schizophrenia treated with typical and atypical antipsychotics. Schizophrenia Res 2006;81:291–300.

76 Prabakaran S, Swatton JE, Ryan MM, et al: Mitochondrial dysfunction in schizophrenia: evidence for compromised brain metabolism and oxidative stress. Mol Psychiatry 2004;9:684–697.

77 Evans DR, Parikh VV, Khan MM, et al: Red blood cell membrane essential fatty acid metabolism in early psychotic patients following antipsychotic drug treatment. Prostaglandins Leukot Essent Fatty Acids 2003;69:393–399.

78 Marchbanks RM, Ryan M, Day IN, et al: A mitochondrial DNA sequence variant associated with schizophrenia and oxidative stress. Schizophrenia Res 2003;65:33–38.

79 Do KQ, Bovet P, Cabungcal JH, et al: Redox dysregulation in schizophrenia: genetic susceptibility and pathophysiological mechanisms; in Lajtha A: Handbook of Neurochemistry and Molecular Neurobiology. New York, Springer, vol 27, 2009.

80 Do KQ, Trabesinger AH, Kirsten-Kruger M, et al: Schizophrenia: glutathione deficit in cerebrospinal fluid and prefrontal cortex in vivo. Eur J Neurosci 2000;12:3721–3728.

81 Yao JK, Leonard S, Reddy R: Altered glutathione redox state in schizophrenia. Dis Markers 2006;22:83–93.

82 Matsuzawa D, Obata T, Shirayama Y, et al: Negative correlation between brain glutathione level and negative symptoms in schizophrenia: a 3T ^{1}H-MRS study. PLoS ONE 2008;3:e1944.

83 Raffa M, Mechri A, Othman LB, et al: Decreased glutathione levels and antioxidant enzyme activities in untreated and treated schizophrenic patients. Prog Neuropsychopharmacol Biol Psychiatry 2009;33:1178–1183.

84 Do KQ, Cabungcal JH, Frank A, Steullet P, Cuenod M: Redox dysregulation neurodevelopment and schizophrenia. Curr Opin Neurobiol 2009;19:220–230.

85 Cabungcal JH, Nicolas D, Kraftsik R, et al: Glutathione deficit during development induces anomalies in the rat anterior cingulate GABAergic neurons: relevance to schizophrenia. Neurobiol Dis 2006;22:624–637.

86 Grima G, Benz B, Parpura V, Cuenod M, Do KQ: Dopamine-induced oxidative stress in neurons with glutathione deficit: implication for schizophrenia. Schizophr Res 2003;62:213–224.

87 Steullet P, Neijt HC, Cuenod M, Do KQ: Synaptic plasticity impairment and hypofunction of NMDA receptors induced by glutathione deficit: relevance to schizophrenia. Neuroscience 2006;137:807–819.

88 Steullet P, Lavoie S, Kraftsik R, et al: A glutathione deficit alters dopamine modulation of L-type calcium channels via D2 and ryanodine receptors in neurons. Free Radic Biol Med 2008;44:1042–1054.

89 Castagne V, Rougemont M, Cuenod M, Do KQ: Low brain glutathione and ascorbic acid associated with dopamine uptake inhibition during rat's development induce long-term cognitive deficit: relevance to schizophrenia. Neurobiol Dis 2004;15:93–105.

90 Castagne VV, Cuenod M, Do KQ: An animal model with relevance to schizophrenia: sex-dependent cognitive deficits in osteogenic disorder: Shionogi rats induced by glutathione synthesis and dopamine uptake inhibition during development. Neuroscience 2004;123:821–834.

91 Cabungcal JH, Preissmann D, Delseth C, et al: Transitory glutathione deficit during brain development induces cognitive impairment in juvenile and adult rats: relevance to schizophrenia. Neurobiol Dis 2007;26:634–645.

92 Piazza PV, Le Moal ML: Pathophysiological basis of vulnerability to drug abuse: role of an interaction between stress glucocorticoids and dopaminergic neurons. Annu Rev Pharmacol Toxicol 1996;36:359–378.

93 Barrot M, Abrous DN, Marinelli M, et al: Influence of glucocorticoids on dopaminergic transmission in the rat dorsolateral striatum. Eur J Neurosci 2001;13:812–818.

94 Ganguli R, Singh A, Brar J, Carter C, Mintun M: Hydrocortisone induced regional cerebral activity changes in schizophrenia: a PET scan study. Schizophrenia Res 2002;56:241–247.

95 Liu J Wang X, Shigenaga MK, Yeo HC, Mori A, Ames BN: Immobilization stress causes oxidative damage to lipid protein and DNA in the brain of rats. FASEB J 1996;10:1532–1538.

96 Harrison PJ: The neuropathology of schizophrenia: a critical review of the data and their interpretation. Brain 1999;122:593–624.

97 Kohr G, Eckardt S, Luddens H, Monyer H, Seeburg PH: NMDA receptor channels: subunit-specific potentiation by reducing agents. Neuron 1994;12: 1031–1040.

98 Krystal JH, Karper LP, Seibyl JP, et al: Subanesthetic effects of the noncompetitive NMDA antagonist ketamine in humans: psychotomimetic perceptual cognitive and neuroendocrine responses. Arch Gen Psychiatry 1994;51:199–214.

99 Kempf L, Nicodemus KK, Kolachana B, et al: Functional polymorphisms in PRODH are associated with risk and protection for schizophrenia and frontostriatal structure and function. PLoS Genet 2008;4:e1000252.

100 Phang JM, Donald SP, Pandhare J, Liu Y: The metabolism of proline a stress substrate modulates carcinogenic pathways. Amino Acids 2008;35:681–690.

101 Fuchs EC, Zivkovic AR, Cunningham MO, et al: Recruitment of parvalbumin-positive interneurons determines hippocampal function and associated behavior. Neuron 2007;53:591–604.

102 Davis KL, Haroutunian V: Global expression-profiling studies and oligodendrocyte dysfunction in schizophrenia and bipolar disorder. Lancet 2003; 362:758.

103 Abekawa T, Ito K, Nakagawa S, Koyama T: Prenatal exposure to an NMDA receptor antagonist MK-801 reduces density of parvalbumin-immunoreactive GABAergic neurons in the medial prefrontal cortex and enhances phencyclidine-induced hyperlocomotion but not behavioral sensitization to methamphetamine in postpubertal rats. Psychopharmacology (Berl) 2007;192:303–316.

104 Rujescu D, Bender A, Keck M, et al: A pharmacological model for psychosis based on N-methyl-D-aspartate receptor hypofunction: molecular cellular functional and behavioral abnormalities. Biol Psychiatry 2006;59:721–729.

105 Wang CZ, Yang SF, Xia Y, Johnson KM: Postnatal phencyclidine administration selectively reduces adult cortical parvalbumin-containing interneurons. Neuropsychopharmacology 2008;33:2442–2455.

106 Behrens MM, Ali SS, Dao DN, et al: Ketamine-induced loss of phenotype of fast-spiking interneurons is mediated by NADPH-oxidase. Science 2007; 318:1645–1647.

107 Bedard K, Krause KH: The NOX family of ROS-generating NADPH oxidases: physiology and pathophysiology. Physiol Rev 2007;87:245–313.

108 Uhlhaas PJ, Linden DE, Singer W, et al: Dysfunctional long-range coordination of neural activity during Gestalt perception in schizophrenia. J Neurosci 2006;26:8168–8175.

109 Li Z, Dong T, Proschel C, Noble M: Chemically diverse toxicants converge on Fyn and c-Cbl to disrupt precursor cell function. PLoS Biol 2007;5:e35

110 Smith J, Ladi E, Mayer-Proschel M, Noble M: Redox state is a central modulator of the balance between self-renewal and differentiation in a dividing glial precursor cell: Proc Natl Acad Sci USA 2000; 97:10032–10037.

111 Robertson GS, Hori SE, Powell KJ: Schizophrenia: an integrative approach to modelling a complex disorder. J Psychiatry Neurosci 2006;31:157–167.

112 O'tuathaigh CM, Babovic D, O'meara G, et al: Susceptibility genes for schizophrenia: characterisation of mutant mouse models at the level of phenotypic behaviour. Neurosci Biobehav Rev 2007;31: 60–78.

113 Rougemont M, Do KQ, Castagne V: A new model of glutathione deficit during development: effect of glutathione deficit on lipid peroxidation in the rat brain. J Neurosci Res 2003;70:774–783.

114 Steullet P, Cabungcal JH, Kulak A, et al: Redox dysregulation affects the ventral but not dorsal hippocampus: impairment of parvalbumin neurons, gamma oscillations and related behaviours. J Neurosci 2010;30:2547–2558.

115 Do KQ, Conus P, Bovet P, et al: developmental critical period in genetic redox dysregulation: animal and human studies in schizophrenia. Schizophr Bull 2009;35:106–107.

116 Behrens MM, Ali SS, Dao DN, et al: Ketamine-induced loss of phenotype of fast-spiking interneurons is mediated by NADPH-oxidase. Science 2007;318:1645–1647.

117 Uhlhaas PJ, Haenschel C, Nikolic D, Singer W: The role of oscillations and synchrony in cortical networks and their putative relevance for the pathophysiology of schizophrenia. Schizophr Bull 2008;34:927–943.

118 Kubicki M, McCarley R, Westin CF, et al: A review of diffusion tensor imaging studies in schizophrenia. J Psychiatr Res 2007;41:15–30.

119 Kyriakopoulos M, Vyas NS, Barker GJ, Chitnis XA, Frangou S: A diffusion tensor imaging study of white matter in early-onset schizophrenia. Biol Psychiatry 2008;63:519–523.

120 Zafarullah M, Li WQ, Sylvester J, Ahmad M: Molecular mechanisms of N-acetylcysteine actions. Cell Mol Life Sci 2003;60:6–20.

121 Tirouvanziam R, Conrad CK, Bottiglieri T, et al: High-dose oral N-acetylcysteine a glutathione prodrug modulates inflammation in cystic fibrosis. Proc Natl Acad Sci USA 2006;103:4628–4633.

122 Decramer M, Rutten-van Molken M, Dekhuijzen PN, et al: Effects of N-acetylcysteine on outcomes in chronic obstructive pulmonary disease (Bronchitis Randomized on NAC Cost-Utility Study, BRONCUS): a randomised placebo-controlled trial. Lancet 2005;365:1552–1560.

123 Arakawa M, Ito Y: N-acetylcysteine and neurodegenerative diseases: basic and clinical pharmacology. Cerebellum 2007;1–7.

124 Adair JC, Knoefel JE, Morgan N: Controlled trial of N-acetylcysteine for patients with probable Alzheimer's disease. Neurology 2001;57:1515–1517.

125 Andreassen OA, Dedeoglu A, Klivenyi P, Beal MF, Bush AI: N-acetyl-L-cysteine improves survival and preserves motor performance in an animal model of familial amyotrophic lateral sclerosis. Clin Neurosci 2000;11:2491–2493.

126 Zhou W, Kalivas PW: N-acetylcysteine reduces extinction responding and induces enduring reductions in cue- and heroin-induced drug-seeking. Biol Psychiatry 2008;63:338–340.

127 Atkuri KR, Mantovani JJ, Herzenberg LA, Herzenberg LA: N-Acetylcysteine: a safe antidote for cysteine/glutathione deficiency. Curr Opin Pharmacol 2007;7:355–359.

128 Cotgreave IA: N-acetylcysteine: pharmacological considerations and experimental and clinical applications. Adv Pharmacol 1997;38:205–227.

129 Berk M, Copolov D, Dean O, et al: N-acetyl cysteine as a glutathione precursor for schizophrenia: a double-blind randomized placebo-controlled trial. Biol Psychiatry 2008;64:361–368.

130 Lavoie S, Murray MM, Deppen P, et al: Glutathione precursor N-acetyl-cysteine improves mismatch negativity in schizophrenia patients. Neuropsychopharmacology 2008;33:2187–2199.

131 Javitt DC, Doneshka P, Zylberman I, Ritter W, Vaughan HG Jr: Impairment of early cortical processing in schizophrenia: an event-related potential confirmation study. Biol Psychiatry 1993;33:513–519.

132 Berk M, Copolov DL, Dean O, et al: N-acetyl cysteine for depressive symptoms in bipolar disorder: a double-blind randomized placebo-controlled trial. Biol Psychiatry 2008;64:468–475.

133 Crow TJ: The continuum of psychosis and its implication for the structure of the gene. Br J Psychiatry 1986;149:419–429.

134 McGorry PD, Yung AR: Early intervention in psychosis: an overdue reform. Aust NZ J Psychiatry 2003;37:393–398.

135 Killackey E, Yung AR, McGorry PD: Early psychosis: where we've been, where we still have to go. Epidemiol Psichiatr Soc 2007;16:102–108.

136 Falloon IR: Early intervention for first episodes of schizophrenia: a preliminary exploration. Psychiatry 1992;55:4–15.

137 Loebel AD, Lieberman JA, Alvir JM, et al: Duration of psychosis and outcome in first-episode schizophrenia. Am J Psychiatry 1992;149:1183–1188.

138 McGlashan TH: Early detection and intervention in schizophrenia: research. Schizophr Bull 1996;22:327–345.

139 McGorry PD, Edwards J, Mihalopoulos C, Harrigan SM, Jackson HJ: EPPIC: an evolving system of early detection and optimal management. Schizophr Bull 1996;22:305–326

140 Yung AR, McGorry PD: The prodromal phase of first-episode psychosis: past and current conceptualizations. Schizophr Bull 1996;22:353–370.

141 Yung AR, Nelson B, Stanford C, et al: Validation of 'prodromal' criteria to detect individuals at ultra high risk of psychosis: 2 year follow-up. Schizophr Res 2008;105:10–17.

142 McGorry PD, Yung AR, Bechdolf A, Amminger P: Back to the future: predicting and reshaping the course of psychotic disorder. Arch Gen Psychiatry 2008;65:25–27.

143 Cannon TD, Cadenhead K, Cornblatt B, et al: Prediction of psychosis in youth at high clinical risk: a multisite longitudinal study in North America. Arch Gen Psychiatry 2008;65:28–37.

144 Birchwood M, Todd P, Jackson C: Early intervention in psychosis: the critical period hypothesis. Br J Psychiatry Suppl 1998;172(suppl 33):53–59.

145 Conus P, Montagrin Y, Bircher R, et al: TIPP-Lausanne first episode psychosis program: patients' baseline characteristics and impact of the program on adherence to psychosocial treatment. Schizophr Res 2008;98(suppl 1):81.

146 McGlashan TH, Miller TJ, Woods SW: Pre-onset detection and intervention research in schizophrenia psychoses: current estimates of benefit and risk. Schizophr Bull 2001;27:563–570.

147 Phillips LJ, McGorry PD, Yung AR, et al: Prepsychotic phase of schizophrenia and related disorders: recent progress and future opportunities. Br J Psychiatry Suppl 2005;48:s33–s44.

148 Bjelland I, Tell GS, Vollset SE, Refsum H, Ueland PM: Folate vitamin B_{12} homocysteine and the MTHFR 677C→T polymorphism in anxiety and depression: the Hordaland Homocysteine Study. Arch Gen Psychiatry 2003;60:618–626.

149 James SJ, Cutler P, Melnyk S, et al: Metabolic biomarkers of increased oxidative stress and impaired methylation capacity in children with autism. Am J Clin Nutr 2004;80:1611–1617.

150 Smythies JR, Gottfries CG, Regland B: Disturbances of one-carbon metabolism in neuropsychiatric disorders: a review. Biol Psychiatry 1997;41:230–233.

151 Muskiet FA, Kemperman RF: Folate and long-chain polyunsaturated fatty acids in psychiatric disease. J Nutr Biochem 2006;17:717–727.

152 Regland B, Johansson BV, Gottfries CG: Homocysteinemia and schizophrenia as a case of methylation deficiency. J Neural Transm Gen Sect 1994;98:143–152.

153 Regland B: Schizophrenia and single-carbon metabolism. Prog Neuropsychopharmacol Biol Psychiatry 2005;29:1124–1132.

154 Park LC, Baldessarini RJ, Kety SS: Methionine effects on chronic schizophrenics. Arch Genet Psychiatry 1965;12:346–351.

155 Deth R, Muratore C, Benzecry J, Power-Charnitsky VA, Waly M: How environmental and genetic factors combine to cause autism: a redox/methylation hypothesis. Neurotoxicology 2008;29:190–201.

156 Connor H, Newton DJ, Preston FE, Woods HF: Oral methionine loading as a cause of acute serum folate deficiency: its relevance to parenteral nutrition. Postgrad Med J 1978;54:318–320.

157 Ventura P, Panini R, Verlato C, Scarpetta G, Salvioli G: Peroxidation indices and total antioxidant capacity in plasma during hyperhomocysteinemia induced by methionine oral loading. Metabolism 2000;49:225–228.

158 Raijmakers MT, Schilders GW, Roes EM, et al: N-acetylcysteine improves the disturbed thiol redox balance after methionine loading. Clin Sci (Lond) 2003;105:173–180.

159 Avila MA, Corrales FJ, Ruiz F, et al: Specific interaction of methionine adenosyltransferase with free radicals. Biofactors 1998;8:27–32.

160 Gomes-Trolin C, Yassin M, Gottfries CG, et al: Erythrocyte and brain methionine adenosyltransferase activities in patients with schizophrenia. J Neural Transm 1998;105:1293–1305.

161 Deth R, Muratore C, Benzecry J, Power-Charnitsky VA, Waly M: How environmental and genetic factors combine to cause autism: a redox/methylation hypothesis. Neurotoxicology 2008;29:190–201.

162 Abdolmaleky HM, Smith CL, Faraone SV, et al: Methylomics in psychiatry: modulation of gene-environment interactions may be through DNA methylation. Am J Med Genet 2004;127B:51–59.

163 Abdolmaleky HM, Cheng KH, Russo A, et al: Hypermethylation of the reelin (RELN) promoter in the brain of schizophrenic patients: a preliminary report. Am J Med Genet B Neuropsychiatr Genet 2005;134:60–66.

164 Godfrey PS, Toone BK, Carney MW, et al: Enhancement of recovery from psychiatric illness by methylfolate. Lancet 1990;336:392–395.

165 Yehuda S, Rabinovitz S, Mostofsky DI: Essential fatty acids are mediators of brain biochemistry and cognitive functions. J Neurosci Res 1999;56:565–570.

166 Simopoulos AP: Importance of the ratio of omega-6/omega-3 essential fatty acids: evolutionary aspects. World Rev Nutr Diet 2003;92:1–22.

167 Keshavan MS, Mallinger AG, Pettegrew JW, Dippold C: Erythrocyte membrane phospholipids in psychotic patients. Psychiatry Res 1993;49:89–95.

168 Reddy RD, Keshavan MS, Yao JK: Reduced red blood cell membrane essential polyunsaturated fatty acids in first episode schizophrenia at neuroleptic-naive baseline. Schizophr Bull 2004;30:901–911.

169 Mahadik SP, Mukherjee S, Correnti EE, et al: Plasma membrane phospholipid and cholesterol distribution of skin fibroblasts from drug-naive patients at the onset of psychosis. Schizophr Res 1994;13:239–247

170 Horrobin DF, Manku MS, Hillman H, Iain A, Glen M : Fatty acid levels in the brains of schizophrenics and normal controls. Biol Psychiatry 1991;30:795–805.

171 Pettegrew JW, Keshavan MS, Panchalingam K, et al: Alterations in brain high-energy phosphate and membrane phospholipid metabolism in first-episode drug-naive schizophrenics: a pilot study of the dorsal prefrontal cortex by in vivo phosphorus 31 nuclear magnetic resonance spectroscopy. Arch Gen Psychiatry 1991;48:563–568.

172 Yao J, Stanley JA, Reddy RD, Keshavan MS, Pettegrew JW: Correlations between peripheral polyunsaturated fatty acid content and in vivo membrane phospholipid metabolites. Biol Psychiatry 2002;52:823–830.

173 Altar CA, Jurata LW, Charles V, et al: Deficient hippocampal neuron expression of proteasome ubiquitin and mitochondrial genes in multiple schizophrenia cohorts. Biol Psychiatry 2005;58:85–96.

174 Freeman MP, Hibbeln JR, Wisner KL, et al: Omega-3 fatty acids: evidence basis for treatment and future research in psychiatry. J Clin Psychiatry 2006;67:1954–1967.

175 Peet M, Horrobin DF: A dose-ranging exploratory study of the effects of ethyl-eicosapentaenoate in patients with persistent schizophrenic symptoms. J Psychiatr Res 2002;36:7–18.

176 Peet M, Horrobin DF: A dose-ranging study of the effects of ethyl-eicosapentaenoate in patients with ongoing depression despite apparently adequate treatment with standard drugs. Arch Gen Psychiatry 2002;59:913–919.

177 Nemets B, Stahl Z, Belmaker RH: Addition of omega-3 fatty acid to maintenance medication treatment for recurrent unipolar depressive disorder. Am J Psychiatry 2002;159:477–479.
178 Su KP, Huang SY, Chiu CC, Shen WW: Omega-3 fatty acids in major depressive disorder: a preliminary double-blind placebo-controlled trial. Eur Neuropsychopharmacol 2003;13:267–271.
179 Ross BM, Seguin J, Sieswerda LE: Omega-3 fatty acids as treatments for mental illness: which disorder and which fatty acid? Lipids Health Dis 2007;6: 21.
180 Bentsen H, Lingjaerde O, Solberg DK, Murck H: A multicentre placebo-controlled trial of eicosapentaenoic acid and antioxidant supplementation in the treatment of schizophrenia and related disorders. Schizophr Res 2006;81:29.
181 Gerster H: High-dose vitamin C: a risk for persons with high iron stores? Int J Vitam Nutr Res 1999; 69:67–82.
182 Podmore ID, Griffiths HR, Herbert KE, et al: Vitamin C exhibits pro-oxidant properties. Nature 1998;392:559.
183 Smythies JR, Gottfries CG, Regland B: Disturbances of one-carbon metabolism in neuropsychiatric disorders: a review. Biol Psychiatry 1997;41:230–233.
184 Handy DE, Zhang Y, Loscalzo J: Homocysteine down-regulates cellular glutathione peroxidase (GPx1) by decreasing translation. J Biol Chem 2005; 280:15518–15525.
185 Vitvitsky V, Prudova A, Stabler S, et al: Testosterone regulation of renal cystathionine beta-synthase: implications for sex-dependent differences in plasma homocysteine levels. Am J Physiol Renal Physiol 2007;293:F594–F600

Dr. Kim Q. Do
Center for Psychiatric Neuroscience, Department of Psychiatry, Lausanne University Hospital
Site de Cery
CH–1008 Prilly-Lausanne (Switzerland)
Tel. +41 21 643 6565, Fax +41 21 643 6562, E-Mail kim.do@chuv.ch

Nutrigenomics and Agriculture: A Perspective

Joseph T. Spence

Beltsville Agricultural Research Center, Agricultural Research Service, U.S. Department of Agriculture, Beltsville, Md., USA

The United States Department of Agriculture (USDA) plays an important role in the nutritional well-being of the country and throughout the world as part of its leadership role related to the production of food. Part of its mission is to conduct research that helps define an optimal and safe diet, to conduct research to enhance agricultural production, and to provide dietary guidance based on the latest research. These activities are carried out largely through the Agricultural Research Service, which is the intramural research arm of the department. In addition, the USDA plays an important role in administering a number of food assistance programs, which in order to be effective must be based on the best nutritional information available. The promise of nutrigenomics holds exceptional opportunities for all of the areas of importance to the department. In this report, I will examine the promise and challenges regarding the use of nutritional genomics in agriculture.

Genomic Prediction in Dairy Cows

The USDA has for over 100 years been active in programs to improve dairy cattle, which today is manifested in the National Cooperative Dairy Herd Improvement Program [1]. This program is aimed at improving the breeding of dairy cows. Through the widespread use of artificial insemination it has been extremely successful in keeping up with the demand for food, improving productivity and breeding, improving the quality of milk, and improving profitability for producers. This program has been of great importance to the dairy industry.

Milk production in dairy cows is a trait that is actually transferred through the male sire. Traditionally, through what is known as prodigy testing, predictions of the value of a bull are based on pedigree and milk production information that was maintained by the Animal Improvement Laboratory at the Beltsville Agricultural Research Center in Beltsville, Md. With the emerging understanding of the bovine genome [2, 3], it has opened up the door for genetic prediction. Working as part of a Cooperative Research and Development Agreement with Illumina Inc., Beltsville scientists and their collaborators began an ambitious examination of single nucleotide polymorphisms (SNPs) in cows. They have developed a commercially available SNP chip that can be used for screening a bull to produce a dairy cow that has the desired characteristics with regard to milk production. This newer method is called genome-enhanced improvement evaluation [4].

A comparison between the 2 methods of evaluating bulls is presented in table 1. The prodigy testing method of prediction is accurate to about 35%, the results are not known until the cow is about 5 years old, and the cost is about USD 50,000. Using an Illumna chip of over 50,000 SNPs, the accuracy of the prediction increases to greater than 70% and the determination can be done at birth of the calf. Significantly, the cost of the analysis is only about $250. This newer approach has changed the dairy industry in a very short time. It will lead to greater increases in productivity and milk production, which as a source of food is of significance for the human population. Beyond the dairy industry, this new approach represents a proof-of-concept of genetic prediction in agriculture. The use of this genomics approach can be used for any traits that one might be interested in. As indicated in the table, it has been used to predict a number of qualities important to the dairy industry. Furthermore, this SNP analysis approach can be used for genetic prediction in other commodities. Scientists at the Beltsville Agricultural Research Center are taking a similar approach to soybeans, by looking at qualities that are traditionally bred into them, such as protein content, disease resistance, yield, drought resistance and their storage characteristics.

Dietary Guidance

In the United States, the Department of Health and Human Services and the Department of Agriculture share the responsibility for development of the *Dietary Guidelines for Americans*. These guidelines form the basis for the government's dietary advice and are revised every 5 years to include the latest nutritional research. In light of the role that nutrition plays in maintaining health and the importance of a proper diet, it is attractive to consider that nutritionally related chronic diseases can be prevented by an improved diet. With the escalation of health care costs, an approach based on prevention is particularly attractive. These guidelines, like much of our nutritional advice, are a population-based recommendation. That is to say, the advice has been 'one size fits all' despite the fact that we know that tremendous variation can exist within the population. Despite this, however, the guidelines do serve a purpose for enlightening people about sound nutritional information. The promise of

Table 1. Comparison of traditional prodigy testing in dairy cows and genomic-enhanced improvement evaluation

	Traditional prodigy testing evaluation	Genome-enhanced improvement
Time of evaluation	5 years	Immediately at birth
Cost	USD 50,000	USD 250
Accuracy of prediction[a]	35%	70%

[a] Predictions determined for net merit, milk produced, fat, protein, productive life, pregnancy rate and calving ease.

nutrigenetics is to develop individualized dietary advice that more accurately represents the risk to an individual with regard to nutritionally related diseases. Today one can see the evolution toward this goal with the availability of information contained on the MyPyramid.gov website, where an individual's lifestyle and basic background can produce an individually tailored dietary pyramid.

As we become more aware of the genes that are involved in health and the polymorphisms associated with those genes, we will be confronted with the need to be able to make meaningful dietary recommendations. The overall approach and pitfalls associated with it are depicted in figure 1. Diets are a complex interaction of a variety of foods, nutrients and non-nutritive components. Changing one or a number of components of the diet will no doubt affect the overall impact of one's diet in ways that we do not fully understand. It is important to recognize that metabolism and interactions between nutrients and genes take place within the metabolic context of a cell or an individual. Many of the diseases that are associated with diet are known to be the results of multiple gene interactions [5, 6]. These interactions are poorly understood and a simple attempt to alter the interaction or to perturb the system might have no effect or even negative effects.

A significant but unknown factor in any discussion of nutrigenomics is the uncertainty of the role that epigenetic influences play in altering the response to diet. These epigenetic influences are likely to be significant in light of the fact that nutrition is the result of a lifetime of ingestion of nutrients and non-nutritive components. It is not clear if there is a threshold of interactions before the biological effects are fixed or are actually observed. Equally unknown is whether the effects of the interactions can be repaired or reversed. Additional research is needed to determine if important nutrient gene interactions occur early in life and if there is significant imprinting of an effect, and what if anything can be done to prevent or reverse the biological effect from occurring.

Fig. 1. Overview of significant interactions between diet and the genome of individuals as related to the development in individualized dietary advice. The shaded boxes highlight some of the concerns and potential problems in the development of the advice.

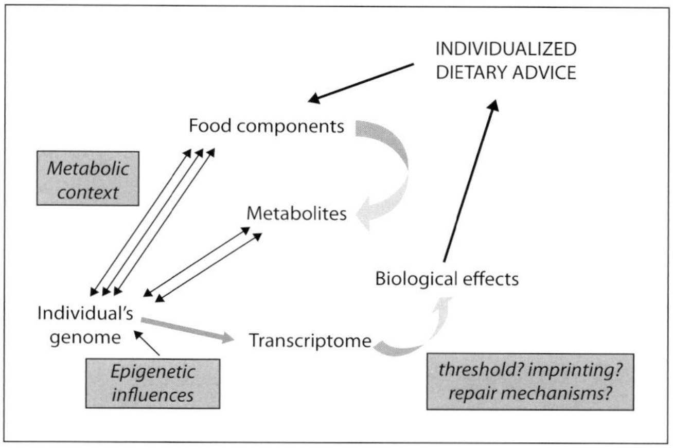

Discussion

The connection between nutrition and agriculture is a relationship that, because it is so fundamental, it is often overlooked or underappreciated. The example of genetic prediction in dairy cows has in a very short period of time changed the dairy industry and demonstrates the potential use of this technology for humans and nutrigenomic approaches to human nutrition. By itself, it demonstrates the value of genomics in making more food available for an expanding population. The ability to expand this approach to other commodities will offer an opportunity to increase yield, improve production and quality.

While genetic prediction might work well in agriculture and certainly reinforces the promise of nutrigenomics in the human population, there are reasons to be cautious. Agriculture has an advantage in that many of the animal and plant commodities are rather homogeneous genetically, while the human population is not. In agriculture, if a product does not meet the desired characteristics it could simply not be used or could be used for other purposes. Significantly, there exists a tremendous amount of phenotypic data for agricultural commodities and ready access to a huge collection of germplasm. Efforts are well underway to develop similar types of information and resources from ongoing nutritional studies and these resources must be available in order to understand and validate nutrigenomic approaches to delivering dietary guidance.

The nutritional status of an individual represents both the recent and lifetime intakes of substances in the diet. It is not clear to what extent the impact of these exposures can be reversed or mitigated. While there are well documented DNA repair mechanisms, their relationship to nutrition is now beginning to be understood [7]. The role of tissue remodeling and the ability to reverse nutritionally related biological effects are not clear. When dealing with genetic transformations, it is possible that imprinting occurs whereby effects on genetic material or gene expression may have long-lasting effects later in life. The role of epigenetic factors in influencing the response of an individual to dietary components will no doubt prove to be significant and need to be explored. The expanding importance and impact of nutrigenomics has the potential to raise some challenging ethical concerns. These and other issues will clearly need to be addressed as research in this important area proceeds.

As seen in the case of dairy production reported herein, the best genetic prediction is not 100% accurate. The guidance of individualized nutrition might be improved, but may never be completely accurate. No doubt the public will hear the terms genomics or individualized nutrition and interpret that as meaning highly accurate or absolute. This could open the door to unethical marketing of products and promises to the consumer or raise expectations that ultimately result in a loss of confidence in dietary guidance.

A significant issue that arises when taking a nutrigenomic approach to the development of dietary guidance is that we may be able to predict genetic predisposition but not know the actual genes that are of importance. It will clearly present a challenge to make meaningful dietary recommendations under such conditions. Even if we can identify the genes, the important point is determining how we can alter the diet in a way that produces the desired beneficial effect. In the simplest case, if we know how a particular dietary component interacts with a gene, then people carrying that gene can be advised to simply avoid that component. However, it is not likely we will be able to do that in many cases, particularly in light of the multiple genes that may be involved in many complex biological processes. Lastly, simply making dietary recommendations and getting people to change their dietary habits based on advice alone is never easy. Effective education programs for individuals, dieticians and health care providers will very much be needed. An important role that agriculture might play would be to develop varieties of commodities that would have desired nutrient profiles that would make it easier to meet the dietary recommendations. A 1998 perspective by Fink [8] highlighted the importance of *Arabidopsis* as a model organism in genetics. He discussed the shortfalls of nutrition and how this model organism might be helpful for studies of nutrition and how the optimal diet would be determined through selective breeding of plants and animals that might better meet our nutritional needs. Clearly we now have the tools to do these types of studies without the use of model systems but we need to have the nutritional rationale for particular studies.

Nutrigenetics/nutrigenomics will no doubt continue to provide information on metabolic processes and nutritional requirements. While the possibility of the development of individualized dietary guidance is becoming a reality, there are concerns and challenges. As we develop the capability to identify nutritional requirements for individuals, it is going to be a challenge to be able to make meaningful changes in a person's diet.

References

1 Wiggans GR: National genetic improvement programs for dairy cattle in the United States. J Anim Sci 1991:69:3853–3860.
2 The Bovine Genome Sequencing and Analysis Consortium, Elsik CG, Tellam RL, Worley KC: The genome sequence of taurine cattle: a window to ruminant biology and evolution. Science 2009:324:522–528.
3 The Bovine HapMap Consortium: Genome-wide survey of SNP variation uncovers the genetic structure of cattle breeds. Science 2009:324:528–532.
4 Wiggans GR, Sonstegard TS, Van Raden PM, et al: Selection of single-nucleotide polymorphisms and quality of genotypes used in genomic evaluation of dairy cattle in the United States and Canada. J Dairy Sci 2009:92:2931–2946.
5 Kraft P, Hunter DJ: Genetic risk prediction: are we there yet? N Engl J Med 2009:360:1701–1703.
6 Janssens AC, van Dujin CM: Genome-based prediction of common diseases: advances and prospects. Hum Mol Genet 2008:17:R166–R173.
7 Mathers JJ, Coxhead JM, Tyson J: Nutrition and DNA repair: potential mechanisms of action. Curr Cancer Drug Targets 2007:7:425–431.
8 Fink GR: Anatomy of a revolution. Genetics 1998:149:473–477.

Joseph T. Spence, PhD
Beltsville Agricultural Research Center, Building 003, Room 238
10300 Baltimore Avenue
Beltsville, MD 20705 (USA)
Tel. +1 301 504 6078, Fax +1 301 504 5863, E-Mail joseph.spence@ars.usda.gov

Opportunities and Challenges in Nutrigenetics/Nutrigenomics: Building Industry-Academia Partnerships

Peter J. Gillies[a] · Penny M. Kris-Etherton[b]

[a]DuPont Applied BioSciences, Wilmington, De., and [b]The Pennsylvania State University, University Park, Pa., USA

The Challenge before Us

Science belongs to society, a public trust that can leverage a wide range of partnerships to achieve shared goals and contribute to the public good. In the context of this article, the word 'partnership' is used to characterize a relationship based on shared ethical values, a passion for scientific excellence, and a dedication to training the next generation of nutrition scientists. More specifically, the word partnership is used to denote a relationship built on trust and mutual benefit rather than the legalities of research collaborations and contracts. The challenge is to build such partnerships in an increasingly skeptical world that is hypervigilant in terms of bias, conflict of interest, and private sector funding [1–3]. While not claiming to be the optimal model, DuPont and Pennsylvania State University (Penn State) may rightfully claim to have nurtured a long-standing and productive partnership centered on the molecular nutrition of omega-3 fatty acids, a partnership that is described herein.

Accelerated Learning Curves

A key measure of the success of a partnership is how far each party moves up the learning curves essential to their organizational or institutional goals. As shown in Box 1, DuPont's association with Penn State enabled them to quickly learn about the complexities of nutripharmacology, the cardiovascular benefits of omega-3 fatty acids, and the specific health benefits of EPA. More importantly, through interactions with the University's Center of Excellence in Nutrigenomics, they were able to glean strategic insights into the differential nutripharmacology of individual omega-3 fatty

> **Box 1. Insights gained by DuPont from their partnership with Penn State**
>
> - Nutrition is about complex mixtures, not single molecules, the effects of which may be additive and/or synergistic in outcome.
> - Omega-3 fatty acids have an extensive nutritional pharmacology; however, not all omega-3 fatty acids are the same.
> - Serum EPA correlates with several emerging cardiovascular biomarkers such as vascular cell adhesion molecule, TNF and C-reactive protein.
> - There is a nutrigenomic basis for the differential health benefits of individual fatty acids.
> - There is an opportunity for biotechnology to provide 'designer oils' as novel health products.

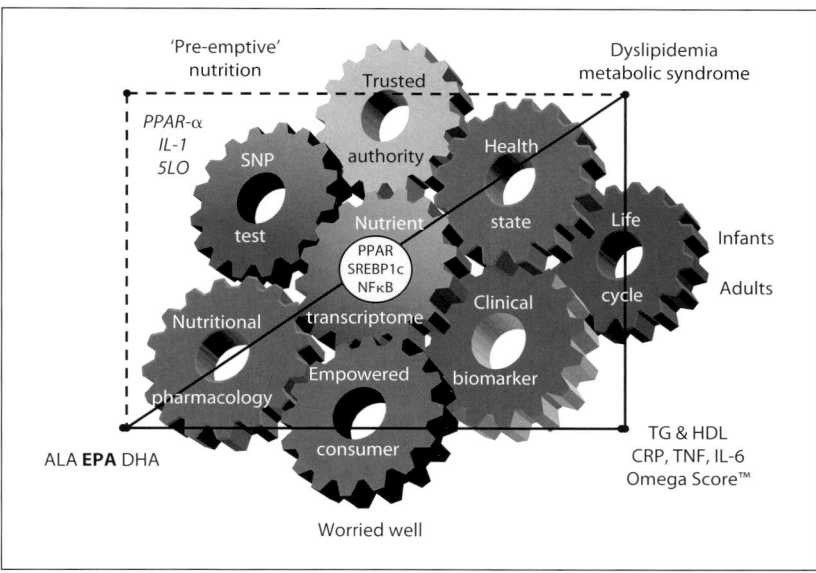

Fig. 1. A nutrigenetc/nutrigenomic model of health based on the emerging science of omega-3 fatty acids. While transcriptomic profiling of nutrients has already been reduced to practice in industry, the genetic testing component remains in its infancy.

acids such as ALA, EPA and DHA. This learning helped DuPont build the business case for developing the technology to produce 'designer oils'. Such oils can provide fatty acid mixtures for a spectrum of nutritional products including functional foods, dietary supplements, medical foods and even pharmaceutical agents. In an era of preemptive nutrition [4, 5], the ability to produce specific mixtures of fatty acids is a key step to enabling personalized nutrition. Figure 1 presents a nutrigenetic/nutrigenomic model of health based on omega-3 fatty acids. While the bottom right side of the model is readily implemented in practice and is applicable to the general population, the upper left side of the model is still unfolding as researchers look to establish

Box 2. Insights gained by Penn State from their partnership with DuPont

- Drugs and nutrients share considerable commonality in their underlying mechanisms of action.
- Profiling of serum fatty acids and the determination of fatty acid indexes can offer new insights into underlying metabolic events.
- Transcriptional regulation of stearoyl-CoA desaturase may be important in the dietary management of cardiometabolic disorders.
- Biotechnology may be important in providing the omega-3 fatty acids needed to meet emerging dietary recommendations.
- The experience and perspectives of private sector scientists represent a unique mentoring opportunity for students.

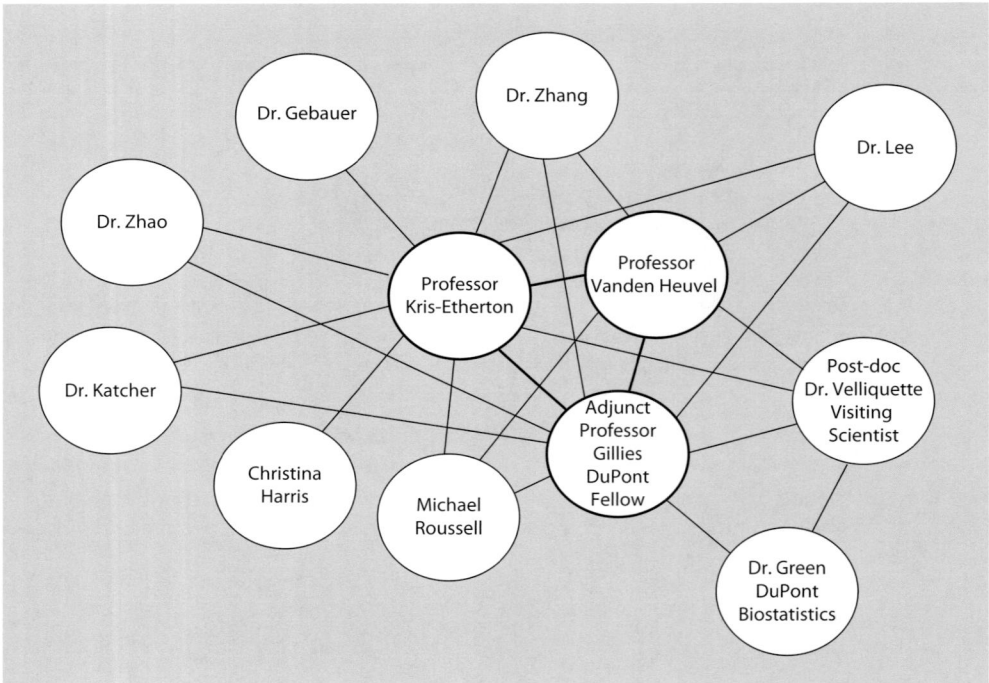

Fig. 2. The training of students and the subsequent development of professional networks is one of the high-value activities of academic-industry partnerships. When this occurs in a nutrigenetic/nutrigenomic paradigm, the future of nutrition science advances in both the public and private sectors.

the impact of different responses of single nucleotide polymorphisms to nutrients, the ethical-legal status of genetic testing is resolved [6] and a business model based on consumer segmentation by genotype is validated.

As shown in Box 2, Penn State's association with DuPont allowed them to tap into expertise in lipid metabolism and clinical pharmacology resulting in a greater appreciation of the mechanistic overlap between drugs and nutrients, to explore stearoyl-CoA desaturase as a potential target for the dietary management of metabolic syndrome through a DuPont visiting scientist, and to become aware of technological advances in the production of novel and healthier oils. Of particular value to its educational mission, Penn State was also able to offer students and postdoctoral fellows experience-based counseling regarding career opportunities in the private sector.

Professional Development and Building Networks

Another measure of partnership success is the extent to which it fosters the development of professional networks. As illustrated in figure 2, the research advisory team of Drs. Kris-Etherton, Vanden Heuvel and Gillies evolved over time into a multidisciplinary training node. Their 'graduates' now have positions in government, academia, industry, and even public-interest groups, organizations to which they bring a familiarity with what is possible at the public-private interface.

Sharing Science

Publications are unquestionably the currency of science. Herein co-authorship is both a reflection of the strength of the professional relationship and an objective measure of the scientific productivity of the partnership (Box 3). To some, such co-authorship raises the specter of bias, conflict of interest and suspect science; however, best-practice policies throughout the publication process from author disclosure, editorial oversight, and professional guidelines on public-private relationships provide powerful counterpoint to such concerns (Box 4) [7–10].

Anatomy of a Partnership Model in Molecular Nutrition

The DuPont-Penn State experience is illustrated in a simple partnership model in figure 3. In sector A on molecular nutrition, there are two special comments to be made. First, omega-3 fatty acids represent yet another example of a bioactive food that is both a nutrient and a drug (other examples being folate, niacin and vitamin A), and underscore the need to bring greater resolution to the 'nutrient-drug' debate [11, 12]. In this regard, nutrigenetics/nutrigenomics has an important role to play in providing a molecular foundation for this dialogue. Second, the partnership was ever mindful of the risks associated with involving students in product development. In sector B on how academia can leverage industrial partners, it should be mentioned that the

> **Box 3. Co-authored publications from DuPont and Penn State**
>
> Zhao G, Etherton TD, Martin KR, West SG, Gillies PJ, Kris-Etherton PM: Dietary alpha-linolenic acid reduces inflammatory and cardiovascular risk factors. J Nutrition 2004;134:2991–2997.
>
> Zhao G, Etherton TD, Martin KR, Vanden Heuvel JP, Gillies PJ, Kris-Etherton PM: Anti-inflammatory effects of polyunsaturated fatty acids in THP-1 Cells. Biochem Biophys Res Comm 2005;336: 909–917.
>
> Katcher HI, Gillies PJ, Kris-Etherton PM: Atherosclerotic cardiovascular disease; in Bowman BA, Russell RM (eds): Present Knowledge in Nutrition. Washington, ILSI Press, 2006, pp 649–668.
>
> Zhao G, Etherton TD, Martin KR, Gillies PJ, West SG, Kris-Etherton PM: Dietary α-linolenic acid inhibits proinflammatory cytokine production by peripheral blood mononuclear cells in hypercholesterolemic subjects. Am J Clin Nutr 2007;85:385–391.
>
> Gebauer S, Gillies P, Vanden Heuvel J, Kris-Etherton P: Integration of molecular biology and nutrition: the role of nutrigenomics in optimizing guidance for dietary fatty acids. Future Lipidol 2007;2:165–171.
>
> Katcher HI, Legro RS, Kunselman AR, Gillies PJ, Demers LM, Bagshaw DM, Kris-Etherton PM: The effectsof a whole grain enriched hypocaloric diet on cardiovascular disease risk factors in men and women with metabolic syndrome. Am J Clin Nutr 2008:87:79–90.
>
> Velliquette R, Gillies P, Kris-Etherton P, Green J, Zhao G, Vanden Heuvel J: Regulation of human stearoyl- CoA desaturase by omega-3 and omega-6 fatty acids: implications for the dietary management of elevated serum triglycerides. J Clin Lipidol 2009;3:281–288.
>
> Gebauer S, Kris-Etherton P, Gillies P: Fatty acid indexes as multifunctional biomarkers. 2009, in preparation.
>
> Zhang J, Kris-Etherton P, Gillies P, Vanden Heuvel J: Decreased expression of stearoyl-CoA desaturase 1 by alpha linolenic acid in macrophage-derived foam cells is responsible for enhanced cholesterol efflux. 2009, in preparation.

relationship evolved over time based on mutual interest in cardiovascular research, common membership in professional societies such as the American Society of Nutrition, the American Heart Association and the National Lipid Association, and a fundamental commitment to student education. Sector C offers a number of ways in which industry can grow the partnership from a relationship between two scientists to a relationship between two organizations. It should be noted that in this sector there is always the possibility of 'duality of interest' as companies move to manage their industry-academic networks in an open innovation model [13]. A duality of interest occurs when declared or undeclared ulterior motives are present even though such motives are not contrary to the interests of the partnership [14]. A duality of interest is not the same thing as conflict of interest, nor is it, a priori, a negative element in a partnership. To the contrary, in a world of leveraged networks, it's quite valuable. The nuanced distinction between conflict of interest and duality of interest is an example of the need for a better vocabulary to describe the relational elements of partnerships. Finally, sector D presents a spectrum of increasingly complex legal arrangements that can exist between industry and academia. Such arrangements fall outside the scope

> **Box 4.** ILSI provides 'guiding principles' for how industry and academia can interact in an open and transparent way. In a nutrigenomic paradigm there is a special need to expand these guidelines to keep pace with the molecular science and to protect consumer rights.
>
> *ILSI's Guiding Principles*
> 1. Conduct or sponsor research that is factual, transparent, and designed objectively and according to accepted principles of scientific inquiry.
> 2. Require control of both study and design research itself to remain with scientific investigators.
> 3. Not offer or accept remuneration geared to the outcome of a research project.
> 4. Ensure, before the commencement of studies, that there is a written agreement that the investigative team has the freedom and obligation to attempt to publish the findings within some specified time frame.
> 5. Require, in publications and conference presentations, full signed disclosure of all financial interests.
> 6. Not participate in undisclosed paid authorship arrangements in industry-sponsored publications or presentations.
> 7. Guarantee accessibility to all data and control of statistical analysis by investigators and appropriate auditors/reviewers.
> 8. Require that academic researchers, when they work in contract research organizations or act as contract researchers, make clear statements of their affiliations; and require that such researchers publish only under the auspices of the contract research organization.
>
> *Some Next Steps*
> - Update the dialogue within the emerging nutrigenomic paradigm.
> - Address issues such as intellectual property in the broader context of genetic tests and nutrigenomic claims.
> - Provide GELS training with attention to key issues of confidentiality, access and privacy.

of the present discussion, other than to note that they all incur a higher liability in terms of conflict of interest and scientific bias, and they are easy prey for the skeptics of industry-academia relations. What is important in sector D is to realize how quickly problems, or the perception thereof, can arise even in the simplest of business relationships. This said, there is clearly a time and place for industry-academic relationships and they can be ethically managed to ensure scientific integrity. The value and importance of such relations is underscored by the existence of the NIH Clinical and Translational Science Awards (CTSA) consortium that has as one of its specific goals 'to stimulate alliances in medical research and research training by identifying opportunities for collaboration among the CTSA members and private-sector organizations' [15]. It is noteworthy that in a recent survey of researchers doing translational science (c.f. nutrigenomics), 61.3% reported ties to industry and believed these ties contributed to their most important scientific work [16]. The key to navigating sector D is to know your relational coordinates. As illustrated in figure 4, one's position is constantly changing regardless of the source of research funding. Thus, the first step is to be aware where you are, the second step is to know how to behave. None of this

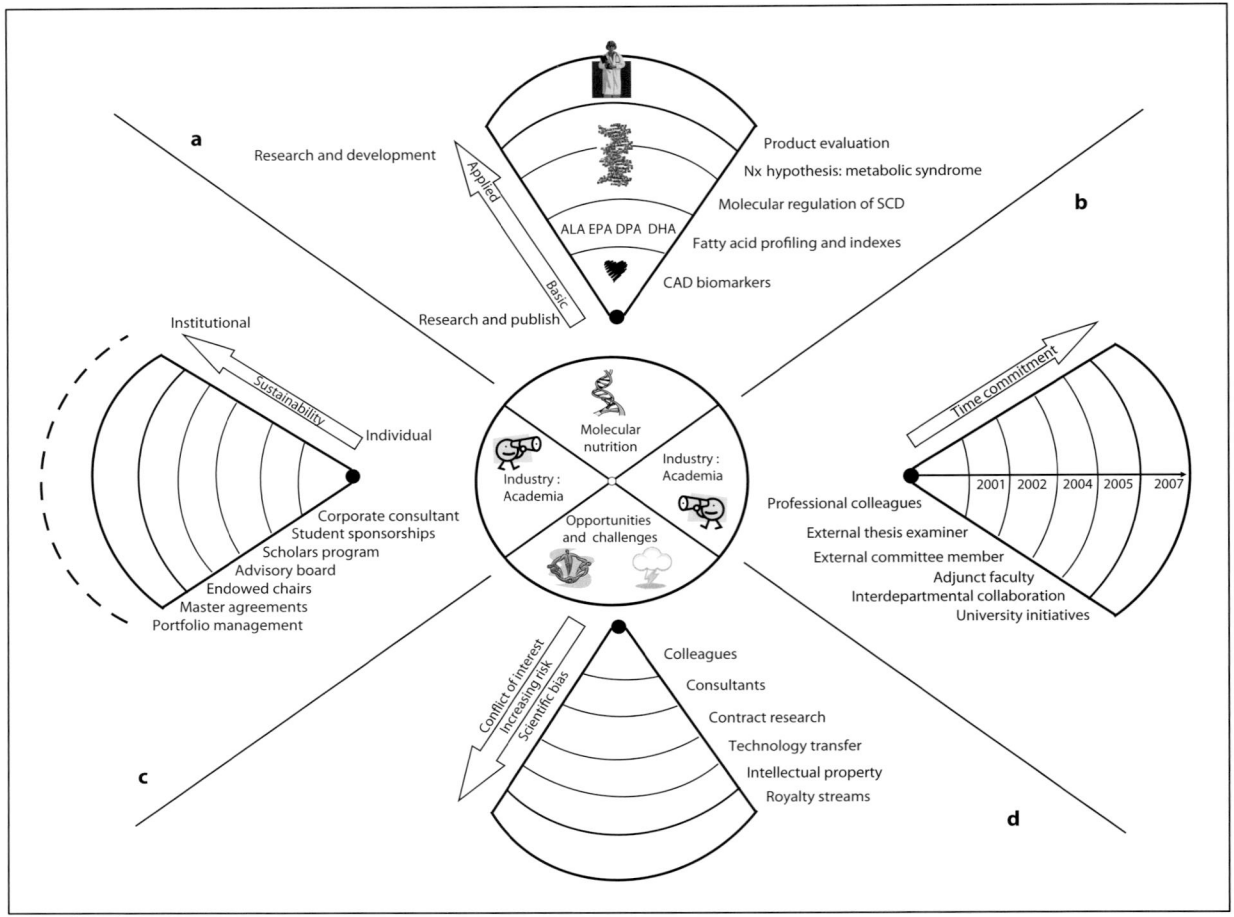

Fig. 3. Partnerships are multifaceted relationships as illustrated in this model. Sector A illustrates how basic research can quickly transition into applied research and product development. Sector B illustrates the different ways in which industry scientists can contribute to university activities. Sector C illustrates the various ways industry and academia can work together in defined relationships. Sector D emphasizes the risk of conflict of interest and duality of interest that can occur as industry and academia combine their resources to work on common projects.

is new territory; on the other hand, the landscape is perhaps more challenging for nutrigenetic/nutrigenomic partnerships. This stems from the over-arching complexity of GELS (Genomics Ethics Law and Society) and the relative lack of GELS training and experience of nutrition scientists and food companies. Given the pressure to seek a return on investment in nutrigenetic/nutrigenomic research and development, coupled with the realities of low-margin food products sold in a competitive, consumer-centric market, ethical quandaries can quickly surface. For this reason, industry scientists need their academic colleagues not only to build the scientific foundation

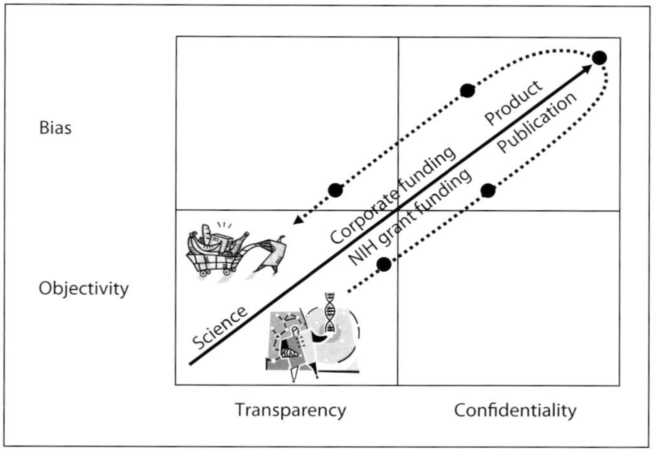

Fig. 4. Relational Coordinates. Research programs, whether supported by private or public funds, transition through different stages that have variable needs for transparency or confidentiality and require that scientists to be both passionate and objective in their research.

of molecular nutrition, but also to vet the credibility and value of industry-academic partnerships. In this regard, industry's investment in nutrigenetic/nutrigenomic partnerships is not only strategic, it is essential for the future of personalized nutrition.

Final Thoughts

There is nothing complicated about building partnerships, it's like playing together in a sandbox. All kids are welcome, but everyone is expected to find their own space, respect the space of others, and to share their toys. Scientists in the nutrigenetic/nutrigenomic sandbox need to:
– build partnerships on the basis of shared values;
– share limited resources;
– hold an open dialogue about scientific bias, conflicts of interest and duality of interest and be sure to engage younger scientists in the conversation;
– institutionalize the emerging guiding principles for funding food science and nutrition research, improve them with respect to issues of intellectual property, and frame them in the modern context of nutrigenetics/nutrigenomics.

Disclosures

Dr. Gillies is employed by DuPont and holds an Adjunct Professorship in the Department of Nutritional Sciences at the Pennsylvania State University.

Dr. Kris-Etherton is a Distinguished Professor in the Department of Nutritional Sciences at the Pennsylvania State University and a consultant to DuPont on a study investigating the effects of omega-3 fatty acids in humans.

References

1 Nestle M: Food company sponsorship of nutrition research and professional activities: a conflict of Interest? Public Health Nutr 2001;4:1015–1022.
2 Lesser LI, Ebbeling CB, Goozner M, Wypij D, Ludwig DS: Relationship between funding source and conclusion among nutrition-related scientific articles. PLoS Med 2007;e5. DOI: 10.1371/journal.pmed.0040005
3 Center for Science in the Public Interest: Integrity in science. www.cspinet.org/integrity/about.html (accessed September 3, 2009).
4 Kaput J, Perlina A, Hatipoglu B, Bartholomew A, Nikolsky Y: Nutrigenomics: concepts and applications to pharmacogenomics and clinical medicine. Pharmacogenomics 2007;8:369–390.
5 Ghosh D, Skinner MA, Lain WA: Pharmacogenomics and nutrigenomics: synergies and differences. Eur J Clin Nutr 2007;61:567–574.
6 Kuehn B.M: Growing calls in United States, Europe to improve regulation of genetic testing. JAMA 2009;302:1405–1408.
7 The American Society for Nutrition: The American Journal of Clinical Nutrition, Authors' Agreement. www.ajcn.org/misc/Authors'_Agreement_Form.pdf (accessed September 3, 2009).
8 The American Society for Nutrition: Journal of Nutrition, Conflict of Interest and Funding Disclosure. http://jn.nutrition.org/misc/ifora_4-ms-prep.shtml#Conflict (accessed September 3, 2009).
9 American Society of Nutrition: Conflict of Interest. www.nutrition.org/about-asn/conflict-of-interest (accessed September 3, 2009).
10 Rowe S, Alexander N, Clydesdale FM, Applebaum RS, Atkinson S, et al: Funding food science and nutrition research: financial conflicts and scientific integrity. Am J Clin Nutr 2009;89:1285–1291.
11 Velliquette RA, Gillies PJ, Kris-Etherton PM, et al: Regulation of human stearoyl-CoA desaturase by omega-3 and omega-6 fatty acids: implications for the dietary management of elevated serum triglycerides. J Clin Lipid 2009;3:281–288.
12 Collins N, Tighe AP, Brunton SA, Kris-Etherton PM: Differences between dietary supplement and prescription drug omega-3 fatty acid formulations: a legislative and regulatory perspective. J Am Coll Nutr 2008;27:659–666.
13 Melese T, Lin SM, Chang JL, Cohen NH: Open innovation networks between academia and industry: an imperative for breakthrough therapies. Nat Med 2009;15:502–507.
14 Personal communication from David Castle, Canada Research Chair in Science and Society, Department of Philosophy, University of Ottawa, Ottawa, Canada.
15 NIH CTSA. www.ctsaweb.org (accessed October 29, 2009).
16 Zinner DE, Campbell EG: Life-science research within US academic medical centers. JAMA 2009;302:969–976.

Dr. Peter J. Gillies
DuPont Applied BioSciences, DuPont Experimental Station, E328/267
Wilmington, DE 19880–0328 (USA)
Tel. +1 302 695 3956, E-Mail peterjgillies@gmail.com

Tailoring Foods to Match People's Genes in New Zealand: Opportunities for Collaboration

Lynnette R. Ferguson[a,c] · Rong Hu[a,c] · Wen Jiun Lam[a,c] · Karen Munday[a,c] · Christopher M. Triggs[b,c]

[a]Discipline of Nutrition and [b]Department of Statistics, The University of Auckland, and [c]Nutrigenomics New Zealand, Auckland, New Zealand

Personalized nutrition according to genotype is based on the premise that optimized dietary advice for one individual may not be appropriate for others, and that optimal health and wellbeing can be tailored according to genotype.

Nutrigenomics New Zealand is a collaboration between The University of Auckland and two Crown Research Institutes: Plant & Food Research and AgResearch [1]. The program involves 55 named individuals, located at 5 different sites across New Zealand. In order to develop the appropriate methodologies and learn how to apply them, we are studying dietary response according to genotype in inflammatory bowel diseases (IBD), especially Crohn's disease (CD), as proof of principle.

IBD are common gastrointestinal disorders, whose incidence appears to be rising in various countries, including New Zealand [2]. Although the diseases are not invariably lethal, the symptoms, which include abdominal cramps and bloody diarrhea, can be debilitating and may result in poor nutrient intakes and severe malabsorption. While there is an apparent familial component to the disease, twin studies have confirmed that genetic variations influence disease susceptibility, rather than inevitably leading to the disease per se [3]. The important observation that diet influences disease but that no single diet suits all [4], makes this an interesting candidate disease in which to study gene-diet interactions. An overview of the approach taken across the program is shown in figure 1.

Role of Genetics in CD in New Zealand

As with other genetic disorders, knowledge of key genes initially depended upon candidate gene studies, and it was not until 2001 that the first gene unequivocally

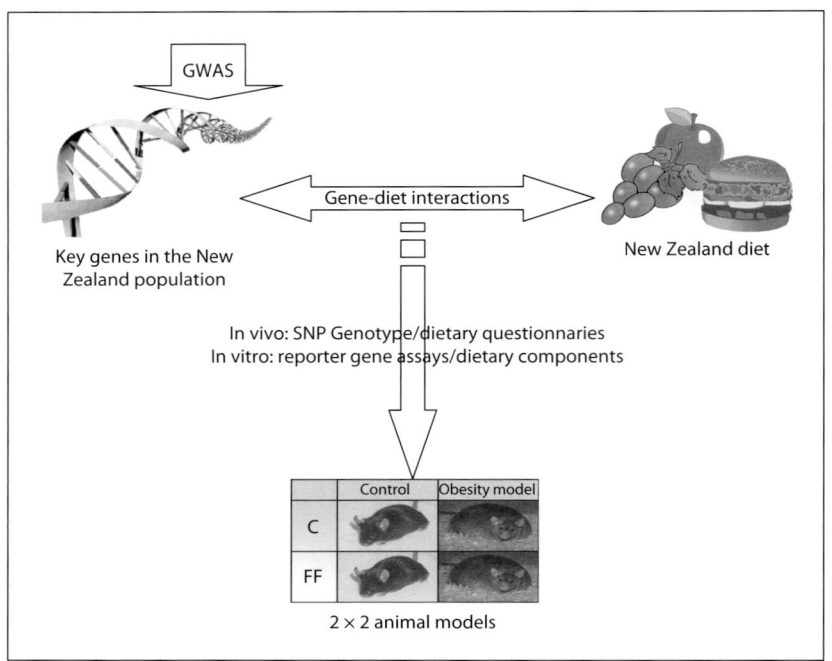

Fig. 1. Outline of the approach used to develop personalized foods, tailored to genotype, by Nutrigenomics New Zealand. Genes associated with specific disease are identified from genetic epidemiology studies, particularly genome-wide association studies (GWAS), and confirmed for importance and relevance to the New Zealand population. The phenotypic effects of those genes which appear particularly important in this country are mimicked in a cell-based reporter gene assay, which is used for testing a wide range of food components and/or food extracts as a high throughput assay. Foods for preferential testing in that assay are identified through matching dietary tolerances or intolerances to specific genotypes (see fig. 2). Those foods that appear to show ability to restore the wild-type phenotype in the mutant reporter gene assay and/or show strong links to genotype from the dietary questionnaires are then tested in animal studies. A systems biology approach in specific animal models is then used to understand how different foods or food compounds might interact with a particular genotype. One output of this approach is a defined set of biomarkers for use in human trials. Human studies utilize subjects stratified according to genotype. Study participants are randomized to a control diet or an experimental diet that includes the food shown to ameliorate the phenotype associated with a particular genotype in animal models. Biomarkers previously identified in those animal studies are monitored to rapidly establish if the experimental diet can restore the non-risk-genotype profile, without the need to follow study participants until the development of disease. Positive results in these studies are considered to provide preliminary evidence to validate the use of that food in subjects carrying the variant genotype.

associated with CD, nucleotide oligomerization domain 2 *(NOD2)*, was identified [5]. The accelerated progress afforded by genome association studies, using high-density arrays (SNP Chips) combined with large population groups and meta-analysis, has now associated more than 30 genes with susceptibility to CD [6]. We have generally not attempted to find novel genes, but confirmed overseas studies in our

Table 1. Examples of genes associated with CD in a Caucasian population from New Zealand

Gene	Abbreviation	SNP	Allelic odds ratio, CD vs. control	Ref.
Drosophila discs large homolog 5	DLG5	rs1248696 rs2289310 rs2289311	1.29 (0.93, 1.78) 0.90 (0.48, 1.66) 0.83 (0.67, 1.03)	[7]
Nucleotide-binding oligomerization domain containing 1	NOD1	rs2075818 rs2075822 rs2907748	0.66 (0.49–0.89) 0.91 (0.69–1.21) 0.84 (0.64–1.10)	[8]
Nucleotide-binding oligomerization domain containing 2	NOD2	rs2066844 rs2066845 rs2066847	2.7 (1.5–5.2) 2.4 (0.94–6.1) 4.4 (1.6–12)	[9]
Toll-like receptor 4	TLR4	rs4986790 rs4986791	1.225 (0.79, 1.91) 1.046 (0.67, 1.63)	[10]
Tumour necrosis factor alpha	TNF-alpha	rs1800629 rs1799724	1.10 (0.72–1.68) 1.09 (0.84–1.42)	[11]
Tumour necrosis factor receptor superfamily, member 1B	TNFRSF1B	rs1061622 rs1061624 rs3397	1.12 (0.87–1.45) 0.98 (0.79–1.22) 0.91 (0.73–1.13)	[12]

New Zealand population group. Examples of key genes in this country are given in table 1 [7–12]. Most of the genes appear to affect immune response and/or bacterial recognition [13]. It is noteworthy that not all genes relevant in other countries are necessarily key genes for susceptibility to this disease in New Zealand, as might be expected [14]. It is also becoming increasingly apparent that risk may associate with gene-gene interactions, rather than a single gene per se [15].

Modeling Genetic Variation in Human CD Populations in vitro

Once a key genotype is established as being important, high throughput screens are developed to test whether selected food components can overcome the phenotype of the functional SNP. For example, Philpott et al. [16] described a reporter gene assay to test effects of foods on the common NOD2 variant, while Danesi et al. [17] have established a screen for IL23R. Robotic systems using 384-well plates enable high numbers of food components to be tested in a given experiment. These then provide leads which may be confirmed by dietary analyses and which can be more extensively studied in animal models.

Food / NOD2		CARD15_2066844 C/C,C/T,T/T		CARD15_2066845 C/C,C/G,G/G		CARD4_2075818 C/C,C/G,G/G		CARD4_2075822 C/C,C/T,T/T		CARD4_2907748 A/A,A/G,G/G	
		Effects	P-value	Effects	P-value	Effects	P-value	Effects	P-value	Effects	P-value
Cream	Better	0.9579	0.114	21.76	1	0.315	0.575	-0.028	0.96631	-0.028	0.96631
	Worse	-0.2271	0.376	-0.108	0.822	-0.15	0.45	-0.15	0.45	-0.367	0.0866
Standard Milk	Better	0.0493	0.863	0.4101	0.439	-0.139	0.531	-0.347	0.144	-0.222	0.348
	Worse	0.4344	0.467	-0.377	0.721	0.8068	0.044	-0.28	0.56444	-0.789	0.09031
Apple	Better	0.3673	0.141	1.865	0.0703	0.0091	0.968	-0.231	0.3154	-0.272	-0.2715
	Worse	-0.6292	0.215	-0.45	0.483	-0.007	0.98	0.4662	0.171	0.643	0.0659
Grape Fruit	Better	0.1072	0.6805	0.6538	0.27	0.1685	0.45146	-0.01	0.968	-0.028	0.905
	Worse	-0.4725	0.628	-5.311	5.55e-11	-0.015	0.978	-0.82	0.10294	-0.439	0.40143
Kiwi Fruit	Better	0.1441	0.56	23.45	1	0.12	0.543	-0.12	0.558	-0.031	0.881
	Worse	-0.7331	0.211	0.2696	0.591	-0.021	0.947	0.4797	0.199	0.333	0.353
Dried Cranberries	Better	-0.0535	0.91	0.3881	0.714	0.3697	0.252	-0.179	0.6132	-0.05	0.889
	Worse	0.2131	0.837	21.15	1	0.0809	0.916	-0.092	0.9107	-0.619	0.4168
Corn	Better	-0.0345	0.8854	0.9521	0.0574	0.1307	0.5071	0.0573	0.772	-0.115	0.564
	Worse	0.4488	0.434	-0.661	0.533	-0.336	0.58	-0.121	0.81636	0.29	0.61686
Cabbage	Better	0.2145	0.3575	1.5169	0.0169	0.1632	0.39157	0.1192	0.555	-0.049	0.809
	Worse	-0.0625	0.914	-0.965	0.215	0.1081	0.783	-0.25	0.53145	-0.158	0.705236
Breadwholegrain	Better	0.2293	0.342	0.4511	0.399	0.2118	0.316	-0.254	0.242	-0.334	0.124
	Worse	0.2661	0.524	-0.543	0.481	-0.783	0.128	0.5304	0.241	0.699	0.13
Rice brown or unpolished	Better	0.0414	0.902	0.6585	0.39	0.2936	0.296	0.0506	0.8687	0.026	0.93237
	Worse	0.2415	0.547	-0.125	0.872	0.1131	0.775	-0.032	0.93785	0.023	0.95748
PorridgeOats	Better	0.3947	0.24	0.0773	0.906	-0.275	0.37	-0.344	0.24642	-0.434	0.143
	Worse	0.3105	0.4	0.2044	0.79	-0.321	0.267	0.2621	0.40393	0.244	0.430139
Breadcorn	Better	0.327	0.30919	0.8334	0.212	-0.114	0.665	-0.385	0.136	-0.293	0.265
	Worse	-0.4666	0.638	-1.499	0.0673	0.2259	0.634	0.3789	0.49635	0.177	0.736355

Fig. 2. Example of a worksheet to identify gene-diet interactions in CD in the New Zealand population. For individuals carrying each of the genetic variants (identified as per fig. 1), we considered self-diagnosed tolerance, neutral effects or intolerance to 269 individual dietary items. We have calculated the probability that each individual food significantly improves or worsens the condition, as previously described [14]. A matrix is then created linking genotype to food tolerance. A section of such a matrix is illustrated.

Estimating the Role of Diet in CD

There is not complete agreement as to what dietary assessment methods are appropriate in epidemiologic studies, and the same is true of nutrigenetic studies. Inevitably there needs to be a compromise between the most accurate record possible and what is practically acceptable to the study population. In particular, many food-frequency questionnaires cluster similar dietary items in order to retain people's attention and not make recording too large a burden. However, in our CD population, we elected to use a much larger list of food items, so that subtle differences in potentially bioactive food components, rather than broad classes of nutrients could be tested [14]. An example of part of the dietary information becoming available for CD is given in figure 2. It can be seen that the same food that is beneficial to one individual may actually trigger symptoms of disease in others.

In the specific case of CD, it is important to realize that food preparation methods may be as important as food components per se. For example, many of our subjects reported that they could tolerate tomatoes, but only when they are peeled and seeded. Ginger ale was typically detrimental, but could be beneficial when allowed to go flat. Kiwifruit eaten as a whole fruit was often detrimental, but a commercially available juice in which the seeds are filtered out could be beneficial. So, knowledge of preparation details may be as important as knowledge of the food items themselves.

Animal Models of IBD

Patients with IBD are a highly sensitive population and it is essential that any potential nutritional therapies are rigorously tested in animal models for in vivo effects before considering human clinical trials. Nutrigenomics New Zealand has utilized 2 different models: the multidrug resistant mouse, and the interleukin-10 knockout mouse [18–23]. A 2 × 2 study design considers the wild-type mouse versus the relevant knockout, in the presence or absence of the dietary item to be tested. The experiments are run for sufficient time for disease (or lack thereof) to be established, the animals euthanized and tissues culled for various endpoints. These range from pathologic assessment of disease presence/absence/severity, to transcriptomics (microarrays), proteomics and/or metabolomics techniques [18–23].

Double-Blind Placebo Controlled Human Clinical Trials

Ultimately, the proof of efficacy of a dietary component in a given genotype or population group depends upon a randomized human clinical trial. Ethical constraints make time to disease an inappropriate endpoint, and biomarkers (or surrogate disease endpoints) become essential. These rely upon collection of a readily accessible tissue (blood, urine, buccal swab or feces) before and after a given period of a defined dietary intervention in a genetically stratified population [24].

There are few published studies of gene-specific approaches to clinical trials. However, Kornman et al. [25] tested effects of their proprietary botanical mixture on inflammation, using C-reactive protein as an endpoint. They showed that the level of C-reactive protein was reduced in the intervention arm of their study, and suggested their preparation would have beneficial effects on inflammation in human populations. This would be likely to relate to chronic human diseases such as cardiovascular disease, but may also be highly relevant to inflammatory disorders such as IBD.

Data Management and Integration

Integral to this study approach are very large datasets. These need to be maintained with confidentiality, but must also have the ability to be interrogated by different individuals with different expertise, working in different locations. In Nutrigenomics New Zealand, we maintain an interdisciplinary wiki that enables cross-disciplinary communication, and enables the analysis of complex multidimensional interactions. Database management, bioinformatics and biostatistics are essential tools whose importance must not be underestimated in a major program of this sort. A relational database may help to reveal relationships among genetic variation, dietary patterns and disease states. A significant analytical challenge remains in reducing the dimensionality of such complex datasets.

The most significant challenge, however, is also common to other nutrigenomics programs. That is, the recognition that adequately powered studies require literally thousands of individuals. This provides numerous opportunities, indeed reflects a necessity, for strategic international alliances for collaboration [26].

Acknowledgments

Nutrigenomics New Zealand is a collaboration between AgResearch, Plant & Food Research and The University of Auckland, and is largely funded by the Foundation for Research, Science and Technology.

References

1 www.nutrigenomics.org.nz
2 Gearry RB, Richardson A, Frampton CM, et al: High incidence of Crohn's disease in Canterbury New Zealand: results of an epidemiologic study. Inflamm Bowel Dis 2006;12:936–943.
3 Spehlmann ME, Begun AZ, Burghardt J, et al: Epidemiology of inflammatory bowel disease in a German twin cohort results of a nationwide study. Inflamm Bowel Dis 2008;7:968–976.
4 Hunter JO: Nutritional factors in inflammatory bowel disease. Eur J Gastroenterol Hepatol 1998;3: 235–237.
5 Hugot JP, Chamaillard M, Zouali H, et al: Thomas Association of NOD2 leucine-rich repeat variants with susceptibility to Crohn's disease. Nature 2001; 411:599–603.
6 Barrett JC, Hansoul S, Nicolae DL, et al: Genome-wide association defines more than 30 distinct susceptibility loci for Crohn's disease. Nat Genet 2008; 40:955–962.
7 Browning BL, Huebner C, Petermann I, et al: Association of *DLG5* variants with inflammatory bowel disease in the New Zealand Caucasian population and meta-analysis of the DLG5 R30Q variant. Inflamm Bowel Dis 2007;13;9:1069–1076.
8 Huebner C, Ferguson LR, Han DY, et al: Nucleotide-binding oligomerization domain containing 1 (NOD1) haplotypes and single nucleotide polymorphisms modify susceptibility to inflammatory bowel diseases in a New Zealand Caucasian population: a case-control study. BMC Res Notes 2009;2:52.
9 Gearry RB, Roberts RL, Burt MJ, et al: Effect of inflammatory bowel disease classification changes on NOD2 genotype-phenotype associations in a population-based cohort. Inflamm Bowel Dis 2007; 13:1220–1227.
10 Browning BL, Huebner C, Petermann I, et al: Has toll-like receptor 4 been prematurely rejected as an inflammatory bowel disease gene? Association study combined with meta-analysis shows strong evidence for association. Am J Gastroenterol 2007;102:2504–2512.

11 Ferguson LR, Huebner C, Petermann I, et al: Single nucleotide polymorphism in the tumor necrosis factor-alpha gene affects inflammatory bowel diseases risk. World J Gastroenterol 2008;14;29:4652–4661.

12 Ferguson LR, Han DY, Huebner C, et al: Tumor necrosis factor receptor superfamily member 1b haplotypes increase or decrease the risk of inflammatory bowel diseases in a New Zealand Caucasian population. Gastroenterol Res Pract 2009, E-pub ahead of print.

13 Baker PI, Love DR, Ferguson LR: Role of gut microbiota in Crohn's disease. Expert Rev Gastroenterol Hepatol 2009;3:535–546.

14 Petermann I, Triggs CM, Huebner C, McCulloch A, Ferguson LR: Mushroom intolerance: a novel diet-gene interaction in Crohn's disease. Br J Nutr 2009; 102:506–508.

15 Petermann I, Huebner C, Browning BL, et al: Interactions among genes influencing bacterial recognition increase IBD risk in a population-based New Zealand cohort. Hum Immunol. 2009;70:440–446.

16 Philpott M, Mackay L, Ferguson LR, Forbes D, Skinner M: Cell culture models in developing nutrigenomics foods for inflammatory bowel disease. Mutation Res 2007;622:94–102.

17 Danesi F, Philpott M, Huebner C, Bordoni A, Ferguson LR: A Screen to test the role of IL-23 receptor in inflammatory bowel diseases. J Nutrigenet Nutrigenom 2008;6:305.

18 Roy NC, Barnett MPG, Knoch B, Dommels Y, McNabb WC: Nutrigenomics applied to an animal model of inflammatory bowel diseases transcriptomic analysis of the effects of eicosapentaenoic acid- and arachidonic acid-enriched diets. Mut 2007;622:103–116.

19 Knoch B, Barnett MP, Zhu S, et al: Genome-wide analysis of dietary eicosapentaenoic acid- and oleic acid-induced modulation of colon inflammation in interleukin-10 gene-deficient mice. J Nutrigenet Nutrigenomics 2009;2;1:9–28.

20 Nones K, Knoch B, Dommels YE, et al: Multidrug resistance gene deficient (mdr1a–/–) mice have an altered caecal microbiota that precedes the onset of intestinal inflammation. J Appl Microbiol 2009;107: 557–566.

21 Dommels YE, Butts CA, Zhu S, et al: Characterization of intestinal inflammation and identification of related gene expression changes in mdr1a(–/–) mice. Genes Nutr 2007;2:209–223.

22 Nones K, Dommels YE, Martell S, et al: The effects of dietary curcumin and rutin on colonic inflammation and gene expression in multidrug resistance gene-deficient (mdr1a–/–) mice, a model of inflammatory bowel diseases. Br J Nutr 2009;101:169–181.

23 Lin HM, Edmunds SI, Helsby NA, Ferguson LR, Rowan DD: Nontargeted urinary metabolite profiling of a mouse model of Crohn's disease. J Proteome Res 2009;8:2045–2057.

24 Ferguson LR: Biomarkers as endpoints in intervention studies; in Vineis P, Sy Garte S, Wild C (eds): Molecular Epidemiology of Chronic Diseases: New Techniques and Approaches. Chichester, John Wiley & Sons, 2008, pp 255–266.

25 Kornman K, Rogus J, Roh-Schmidt H, et al: Interleukin-1 genotype-selective inhibition of inflammatory mediators by a botanical a nutrigenetics proof of concept. Nutrition 2007;23:844–852.

26 Kaput J, Allen L, Ames BN, et al: The case for strategic international alliances to harness nutritional genomics for public and personal health. Br J Nutr 2005;94:623–632.

Lynnette R. Ferguson
Discipline of Nutrition, The University of Auckland
Auckland 1142 (New Zealand)
Tel. +64 9 373 7599 ext 86372, Fax +64 9 303 5963, E-Mail l.ferguson@auckland.ac.nz

Author Index

Ahn, J. 34

Beland, F.A. 123
Berndt, S.I. 34
Burdge, G.C. 56

Carlsson, L.M.S. 103
Chanock, S.J. 34
Chung, S. 84
Conus, P. 131
Cross, A.J. 34
Cuenod, M. 131

Dashwood, R.H. 95
De Caterina, R. 1
Do, K.Q. 131

Ferguson, L.R. 8, 169
Ferrucci, L.M. 34

Gillies, P.J. 160
Goyenechea, E. 21
Graubard, B.I. 34
Gummesson, A. 103
Gunter, M.J. 34

Hayes, R.B. 34
Ho, E. 95
Huang, W.-Y. 34
Hunt, S.C. 46
Hu, R. 169

Jackson, A.A. 56

Kosyk, O. 123
Kris-Etherton, P.M. 160

Lam, W.J. 169
Lillycrop, K.A. 56

Manku, M.S. 15
Marti, A. 21
Martínez, J.A. 21
Ma, X. 34
Mayne, S.T. 34
Milner, J.A. XI
Munday, K. 169

Pogribny, I.P. 123
Puri, B.K. 15

Rahman, I. 84
Ross, S.R. 123
Rusyn, I. 123

Simopoulos, A.P. XI
Sinha, R. 34
Sjöholm, K. 103
Spence, J.T. 154
Starlard-Davenport, A. 123
Svensson, P.-A. 103

Thompson, K. 115
Triggs, C.M. 169
Tryndyak, V. 123

Yeager, M. 34

Zeisel, S.H. 73

Subject Index

N-Acetyl cysteine (NAC), schizophrenia
    trials 141–143
Activin receptor-like kinase (ALK), expression
    in obesity 110, 111
Adiponectin, gene polymorphisms in
    obesity 28
Adipose tissue
    expression profiling in diet-induced weight
        loss 105–111
    types 104, 105
Adrenergic receptor 2 protein (ADBR2), gene
    polymorphisms in obesity 24, 28
Agriculture, nutrigenomic approach to dietary
    guidance 154–158
Angiotensin II type 1 receptor (AT1R), gene
    polymorphisms in hypertension 49, 50
Angiotensinogen (AGT), gene polymorphisms
    in hypertension 51–53
Apolipoprotein A5 (APOA5), gene
    polymorphisms in obesity 24, 27
Asthma, oxidative stress 84

Birth weight, influence on adult disease 62, 63
Butyrate, histone deacetylases inhibition
    90, 99

Cancer
    colorectal adenoma, see Meat
    epigenetics 67
    fetal origins hypothesis 59, 60
    histone deacetylase inhibitors
        prevention 95–97
    microRNA expression
        liver carcinogenesis role
            dysregulated microRNA
                functions 125–129
            methyl-deficient diet effects 125

study design 124
overview 121
Catechins, see Polyphenols
Choline
    deficiency
        consequences in humans 76, 77, 80
        epigenetic effects 79
        fetal deficiency and long-lasting
            consequences 79, 80
        neural development studies in
            animals 78, 79
        nutrigenetics/nutrigenomics prototype
            experiment 75
    gene polymorphisms and dietary
        requirements 78
    metabolism 75, 76
Chromatin remodeling
    chronic obstructive pulmonary disease 84
    histone deacetylases
        inflammation
            HDAC2 and steroid resistance 87, 88
            sirtuins and epigenetic changes
                87, 88
        inhibitors
            cancer prevention 95–97
            dietary sources 97–99
        polyphenol modulation
            inhibitors 90, 91
            mechanisms 91
            SIRT1 89, 90
Chronic obstructive pulmonary disease
    (COPD)
    chromatin remodeling 84
    oxidative stress 84
CIDEs, diet-induced weight loss effects 109, 110
Clinical and Translational Science Awards
    (CTSA) 165

177

Cobalamin, schizophrenia trials 145
Colorectal adenoma, *see* Meat
Copy number variation (CNV), ethyl-eicosapentaenoic acid action effects in disease 15, 17, 18
Crohn's disease (CD)
    animal models 173
    candidate genes 11, 161, 170
    end points in clinical trials 173
    gene-diet interactions 12, 13, 172, 173
    genetic variant modeling in vitro 171
    Nutrigenomics New Zealand data management 174
Curcumin, *see* Polyphenols

Dairy cattle, prodigy testing 154–156
Dietary Guidelines for Americans 155
DNA microarray
    genome-wide association studies 10
    noise sources 117–119
    phenotypic anchoring 119, 120
    reference materials for performance assessment 116, 117, 120
DuPont, Penn State partnership 163–167
Dutch famine, fetal origins hypothesis 58, 59

Eicosapentaenoic acid (EPA)
    benefits in neurological disease
        Huntington's disease 16, 17
        myalgic encephalomyelitis 17, 18
    ethyl-eicosapentaenoic acid, *see* Ethyl-eicosapentaenoic acid
Epigenetics, *see also* Chromatin remodeling
    choline deficiency effects 79
    DNA methyltransferase 66
    fetal origins hypothesis
        adult disease 65, 66
        cancer 67
Estrogen response element (ERE), *PEMT* 77
Ethyl-eicosapentaenoic acid
    benefits in neurological disease
        copy number variation in mechanism 15, 17, 18
        Huntington's disease 17
        myalgic encephalomyelitis 18
    metabolism 15, 16

Fetal origins hypothesis
    animal models 63–67
    cancer
        epigenetics 67
        risk 59, 60
    developmental plasticity 63
    Dutch famine 58, 59
    overview 57
FTO, gene polymorphisms in obesity 24, 25

Garlic, histone deacetylases inhibition 90, 99
Genome-wide association studies (GWAS)
    Crohn's disease
        candidate genes 11
        gene-diet interactions 12, 13
    DNA microarray 10
    growth in research 8, 9
    hypertension 47, 52, 53
    monogenetic disorders versus complex diseases 9
    personalized health predictions 11, 12
    rationale for study 10, 11
Genomics Ethics Law and Society (GELS) 166
Glucocorticoid receptor (GR), pregnancy and fetal epigenetics 65, 66
Glutathione deficiency, *see* Schizophrenia
Growth pattern, influence on adult disease 60–62

Hepatic lipase, gene polymorphisms in obesity 27, 28
Histone deacetylases, *see* Chromatin remodeling
Huntington's disease, eicosapentaenoic acid therapy 16, 17
Hypertension
    gene detection
        intervention selection 48
        intervention studies 51, 52
        study time windows 48, 49
        subject selection 47
        tissue versus central phenotype measurement 49–51
    genome-wide association studies 47, 52, 53

Inflammation
    histone deacetylases and inflammation
        HDAC2 and steroid resistance 87, 88
        sirtuins and epigenetic changes 87, 88
    polyphenol modulation
        catechins 86, 87
        curcumin 86
        resveratrol 85, 86
    serum amyloid A expression 108, 109

Inflammatory bowel disease, *see* Crohn's
disease
Inhibin, expression in obesity 110

Leptin
    gene polymorphisms in obesity 25
    receptor polymorphisms and diet
        interactions 28, 29
Liver carcinogenesis, *see* Cancer

Meat
    carcinogen metabolic activation 34, 38
    colorectal adenoma screening study
        gene selection and genotyping 35, 36,
            38–41
        nitrate/nitrite intake estimation 36
        population characteristics 35, 37
        statistical analysis 36
    cooking and carcinogen formation 34
Melanocortin receptor 3 (MC3R), gene
    polymorphisms in obesity 25
Melanocortin receptor 4 (MC4R), gene
    polymorphisms in obesity 22
Methionine, schizophrenia trials 143
Methylene tetrahydrofolate, metabolizing gene
    polymorphisms and choline
    requirements 78
Methylfolate, schizophrenia trials 145
MicroRNA
    liver carcinogenesis role
        dysregulated microRNA functions
            125–129
        methyl-deficient diet effects 125
        study design 124
        tumor expression 121
Milk, prodigy testing in dairy cattle 154–156
Myalgic encephalomyelitis, eicosapentaenoic
    acid therapy 17, 18

Nutrigenetics/nutrigenomics
    challenges
        ethical and legal implications 5, 6
        meeting challenges 6
        polymorphism variety 75
        premature health claims 5
        study size 73, 74
        surrogate endpoints 4, 5
    choline deficiency, *see* Choline
    dietary guidance 155, 156
    genome-wide association studies, *see*
        Genome-wide association studies

    industry-academia partnerships
        DuPont-Penn State partnership
            163–167
        learning curve 160–163
        omega-3 fatty acids 160, 161
        professional development and
            networks 163
        publications 163, 164
    obesity personalized nutritional therapy, *see*
        Obesity
    opportunities 2–4
    rationale for study 1, 2

Obesity
    adipose tissue expression profiling in
        diet-induced weight loss 105–111
    candidate genes 21, 22
    CIDE family expression 109, 110
    definition 103
    epidemiology 21
    gene-nutrient interactions
        interventional studies 25–28
        nutritional studies concerning
            gene-dependent effects on
            obesity-related manifestations
            28–30
        observational studies 22–25
        weight gain genes
            adipogenesis genes 24, 25
            food/energy intake genes 22, 24
            lipid utilization genes 24
        weight loss and maintenance genes
            adipocyte metabolism genes 28
            food/energy intake genes 25
            lipid utilization and adipogenesis
                genes 27, 28
            thermogenesis genes 28
    inhibin expression 110
    metabolic syndrome 101
    serum amyloid A expression 108, 109
    treatments 21, 104
Oxidative stress, *see* Schizophrenia

Penn State, DuPont partnership 163–167
Perilipin, gene polymorphisms in obesity 27
Peroxisome proliferator-activated receptor-α
    (PPARA), pregnancy and fetal
    epigenetics 65, 66
Peroxisome proliferator-activated receptor-γ
    (PPARG), gene polymorphisms in
    obesity 24, 25

Phosphatidylethanolamine-*N*-
methyltransferase (PEMT)
  choline metabolism 76
  estrogen response element 77
  gene polymorphisms and choline
    requirements 78
Polyphenols
  histone deacetylase modulation
    inhibitors 90, 91
    mechanisms 91
    SIRT1 89, 90
  inflammation modulation
    catechins 86, 87
    curcumin 86
    resveratrol 85, 86
  overview 85
Polyunsaturated fatty acids (PUFAs),
  schizophrenia trials 145, 146

Resveratrol, *see* Polyphenols

Schizophrenia
  brain connectivity impairments 133, 134
  developmental factors 132, 133
  environmental factors 132
  epidemiology 131
  genetic factors 132
  glutathione deficiency
    butyl sulfoximide induction in animal
      models 139
    cell morphology effects 138, 139
    etiology 137
    glutamate receptor response effects 137
    glutamate:cysteine ligase knockout
      mice 140, 141
    myelination defects 138

one-carbon metabolism effects 143–145
overview 134–136
parvalbumin-containing neuron
  reduction in prefrontal cortex
  137, 138
neurotransmission dysfunction 133
oxidative stress
  developmental animal models of
    dysregulation 138–141
  therapeutic targeting
    N-acetyl cysteine 141–143
    cobalamin 145
    early intervention 142, 143
    methionine 143
    methylfolate 145
    polyunsaturated fatty acids 145, 146
  vulnerability factor 134
symptoms 131
Serum amyloid A (SAA)
  diet-induced weight loss effects 108
  expression in obesity 108, 109
Sirtuins, *see* Chromatin remodeling
Sulforaphane (SFN), histone deacetylase
  inhibition 90, 91, 97–99

Toxicogenomics
  interpretation of adverse versus adaptive
    effects 120
  noise sources in expression studies
    117–119
  phenotypic anchoring 119, 120
  reference materials for microarray
    performance assessment 116, 117, 120

Uncoupling protein 3 (UCP3), gene
  polymorphisms in obesity 28

RETURN TO PUBLIC HEALTH LIBRARY